Suicide and Society in India

In India about 123,000 people take their own lives each year, the second highest total in the world. There is a suicide death in India almost every four minutes, and it is the leading cause of death for rural Indians, especially women, in early adulthood. This book presents a comprehensive analysis of suicide in India based on original research as well as existing studies, and looks at the issue in an international, sociological and historical context.

The author looks at the reliability of suicide data in India, and goes on to discuss various factors relating to suicide, including age, gender, education and marriage. Among its findings, the book exposes a hidden youth suicide 'crisis' in India, which is argued to be far more serious than the better known crisis of farmer suicides. The book dispels many myths that are commonly associated with suicide, and highlights a neglected public health problem. Suicide in the region of Pondicherry is examined in detail, as well as in the Indian Diaspora. This book is a useful contribution to South Asian studies, as well as studies in mental health and sociology.

Peter Mayer is Associate Professor in Politics at the University of Adelaide. His research interests include suicide in India; the privatisation of state-owned enterprises; the masculinisation of the Indian population; civic engagement and social capital in human development and state weakness in South Asia. He is series editor for the Routledge/ASAA South Asian Publications Series.

Routledge/ASAA South Asian Publications Series
Edited by Peter Mayer, *Politics Department, University of Adelaide, Australia*

Published in Association with the Australian Studies Association of Australia (ASAA), represented by Maria Roces, chair of the ASAA Publications Committee, University of New South Wales, Australia.

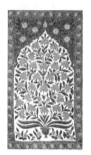

Founded in 1986 to publish outstanding work in the social sciences and humanities, the SAPS entered a new phase in 2010 when it joined with Routledge to continue a notable tradition of Australian-based research about South Asia. Works in the series are published in both UK and Indian editions.

SAPS publishes outstanding research on the countries and peoples of South Asia across a wide range of disciplines including history, politics and political economy, anthropology, geography, literature, sociology and the fields of cultural studies, communication studies and gender studies. Interdisciplinary and comparative research is encouraged.

SAPS is edited by Dr Peter Mayer (University of Adelaide: peter.mayer@ adelaide.edu.au) who welcomes any inquiries. Prospective authors, including PhD candidates, are encouraged to submit a one-to-three page abstract plus annotated chapter outline, a sample chapter and a curriculum vitae copy for initial consideration.

1. Suicide and Society in India
Peter Mayer

Suicide and Society in India

Peter Mayer

With
Clare Bradley
Della Steen
Tahereh Ziaian

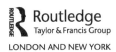
Routledge
Taylor & Francis Group

LONDON AND NEW YORK

First published 2011
by Routledge
2 Park Square, Milton Park, Abingdon, Oxfordshire OX14 4RN

Simultaneously published in the USA and Canada
by Routledge
711 Third Avenue, New York, NY 10017

First issued in paperback 2015

*Routledge is an imprint of the Taylor & Francis Group, an
informa business*

Typeset in Times by RefineCatch Limited, Bungay, Suffolk

British Library Cataloguing in Publication Data
A catalogue record for this book is available
from the British Library

Library of Congress Cataloging-in-Publication Data
Mayer, Peter.
    Suicide and society in India / Peter Mayer.
       p. cm. — (Routledge/ASAA South Asian series; 1)
    Includes bibliographical references and index.
    ISBN 978–0–415–58938–3 (hardback) — ISBN 978–0–203–84008–5
    (ebook) 1. Suicide—India. 2. Suicide—Sociological aspects. I. Title.
    HV6548.I5M39 2010
    362.280954—dc22
    2010018637

ISBN 13: 978-0-415-68381-4 (pbk)
ISBN 13: 978-0-415-58938-3 (hbk)

For Eddie and Kay
Braha
Lata, Asha & Janak

Contents

Figures

Tables

Acknowledgements

It is not only well-prepared minds, as Pasteur had it, that are smiled upon by Chance. Sometimes Fortuna roughly grabs the unprepared scholar by the collar, as she did in my case, and insists that a hitherto ignored subject be investigated.

This study began in the unlikely fields of India's Green Revolution, in an exploration of the causes of atrocities on Untouchables and the proposition that those attacks were evidence of growing class tensions in the countryside. The data I collected from time to time never produced a plausible explanation of rural violence, but it did, in time lead me to investigate the broader issue of the causes of homicide. In 1996 I visited the wellspring of national data on murder in India, the National Crime Records Bureau in New Delhi. The Director of the Bureau at that time, Mr L. C. Amernathan, welcomed me, and after tea and an illuminating discussion offered me a copy of 'their latest publication'. I did my best to conceal my dismay when it proved to be, not *Crime in India* with its bloodless accounting of grisly murders, rapes and assaults, but instead the 1994 volume of *Accidental Deaths and Suicides*. I duly packed the volume away and brought it back with me to Australia, where it remained, unread, on my bookshelf.

About two years later, my colleague Professor Robert Goldney gave a professorial lecture at the University of Adelaide on the topic of youth suicide. As Bob spoke of what we know of the aetiology of youth suicide, especially the suicides of young males, questions flooded into my mind about whether the situation and causes were comparable in India. That evening I reached for the neglected copy of *Accidental Deaths and Suicides*. I found rich and promising data there. A little browsing of journal abstracts showed that there appeared to be little sociological study of this major issue. A project, which a day before had never even crossed my mind, now demanded my commitment for the next decade.

Not long afterwards, I applied for, and received, a grant from the University of Adelaide to assist me to begin to work on the social origins of suicide in India. My colleague Professor Andrew Watson, who had seen that application, suggested that I should develop it into a request for a major grant from the Australian Research Council. In late 1999 I learned that I had won funding for the next three years to conduct the project. I wish to acknowledge here the extent of my debt to the ARC. Without their support, this volume would never have existed.

At different stages, three talented researchers – Tahereh Ziaian, Della Steen and Clare Bradley – worked with me on the project, mining the literature, grinding through the intricacies of the data, writing papers and publications; they are all listed as associated authors of this book.

Along the winding path that has led to this book, I have incurred other debts. At the Indian Institute of Public Administration Dr S. N. Suri assisted me to obtain photocopies of past volumes of *Accidental Deaths and Suicides*. Colleagues at the Rajya Sabha were kind enough to help me fill a few of the gaps in the records. Sri S. C. Sharma, IPS, Inspector General of Police for Tamil Nadu, and Sri J. P. Singh, IPS Inspector General of Police for Pondicherry, extended assistance to us in our study of suicide records in Tamil Nadu and Pondicherry. Sub-Inspector A. Sabibulla of Reddi Chavri Police Station, Cuddalore in Tamil Nadu cheerfully endured a boring morning going over several years of accidental death and suicide First Information Reports (FIRs). In Pondicherry (now Puducherry) Dr. S. Vaidyanathan and Mr. S. Radjagopalane of Maitreyi, Befrienders India Centre assisted in understanding the reasons for the very high suicide rates in the Territory.

At many points the data in the book rely on a special analysis of the data for 1997, the most recent year available during the tenure of the ARC grant. I am indebted to Sri Sharda Prasad, then Director of the National Crime Records Bureau, for his assistance in providing this important information.

I wish to thank The Samaritans, UK for permission to use material from their guidance to the media in Appendix II.

I am also obliged to Robert Goldney and Riaz Hassan for reading a draft of this book and for their comments and encouragement.

Finally, my wife Lata, who first introduced me to India, in all things made this book possible.

Part I

1 Introduction

To her husband

My Raja [king]

I am going away. Forgive me. You always used to complain that I did not write letters to you, so now I am writing to you.

Ever since I came into your house, your family has had difficulties. My coming into your house was not auspicious for you. So I am going away. I will make every effort to see that I do not survive, because if I do, not only will my life be ruined but so will yours. Do not take me to hospital.

I hope you will accede to one request of mine. Marry again very soon. But examine the girl very carefully, first. See that she knows good English. See that the family members respect everyone in your family very much. Especially that they respect you . . .

When the new bride comes, try and listen to what she says, and do not quarrel with her. Even if her relatives do not pay much attention to you, you should try to stay happy . . . [If] she talks to you privately about anything, never tell anyone else in the house what she says. Now I am going. If I survive, do not come to see me because you will not be able to stand the sight. If such a situation arises, you should give me poison so that I do not suffer much before I die . . . .

Only your
Tato
(Kishwar and Vanita 1984: 204–205)

Agriculture here [in Ananthapur, A.P.] faces a huge crisis. The crash in groundnut prices has shattered thousands of households. And debt has broken the spirit of many. Between 1997 and the end of 2000, 1,826 people, mainly farmers, committed suicide in this district. Hundreds did so by swallowing poison. Mainly pesticide. But the data was fudged. As many as 1,061 – over 58 per cent – of these were recorded as having taken their lives because of 'sickness'. Indeed, hundreds of these deaths went into the records as people killing themselves due to 'unbearable stomach ache'. This helped conceal the fact that the suicides were mostly of small farmers, pushed over the brink by economic distress. (Sainath 2001a)

Introduction

Every suicide is an individual tragedy whose origins can never be said to be fully understood. In *The Myth of Sisyphus* Albert Camus based his version of Existentialism on the intimate, personal choice made between life and death.

> There is but one truly serious philosophical problem, and that is suicide. Judging whether life is or is not worth living amounts to answering the fundamental question of philosophy. All the rest – whether or not the world has three dimensions, whether the mind has nine or twelve categories – comes afterwards.
>
> (Camus 1955: 3)

Every family touched by suicide is devastated by the experience and searches, as mankind has for centuries, to understand the reasons for this most unfathomable of human actions. The decision to end one's life is undeniably the ultimate individual act, the study of which occupies the realm of psychiatry.

Yet there is a paradox, first noted by nineteenth-century sociologists – most notably Emil Durkheim – that there is such a regularity in different societies in the annual numbers and kinds of individuals making the decision to end life that suicide must also be seen as a social phenomenon. Changes in society and economy seem to be the most potent explanations for both major regional differences in the incidence of suicide within nations and for changes in rates over time within societies. This book considers suicide in India primarily through a social lens incorporating insights from disciplines as diverse as sociology, history, political science, anthropology and agricultural economics. It focuses principally on the impact of such things as gender, age, marital status and occupation.

Powerful though social forces are in understanding the differential and changing impact of suicide, we must never lose sight of the fact that these social forces act on everyone in a society. The decision to end one's life is made, however, only by a comparative handful of individuals. When we seek to understand why social forces – which the majority of the population are able to cope with – lead a troubled minority to take their own lives, we must turn for insights to other social disciplines which take individual behaviour as their domain, especially psychology and psychiatry. The all-important tasks of developing effective strategies for suicide prevention and counselling and the identification of at-risk individuals must necessarily draw most heavily on those disciplines.

Comparative international statistics

Suicides are relatively rare causes of death. Worldwide, suicides constitute just over 1.5 per cent of all causes of death (Figure 1.1), far fewer than the deaths caused by non-communicable conditions and by communicable diseases.

Diseases of the heart (29.2 per cent), malignant cancers (12.5 per cent) and HIV/AIDS (4.9 per cent) are the most significant causes of death worldwide (Figure 1.2). The incidence of suicide (1.6 per cent) (roughly the same as the

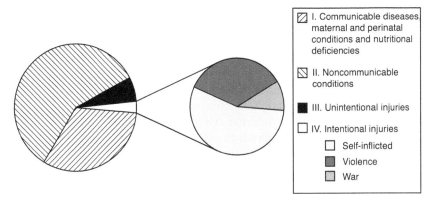

Figure 1.1 Worldwide deaths by cause (%).

Source: Compiled from World Health Organisation 2003, annex table 2.

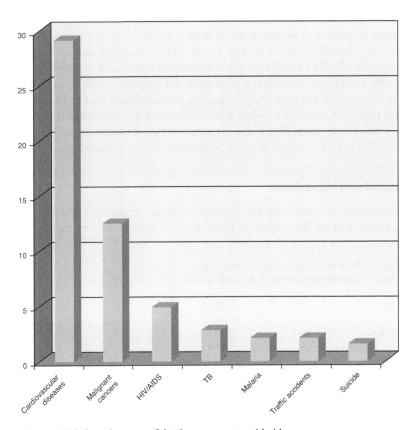

Figure 1.2 Selected causes of death – per cent worldwide.

Source: Compiled from World Health Organisation 2003, annex table 2.

WHO's category of self-inflicted intentional injury) is slightly less than that of malaria (2.1 per cent) and deaths due to traffic injuries (2.1 per cent).

Suicides are so infrequent a cause of death that we customarily report rates of suicides per 100,000 of the population. Nevertheless in some age groups the impact of suicide is very high. For rural Indians aged between 15 and 34, suicide is the leading cause of death and it is the second most frequent cause of death, after tuberculosis, for those aged between 35 and 44 (Registrar General 2002, Statement 7). India's Registrar General reported that in 1998 'deaths due to *Suicide* in females [in the] reproductive age group [viz. 15–44] has been reported as [the] top killer in India' [emphasis in original] (Registrar General 2002: 35).

Each year approximately 123,000 Indians – equivalent to the population of a medium-sized town – take their own lives (based on 2007 figures). Put in other terms, every four-and-a-quarter minutes of every day an Indian takes his or her own life. This is the second largest national total in the world; only in China is the total larger. Between them, India and China account for about 30 per cent of world suicide deaths. As can be seen from the international comparison compiled by the WHO (which uses Indian data from 1995) in Table 1.1, annual Indian suicide deaths are roughly equal to the total of those of the next seven countries combined.

The huge magnitude of suicide deaths in India is a stark indication of the gravity of the country's suicide burden. The large suicide total is, however, also a reflection of the huge size of India's population. For purposes of international comparison, we must control for the size of a nation's population and consider suicide rates. When countries are grouped into three broad categories, India falls into the middle grouping which includes Canada, the United States of America and the United Kingdom (World Health Organisation 2005). This is confirmed by a detailed comparison with 84 nations (Table 1.2), in which India sits in the very middle at number 43.

Region and suicide in India

Interesting though they are, national rankings are based on averages and thus tell us little about regional disparities. In India the differences between regions are

Table 1.1 Ranking of the top ten countries by number of suicides (estimated by the year 2000)

China	195,000
India	87,000
Russia	52,500
USA	31,000
Japan	20,000
Germany	12,500
France	11,600
Ukraine	11,000
Brazil	5,400
Sri Lanka	5,400

Source: WHO 1999: viii.

Table 1.2 World suicide rates (per 100,000)

Country	Total
Lithuania	38.4
Russian Federation	32.1
Belarus	30.9
Estonia	28.1
Kazakhstan	27.9
Latvia	27
Hungary	26.9
Ukraine	25.2
Slovenia	24.6
Sri Lanka	21.5
Finland	21.1
Croatia	18.5
Belgium	17.9
Cuba	17.1
Switzerland	16.7
Austria	15.5
Republic of Moldova	15.5
Yugoslavia	15.3
New Zealand	15
France	14.8
Luxembourg	14.7
Japan	14.5
Mauritius	14.3
Kyrgyzstan	14
China (selected areas)	13.7
Denmark	13.6
Poland	13.4
Australia	13.3
Seychelles	13.2
Czech Republic	13
Republic of Korea	12.8
Trinidad and Tobago	12.6
Guyana	12.5
Ireland	12.5
Bulgaria	12.3
Suriname	11.9
Sweden	11.8
Singapore	11.7
Slovakia	11.5
Bosnia/Herzegovina	11.3
Canada	11.3
China (Hong Kong SAR)	11.2
India	**11.2**
Norway	10.9
Romania	10.8
Germany	10.6
Iceland	10.4
Turkmenistan	10.4

(Continued Overleaf)

Table 1.2 (Continued)

Country	Total
United States of America	10.4
Uruguay	9.6
El Salvador	8.5
Netherlands	8.3
Puerto Rico	8.1
Uzbekistan	8
Zimbabwe	7.9
United Kingdom	6.8
Costa Rica	6.6
Argentina	6.5
Israel	6.5
Spain	6.5
Italy	6.2
Chile	6.1
Venezuela	6.1
Nicaragua	5.9
Panama	5.8
Ecuador	5.5
Albania	5.3
Tajikistan	5.2
Brazil	4.7
Thailand	4.1
Portugal	4
Georgia	3.9
Mexico	3.9
Colombia	3.4
Paraguay	3.2
Greece	3.1
Armenia	1.7
Kuwait	1.5
Philippines	1.5
Azerbaijan	0.8
Peru	0.6
Jamaica	0.3
Iran	0.2
Syrian Arab Republic	0.1

Source: Data from Krug, Dahlberg *et al.* 2002 for all countries except Iran, Peru, Seychelles, Sri Lanka, Suriname, Syria, Yugoslavia, Zimbabwe, which are taken from World Health Organisation 1999.

truly vast. If we treat the Indian states (and two large Union Territories (UT)) as though they were individual nations – and most are far larger than many nations with seats in the UN General Assembly – the magnitude of those differences in the incidence of suicide becomes starkly apparent (Table 1.3). Some states and territories have suicide rates that place them amongst the very highest worldwide. Seven of the 20 states/nations with the world's highest suicide rates are in India. These include the larger states of Kerala, Karnataka, Tamil Nadu and West Bengal

Table 1.3 Indian and world suicide rates (per 100,000)

Country	Year	Total
Pondicherry (UT)	1999	**58.3**
Lithuania	1999	38.4
Russian Federation	1998	32.1
Belarus	1999	30.9
Kerala	1999	**30.5**
Estonia	1999	28.1
Kazakhstan	1999	27.9
Latvia	1999	27
Hungary	1999	26.9
Tripura	1999	**25.3**
Ukraine	1999	25.2
Slovenia	1999	24.6
Sri Lanka	1995	21.5
Karnataka	1999	**24.2**
Finland	1998	21.1
Sikkim	1999	**19.7**
Tamil Nadu	1999	**18.6**
Croatia	1999	18.5
Belgium	1995	17.9
West Bengal	1999	**17.7**
Cuba	1996	17.1
Goa	1999	16.4
Switzerland	1996	16.7
Austria	1999	15.5
Republic of Moldova	1999	15.5
Yugoslavia	1990	15.3
Maharashtra	1999	**15**
New Zealand	1998	15
France	1997	14.8
Luxembourg	1997	14.7
Japan	1997	14.5
Mauritius	1998	14.3
Kyrgyzstan	1999	14
China (selected areas)	1998	13.7
Andhra Pradesh	1999	**13.6**
Denmark	1996	13.6
Poland	1996	13.4
Australia	1997	13.3
Seychelles	1998	13.2
Czech Republic	1999	13
Republic of Korea	1997	12.8
Trinidad and Tobago	1994	12.6
Guyana	1994	12.5
Ireland	1996	12.5
Madhya Pradesh	1999	**12.3**
Bulgaria	1999	12.3
Suriname	1995	11.9
Sweden	1996	11.8

(Continued Overleaf)

Table 1.3 (Continued)

Country	Year	Total
Haryana	1999	11.7
Singapore	1998	11.7
Slovakia	1999	11.5
Bosnia/Herzegovina	1991	11.3
Canada	1997	11.3
China (Hong Kong SAR)	1996	11.2
India	1999	**11.2**
Norway	1997	10.9
Romania	1999	10.8
Germany	1998	10.6
Gujarat	1999	**10.4**
Iceland	1996	10.4
Turkmenistan	1998	10.4
United States of America	1998	10.4
Orissa	1999	**10.3**
Assam	1999	**9.8**
Uruguay	1990	9.6
El Salvador	1993	8.5
Netherlands	1997	8.3
Puerto Rico	1992	8.1
Uzbekistan	1998	8
Zimbabwe	1990	7.9
Delhi (UT)	1999	**7.6**
Rajasthan	1999	**7.1**
United Kingdom	1998	6.8
Costa Rica	1995	6.6
Argentina	1996	6.5
Israel	1997	6.5
Spain	1997	6.5
Arunachal Pradesh	1999	**6.3**
Italy	1997	6.2
Chile	1994	6.1
Venezuela	1994	6.1
Nicaragua	1994	5.9
Panama	1987	5.8
Ecuador	1995	5.5
Albania	1998	5.3
Tajikistan	1995	5.2
Himachal Pradesh	1999	**4.9**
Brazil	1995	4.7
Thailand	1994	4.1
Punjab	1999	**4.2**
Portugal	1998	4
Georgia	1992	3.9
Mexico	1995	3.9
Uttar Pradesh	1999	**3.3**
Colombia	1994	3.4
Paraguay	1994	3.2
Greece	1998	3.1

(Continued Overleaf)

Table 1.3 (Continued)

Country	Year	Total
Mizoram	1999	**3**
Meghalaya	1999	**2.4**
Bihar	1999	**1.8**
Jammu & Kashmir	1999	**1**
Armenia	1999	1.7
Kuwait	1999	1.5
Philippines	1993	1.5
Nagaland	1999	**0.9**
Azerbaijan	1999	0.8
Peru	1989	0.6
Jamaica	1985	0.3
Iran	1991	0.2
Syrian Arab Republic	1985	0.1

Source: Adapted from World Health Organisation 1999: iv, figure 1 and p. 43.

as well as smaller states and territories including Pondicherry, Tripura and Sikkim. Indeed, suicide rates in Pondicherry are far higher than in any actual nation state recorded by the World Health Organisation.

If some Indian states have rates that place them among the highest in the world, others have very low rates. Of the 25 states/nations with the world's lowest suicide rates, eight are Indian states. These include the major states of Punjab, Bihar, Assam and Uttar Pradesh as well as the smaller states of Mizoram, Meghalaya, Jammu & Kashmir and Nagaland.

Not only are there great differences between suicide rates in the Indian states that are unmistakeable in international comparisons but there is also a striking pattern to the geographical distribution of the differences (Figure 1.3).

Leaving aside for a moment West Bengal and the small northeast Indian states, we observe broad bands of increasing incidence of suicide as we move south from the Gangetic plain where suicides are lowest (less than 5 per 100,000). There is an intermediate zone with higher levels between 5 and 15 per 100,000 in the Deccan (broadly construed to include the Union Territory of Delhi, Haryana, Rajasthan and Gujarat as well as the Deccan proper: Maharashtra, Madhya Pradesh, Orissa and Andhra Pradesh). The highest levels (over 15 per 100,000) are found in the third band in the south of the Indian peninsula. As we have already noted, the most extreme rates are in Kerala and Pondicherry. Since these bands broadly correspond to very ancient linguistic regions (Indo-European in the north and Dravidian in the south) and the intermediate zones of contact between them, it is tempting to speculate that the regional differences we find can in part be traced to pre-colonial origins (for a discussion of these regions, see Dyson and Moore 1983).

West Bengal clearly does not fit readily into these bands. Its elevated suicide levels make it similar to those in the southernmost band. There is also no simple geographic explanation for the variations in suicide rates we find in the small hill states of northeastern India, which seem to reflect instead specific cultural

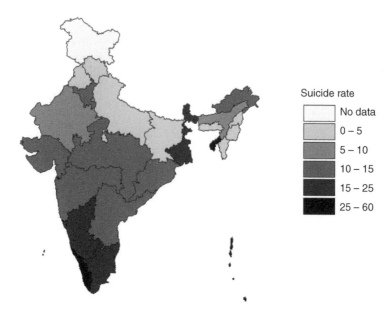

Suicide rate

☐	No data
☐	0 – 5
☐	5 – 10
☐	10 – 15
☐	15 – 25
☐	25 – 60

Figure 1.3 Suicide rates per 100,000 in India, 1999.

characteristics of the societies in each state. Rates are very high in Tripura, moderately high in Arunachal Pradesh and Assam, but very low in Nagaland, Meghalaya and Mizoram.

Suicide trends

Around the world, suicide rates have increased over the past half-century (Figure 1.4), especially among males. We will consider the trend of Indian suicides in detail in Chapter 6. Since the 1980s Indian suicide rates have risen steadily – and more rapidly than the global trend. In Chapter 6, in addition to exploring what light evidence from the nineteenth and early twentieth centuries throws on the contemporary situation, we will also see that there are puzzles in the past four decades that are not apparent in more recent trend figures. In addition we shall see that there are major regional differences in changes over time.

Indian attitudes toward suicide

Let us turn now to more subjective aspects of how Indians perceive suicide. In Chapter 2 we will consider what can be gleaned from written sources about attitudes in ancient and medieval times. It is clear from a number of small, local studies that the overwhelming majority of Indians believe that suicide is never permissible. Bhalla and his colleagues, for example, reported that in the Punjab almost 90 per cent of respondents disapproved of suicide (Bhalla, Sharma *et al.*

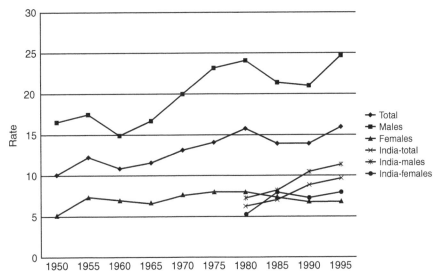

Figure 1.4 Trend in global and Indian suicide rates (per 100,000), by gender, 1950–1995.
Source: Adapted from World Health Organisation 1999: iv, figure 1 and p. 43.

1998: 78). The most comprehensive evidence about Indian attitudes to suicide comes from the World Values Survey conducted by Ronald Ingelhart of the University of Michigan. In interviews conducted in a large number of countries and regions between 1995 and 2000, one question asked 'Please tell me . . . whether you think [suicide] can always be justified, never be justified, or something in between'. The results summarized from over 78,500 interviews are presented in Figure 1.5.[1] Consistent with the broader findings of the World Values Surveys, disapproval of suicide is highest in developing countries and lowest in some former Soviet-bloc countries and countries in northern Europe. More than two-thirds of Indian respondents said that suicide can never be justified. In this respect, Indian attitudes are very similar to those of citizens in South Africa, Russia, the Philippines and the United States.

The role of media coverage

Despite the very large number of suicides in India and the worryingly high rates of suicide in parts of India, there is little serious coverage of the broader issue of suicide and suicide prevention in the Indian media. Reports of suicides, of course, appear relatively frequently in the press but with few exceptions these are presented by the media in terms of a few stereotyped genres. Because the media report only a small fraction of all suicide deaths and concentrate disproportionate attention on a few categories of suicides, popular understanding of and policy responses to suicide in India tend to be ill informed.

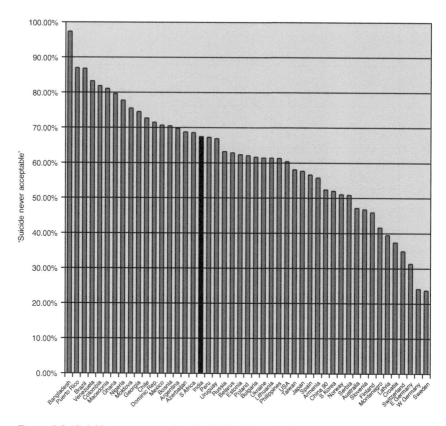

Figure 1.5 'Suicide can never be justified': World Values Survey, 1995–1996.

Ordinary suicides

Every day over 300 Indians choose to end their lives. Only a fraction of these receive even cursory mention in the daily press. At whatever period they have been collected, there is a sad similarity to most of these brief accounts. A handful of examples from the papers of Tamil Nadu collected by C. J. James in 1981 are indistinguishable from those of virtually any year in the past two decades.

> A newly married doctor couple committed suicide in Coimbatore District due to domestic unhappiness. This young couple aged 20 and 30 married only two months earlier by registered marriage as their parents did not approve of it. One evening the doctor and his new bride committed suicide in their residence by pouring kerosene. Another couple aged 20 and 25 at Tirupur were found dead in a lodge. A letter believed to have been written by the couple said they were suffering from ailments and therefore putting an end to their life. Another case is reported from Coimbatore in which a 13 year old girl

committed suicide at her residence by setting fire to herself. It is alleged that her father was humiliated by some persons in her presence. Unable to bear the humiliation, the young girl set herself on fire.

(James 1983: 53–54)

A brief but typical article from *The Hindu* of 9 April 2002 reports three suicides in New Delhi. The first death, by burning, was of an unemployed 30-year-old man living with his wife and brother. The second was a death by hanging of a 35-year-old man about whom nothing else is reported. The third, also a hanging, was of an unidentified man of about 30 years of age (*The Hindu* 2002).

A common topic of media coverage of 'ordinary' suicides is of the suicides of entire families.

> In a suicide pact, five members of a businessman's family, including his wife and three daughters, died by consuming pesticide on Monday in Suryapet town of Nalgonda district.
>
> A suicide note signed by the five stated that they resorted to the extreme step due to financial problems.
>
> (*The Hindu* 2002b)

> Nine members of a family committed suicide in Marakal village, near Hillur in Ankola Taluk on Friday . . . All the members of the family were said to be dejected with the behaviour of [the family head], who allegedly had a criminal background.
>
> (*The Hindu* 2001a)

> Two members of a family of Saidabad have committed suicide allegedly over a dispute arising out of their failure to get back the Rs. 4 lakhs deposited in the now defunct Charminar Cooperative Urban Bank.
>
> (Our Staff Reporter 2002)

> A young [Hyderabad] couple attempted suicide last night by consuming sleeping pills allegedly due to financial problems . . .
>
> (*The Hindu* 2002c)

In one of the few systematic examinations of media coverage of ordinary suicides, Gururaj and Isaac estimated that only one suicide in nine registered by the police in Bangalore was reported by newspapers in the city (Gururaj and Isaac 2001: 51). (We infer that an even smaller fraction of rural suicides receives press coverage) Gururaj and Isaac note some recurrent features of this genre of media coverage:

- 'a tendency to "sensationalise" the act with catchy and attractive captions';
- a focus on poverty related issues;
- disproportionate coverage of suicides of a number of individuals at one time;
- greater coverage of unusual events;
- greater coverage of mysterious deaths (Gururaj and Isaac 2001: 45).

Celebrity suicides

At the other end of the spectrum is coverage of the suicide deaths of celebrities. These are placed, not amongst the municipal and police items, but receive far greater prominence near the front of the paper or magazine. Sometimes, as in the death of the Tamil film producer, G. V. Ventkateswaran, the story is picked up by foreign media such as the US trade paper *Variety* (Pearson 2003). The death of Anju Illyasi, wife of TV-personality Suhaib Illyasi in 2000, apparently a case of suicide by stabbing, received repeated coverage over an extended period (for example, Service 2000; Subramanyam 2004).

Other examples of the relatively more prominent coverage of celebrity suicides are: the death by jumping from the fifth story of a five star hotel in New Delhi of media personality and news reader Bhaskar Bhattacharya in 2000 (Kant 2000), the death of Tamil filmstar Revathisree in Chennai in 2003 (India 2003), the death of Bangalore model Rakhee Choudhari in Mumbai in 2002 (Deccan Herald 2002) and of contemporary dancer Ranjabati Chaki Sircar in Calcutta in 1999 (Kalidas 1999).

Exam failures

Another genre, especially prominent between March and June when examinations are in progress, are stories of students taking their own lives. An almost archetypical story is one from Mumbai in 1998:

> A 17-year-old girl student who failed in the HSC examinations for the second consecutive time this year leapt off the second floor of her college building in Parel this evening and died.
>
> (Indian Express 1998)

Sometimes no cause is given for a student's death (Our Staff Reporter 2002). Other stories probe more deeply into education policy changes that place families in debt to pay for their children's education (Nair 2004) or report on official investigations following a spate of suicide deaths (Das 2001) or on the work of NGOs such as Kerala's Maithri (George 2002). Others look more broadly at the phenomenon of student suicides, such as a thoughtful article on the situation in Kerala by Leela Menon in *The Hindu* in 2002, which reported that:

> Kerala, the suicide capital of India, witnesses a wave of suicide mania sweeping over the adolescent scene in the post-SSLC scenario every year. It was no different this year with the suicide trend gripping even the new teens. Both the suicide prevention centre 'Maithri' and the adolescent helpline, 'Childline' reported a flood [of] calls prior to the announcement of the result and in the aftermath of the announcement. Strangely, the calls were not exclusively from children but also from desperate parents, neighbours, friends, and even from teachers. Which testifies to the anxiety, expectations and frustrations that mark the educational scenario in Kerala.
>
> (Menon 2002)

Indian student suicides occasionally feature in the international media as happened in 2002 when the Saudi press picked up a story – then reprinted in the USA – of the suicide of a student who had actually passed the second-year exam but who took his life before it was found that his name was inadvertently left off the university list (Washington Report on Middle East Affairs 2002).

Female suicides

Although the ratio of female to male suicides is relatively high in India, media coverage of female suicides tends to focus on a few prominent themes. Suicides attributed to a family's inability to afford dowry for its daughters (Sethi and Anand 1988) and as a result of harassment from in-laws for additional payment of dowry (Kishwar and Vanita 1984: 203–205) receive detailed coverage, especially from feminist journals such as *Manushi*.

One significant report was that of Prabhjot Singh, who reported in *The Tribune* in 2000 that 'harassment by in-laws for various reasons, including insufficient dowry, accounts for 80 per cent of suicides by women in Punjab, where the incidence of ending one's own life has been alarmingly on the rise in the recent past' (Singh 2000). The report continued that in the first half of 2000 there had been 77 cases of suicide in the Punjab, two-thirds of which were by women. 'Though doctors hold that changing lifestyles, stress both at the place of work and at home and financial frustrations are the main reasons for the high incidence of suicide in Punjab, they could not explain why more women than men take this drastic step' (Singh 2000).

On occasion, newspaper reports highlight suicides that illustrate other abuses of women, such as the suicide of a young Gond woman in 2002 following her 'sale' at auction as punishment for allegedly being 'caught' with a boy (Dhar 2002).

Economic suicides

The largest, and in many respects the most complex genre, is that which reports on the suicides attributed to economic distress, particularly among weavers and farmers. What distinguishes the articles belonging to this genre is the focus on economic issues, which in most cases are linked to policy changes that have taken place in the post-1991 era of economic reforms. In almost all cases in this genre, suicides are reported, not as the principal subject of the article, but as a routine journalistic device, at times almost a cliché, used to highlight the hardships experienced by a broader class of workers. In this genre, vignettes of worker suicides – frequently with a photo of surviving relatives – are an almost obligatory feature, used in much the same way that pictures of severely malnourished children are in articles on famine in Africa (for general discussions of the selective attention of the media to development issues, see Bennett and Daniel 2002; Sainath 2002).

Weaver suicides

In 2001 and 2002 a number of articles appeared that highlighted the plight of powerloom weavers in Andhra Pradesh (see for example, Our Staff Reporter 2001; Farooq 2001; Dayashankar 2001, 2001; Reddy 2002). Farooq's report, which was run by the BBC, is typical:

> A crisis in the weaving industry in the southern Indian state of Andhra Pradesh is forcing workers there to resort to a drastic solution – taking their own lives. As many as 90 weavers have committed suicide in the past four years – half of them during the last 18 months alone. This in a state at the forefront of an ambitious economic reform programme, which some analysts argue has contributed to the crisis.
>
> (Farooq 2001)

The most extensive and in-depth examination of the condition of weavers in Andhra that we have seen is the series of articles written by Asha Krishnakumar in 2001 (Krishnakumar 2001a, 2001b, 2001c, 2001d, 2001e, 2001f, 2001g).[2] Krishnakumar outlines a series of policy changes since 1985 as well as changes in the national and international market that have led to an economic crisis for both handloom and powerloom weavers in the state (see especially Krishnakumar 2001b, 2001d). These changes include: the emergence of competing powerloom centres in Maharashtra that have lower costs of production and higher product- ivity and that more recently have introduced jet looms,[3] liberalisation policies, which promoted the export of cotton and yarn, increased electricity charges and excise on yarn, and the removal of import restrictions, which has led to dumping of cloth by Thailand and China.

   At the end of several of Krishnakumar's articles are poignant case studies of weaver suicides that trace a common, distressing history of loss of income, lack of alternative work, mounting debt and family distress and finally a decision to end life (Krishnakumar 2001a, 2001b, 2001e). One further feature sets Krishna- kumar's articles on weaver suicides apart from almost all other discussions of suicides arising from economic causes in the Indian media: a relatively informed discussion about the causal factors that lead a tiny minority of affected individuals to choose death.

Farmer suicides

The largest body of reports on suicides with economic causes are those that cover farmer suicides. As with weavers, coverage of farmer suicides tends to focus on the economic distress of the individual. Some accounts are brief and relatively factual, much like the coverage of 'ordinary' suicides (for example, The Hindu 1998; Our Principal Correspondent 1998; Siddiq 2000; Sharma 2002). Most stories use farmer suicides as a stock journalistic device for highlighting agricul- tural distress in a district or region (for example, David 1998; Nautiyal 2002;

Deshpande 2003). In these reports the vulnerable rain-fed agricultural regions of the Deccan feature prominently.

A number of articles locate the causes for farmer distress in the intersection of adverse weather, government policy failures and inappropriate crop choices. In 2004 Vivek Deshpande reported on the distress experienced by cotton farmers in Maharashtra's Vidharba region arising in part from failures in official procurement mechanisms (Deshpande 2004). Samar Harlankar surveyed the situation in Karnataka, Andhra and Maharashtra, concluding that the agricultural crisis could be traced to a headlong rush by farmers to embrace cash crops:

> All of the farmers who died were trying to speed along the fast lane of agricultural success. Most of them had replaced traditional crops with lucrative cash crops, little realising that raising them is a costly and precise science. This requirement was impossible to meet, given that the farmers today are ignored by the agricultural credit system of banking, squeezed dry by moneylenders and abandoned by the complete breakdown in the Government's agricultural extension services. Their life is like a house of cards: built on paper-thin supports. Take one away – like a failed monsoon, an overdose of pesticides and everything comes crashing down.
>
> (Harlankar 1998; a similar assessment was made by Iyer 1998)

Stories about agrarian distress and farmer suicides in India are occasionally picked up by the international media who report matters in much the same terms as appear in the Indian press (for example, Time International 1998; Waldman 2004).

As with weaver suicides, a few journalists have probed the issues in greater depth or with greater persistence. In a companion piece to Krishnakumar's articles on weaver suicides, Parvathi Menon wrote an in-depth study of suicides by groundnut (peanut) farmers in Andhra's Anantapur District. Menon found that drought, as well as market changes brought about by economic liberalisation – higher costs for electricity, fertilisers, seeds and low prices because of cheap imported edible oil – had all pushed families into debt (Menon 2001a, 2001b).

Among those who have reported for many years on all aspects of Indian rural life, including farmer suicides, perhaps none is more distinguished than the rural affairs reporter of *The Hindu* P. Sainath (Sainath's investigations of rural poverty in the 1990s were summarised in Sainath 1999; for more recent reports on farmer suicides, see, for example, Sainath 2001a, 2001b; Sainath 2005a, 2005b, 2005c, 2005d, 2005e).[4] In many of Sainath's articles a farmer suicide (often accentuated by a poignant photograph taken by the journalist) is used to frame an acute investigation of the broader issues facing farmers. An article on the situation in Maharashtra's Vidharba region in 2005, for example, found that drought, lack of access to credit, failures of cotton cooperatives to pay farmers, rising input costs and falling prices have plunged farmers into mounting debt.

> Other reasons driving the crisis are the same as those in Andhra Pradesh or Kerala. Input prices are rising and output prices crashing. Debt is soaring. 'Not

only is the cost of production going up,' says [Warda farmers' leader] Vijay Jawandia, 'so is the cost of living. Health, transport, all other items. Globalisation and liberalisation have had a deadly impact. Earlier when production failed, prices rose. Now, even when the crop fails, prices go down . . . Rural credit has collapsed . . . [T]he state has turned its back on the farmer'.

(Sainath 2005c)

The politics of farmer suicides

The media also occasionally covers the politics of farmer suicides, for example, speculation on the impact of farmer suicides on impending elections (Reddy 1998; Datta 2003) or reports of official investigations into the causes of farmer suicides (*The Hindu* 2001c).

Economic commentators have also used farmer suicides to highlight policy changes that they feel are necessary. In 1998, Jairam Ramesh, an economist affiliated with the Congress Party, noted that differing explanations had been offered for the suicides of cotton farmers in Andhra in that year: media exaggeration, imitation and the risks of farming in arid and semi-arid regions. Ramesh went on to argue that cotton farmers had been hurt less by economic reforms than by policy failures. In addition to the collapse of state supported credit and the provision of agricultural extension, the failure to give cotton farmers consistent access to world markets had also hurt them.

> Trade policy has gone against cotton farmers. Stop-go and restrictive export policies have contributed to low growth rates in productivity. What we have done by denying our farmers free access to world markets is provide an implicit subsidy to our organised textile mill owners.
>
> (Ramesh 1998)

More commonly, though, suicide deaths among weavers and farmers have also been utilised by activists as a means of dramatising their opposition to economic liberalisation, globalism and intellectual property regimes promoted by the international bodies such as the World Trade Organisation. In her 2000 Reith Lecture for the BBC, the prominent environmentalist Vandana Shiva introduced her argument that 'industrialisation and genetic engineering of food and globalisation of trade in agriculture are recipes for creating hunger, not for feeding the poor' by a reference to farmer suicides:

> Recently, I was visiting Bhatinda in Punjab because of an epidemic of farmers suicides. Punjab used to be the most prosperous agricultural region in India. Today every farmer is in debt and despair. Vast stretches of land have become water-logged desert. And as an old farmer pointed out, even the trees have stopped bearing fruit because heavy use of pesticides have killed the pollinators – the bees and butterflies.
>
> (Shiva 2000)

As we will see in Chapter 11, a rigorous academic study of farmer suicides investigated the situation in the Punjab, concluding that on the whole, Punjab has a very low number of suicides, and 'that politicians and the mainstream media misrepresented the scale and causes of what they claimed were debt-driven suicides by farmers in the Punjab'. Rather, dowry 'and expenditure on narcotics and alcohol' were the major causes of debt (Swami 1998). Vandana Shiva has highlighted farmer suicides in other parts of India to illustrate her arguments about the harm being done to small farmers by trade liberalisation and the entry into India of giant international seed corporations (see for example, Shiva, Jafri *et al.* 2002; Shiva 2004a, 2004b).

Another prominent environmental activist who has highlighted farmer suicides to criticise harmful aspects of globalisation is the journalist Devinder Sharma. Commenting on the agricultural situation after the defeat of the Chandrababu Naidu government in Andhra in 2004, Sharma observed that:

> . . . governments are clueless of the reasons that force farmers to commit suicides . . . The reason is obvious. No one has the political courage to point a finger at the real villain – industrial farming model that shifts the focus on cash crops and thereby plays havoc with sustainable livelihoods.
>
> (Sharma 2005)

The most sweeping linkage of Indian farmer suicides with economic liberalisation has been a report issued by Christian Aid 'The Damage Done: Aid, Death and Dogma' (Christian Aid 2005). The report argued that the real origins of the agrarian crisis in Andhra Pradesh lie outside India. (An Indian NGO introduced the report with the headline 'Britain blamed for Indian Suicides'). The crisis:

> . . . was caused by a zealous programme of liberalisation and privatisation brought about by the World Bank, and the International Monetary Fund – with the active support of the UK government.
>
> (Christian Aid 2005: 14)

The Christian Aid report concluded:

> The number of farmers taking their own lives in Andhra Pradesh is shocking and indicates that something has gone terribly wrong with the agricultural sector. These are not deaths from just one area or from just one type of farming. This is suicide on a scale that is surely unique in modern times.
>
> The immediate cause of these deaths is debt. This debt was brought on by a number of factors, all of which, except for the weather, can be ascribed to liberalisation. These liberalising factors at both national and state level, were the results of policies made by India's central government, the Andhra Pradesh state government of Chandrababu Naidu, the IMF, the World Bank and [UK development agency] DFID . . . . [H]ow many more years will it take for the world to wake up to the fact that wholesale liberalisation of agriculture

and the privatisation of the support mechanisms that sustain it are killing farmers?

(Christian Aid 2005: 29–30)

In Chapter 11 we consider what can be determined about the relationship between occupation and suicide. We will argue there that farmers are not at elevated risk of suicide and that the rates of farmer suicides in states that have received intense media coverage such as Andhra Pradesh are actually considerably lower than those in other states that have received relatively little media coverage.

Political suicide

There is one further category of suicides whose media coverage is significant: those intended to draw attention to an issue or cause. While relatively rare, these very political suicides often receive prominent coverage.

One of the first and most famous of the post-Independence political suicides was the fast-unto-death of Potti Srirumalu. Sriramulu, a Gandhian Congress Party Freedom Fighter commenced his fast on 19 October 1952 to underscore the demand for the creation of a separate Telugu-speaking state out of the colonial Madras Presidency. Prime Minister Nehru, fearing that accepting the division of Madras would precipitate the Balkanisation of India, refused to create a new linguistic state. After 58 days of fasting, Sriramulu died. His death precipitated mass demonstrations in the Telugu-speaking districts and four days later, Nehru agreed to divide Madras into separate linguistically based states (B.M.G. 2002; Harrison 1960: 17).

Another episode of political suicides occurred in Tamil Nadu in the mid-1960s during the anti-Hindi agitations. Sumathi Ramaswamy begins her major study of the devotion to the Tamil language with an account of some of those suicides:

It was a quiet cool January dawn in the South Indian city of Tiruchirapalli in the year 1964. A can in his hand, a man named Chinnaswami left his home – leaving behind his aging mother, young wife, and infant daughter – and walked to the city's railway station. On reaching there, he doused himself with its contents and set himself on fire, shouting out aloud . . . (Death to Hindi! May Tamil flourish!). Chinnasami's example was not lost. A year later, to the date, history epeated itself . . .: five other men burned themselves alive 'at the altar of Tamil'. Three others died just as painfully – not in a raging blaze, but by swallowing insecticide – also for the sake of Tamil, as they declared in their own last words. These dramatic acts were reported by the mainstream news media in India, sometimes in a matter-of-fact fashion, sometimes with derision, but invariably as yet another example of the 'frenzy' and 'fanaticism' that speakers of Tamil habitually display when it comes to their language.[5]

(Ramaswamy 1997: 1)

Similar acts of public suicide occurred in Tamil Nadu when the popular DMK leader C. N. Annadurai died in February 1969. In 1982 when DMK leader M. Karunanidhi was arrested, five activists took their lives. When Tamil film star and All-India Anna Dravida Munnetra Kazhagam (AIADMK) leader M.G. Ramachandran (MGR) became ill in 1984 there were 12 self-immolations; when he became critically ill in 1987, 22 individuals killed themselves and 26 others committed suicide following his death in 1987 (Sethi 1991: 69; upperstall.com 2004). Following findings of corruption against MGR's lover and political successor, Tamil Nadu Chief Minister Jayalalita, in February 2000 at least one party volunteer died after setting himself alight (Reporter 2000).

The most recent significant episode of political suicides was that which accompanied the 'anti-Mandal' agitations in 1990. The widespread public agitations in north India followed the announcement by Prime Minister V.P. Singh that government would implement the long-neglected recommendations of the Mandal Commission and increase the number of jobs and university places reserved for candidates from backward castes. Students from upper castes, irate that their future opportunities were to be restricted, took to the streets. The first student to take his life, Rajeev Goswami, apparently did so unintentionally when a mock self-immolation went wrong (Pachauri, George *et al.* 1990: 15). Goswami's example on 19 September, 1990 was rapidly imitated by angry, suddenly politicised young people in cities across north India (Pachauri, George *et al.* 1990: 16). By the end of October 159 people had attempted to take their own lives, 63 successfully (Baweja, Singh *et al.* 1990: 10). By the end of the agitation, there had been 202 attempts and 112 completed suicides, one-third of them women (Sethi 1991: 69 and 71; see also, Bhugra 1991). Naturally these protest suicides received extensive coverage by the media. Perhaps because most of those who attempted or died were students, there was a noticeable tendency to explain the psychological as well as the palpably political causes of the suicides that sets these reports apart from almost all others.[6] In a critical examination of the anti-Mandal suicides, Harsh Sethi stated:

> it can be broadly argued that the archetypical victim is either a young student, or a semi-educated, semi-skilled unemployed or inefficiently employed youth [for whom the decision to implement the Mandal recommendations represented a significant denial of opportunity for employment]. There is some evidence to suggest that many of the victims were not just relatively poor and harassed, they suffered from a troubled background and could count on low family/social support. In short, many of them would well fit the textbook category of potential suicide victims.
>
> (Sethi 1991: 70)

Sethi argued that media coverage actually increased the number of suicides:

> instead of advising restraint or condemning them as anti-democratic acts, the general refrain was one of glorifying them as acts of self-sacrifice and martyrdom in the national interest.
>
> (Sethi 1991: 70)

Sethi argues that the high percentage (57 per cent) of deaths by burning had a clear cultural component and:

> ... needs to be located in the cultural repertoire of inwardly directed protest in our society: fasting to death or self-immolation probably fit better into this framework, more so since they also carry an association of purification. Since fasting has been 'overused' as a political weapon in recent decades, its appeal has somewhat declined. In self-immolation, undoubtedly as an extremely painful way to court death, the symbolic protest probably gains in strength.
>
> (Sethi 1991: 72)

An *India Today* article by Harinder Baweja reported an interview with Dr D. Mohan, Head of the Psychology Department in the All-India Institute of Medical Sciences, who commented on the role of imitation and media in the anti-Mandal suicides:

> 'The otherwise lost souls started finding mention in newspapers. In an epidemic, the degree of exposure you get overtakes pain, the thought of death or even rational thinking.' He isn't exaggerating. The first question that Monica Chadha, 19 [who set herself ablaze in New Delhi], asked her mother a day after her suicide attempt was: 'Has my photograph appeared in the newspapers?'
>
> (Baweja, Singh *et al.* 1990: 12)

Unique among the dozens of media articles covering suicides in India, Baweja's article included information on the early warning signs of suicide and advice on what others can do to prevent a person from acting on suicidal ideas (Baweja, Singh *et al.* 1990: 12).

Plan of the book

There are two broad parts to the book. Part I, which presents background to the detailed investigations that follow, comprises Chapters 2 to 6. In Chapter 2 we survey the history of Indian attitudes to suicide, considering what can be gleaned from classical sources and religious texts about attitudes to suicide in ancient and medieval times. The chapter also considers the theological attitudes expressed toward suicide by India's major religions, noting in particular the relatively more permissive attitudes of Hindusim and Jainism. Chapter 2 concludes with a survey of the existing literature, which analyses the Indian experience of suicide from the colonial period to the present day. Chapter 3 considers the legal and administrative context in which official data on suicides are collected and reports on eight different tests of the validity of the data that lead us to reject the frequently made assertion that official data seriously understate the number of suicides in India. In Chapter 4 the aetiology of India suicides is examined. We argue there that it is possible to identify two major types of crises in the data, those of human development and those of personal relationships. In Chapter 5 we examine the significance in changes in the methods that Indians have utilised to take their own lives. One of the most striking changes has been the rapid rise in the use of agricultural poisons since the late 1960s. The trend of suicides in India, beginning with data from the colonial period, is presented in Chapter 6. During the colonial period, suicide peaks appear to have been associated with major famines and outbreaks of disease. In independent India, there has been a steady rise in suicide rates, with one puzzling dip in the mid 1970s, which receives detailed consideration.

Part II, comprising Chapters 7 to 16, presents the results of detailed investigations of the impact of a range of social factors on the Indian experience of suicide. In Chapter 7 we study the impact of gender on suicide. We find that women in India are at a relatively far higher risk of suicide than women in industrialised societies, a difference that does not seem to be related to changes in either equality or modernisation. Chapter 8 broadens the survey to include the influence of age. Here we find the widest diversity in age patterns between the Indian states. In general, Indian women are at highest risk between the ages of 15 and 29; for men, the years of maximum risk are 30 to 44. We argue that India has an emerging youth and young adult suicide crisis that has yet to be either recognised or to receive the urgent policy responses it demands. Chapter 9 investigates the impact of urbanisation on suicide. We find a complex relationship, with lower urban than rural suicide rates in south India, but higher urban rates in some north Indian cities. In Chapter 10 we report on the relationship between increasing levels of education and suicide, finding that suicide rates tend to rise with each increment in formal education, except for university graduates. The impact of occupation on suicide rates is the subject of Chapter 11. These findings present a picture with is frequently at variance with the impressions created by media reporting of suicide. The consequences of different marital statuses are reported in Chapter 12. In contrast with the experience of industrialised societies, in India marriage confers little or no protection from suicide; between half and three-quarters of all those who take their lives in India are married. Chapter 13 examines the impact of alcohol consumption on suicide rates in India finding that, unlike the experience in European societies, there is little discernible relationship between levels of alcohol consumption and suicide. In Chapter 14 we survey the suicide experience of the approximately 9 million members of the Indian diaspora. Indians, like other migrants, appear to take both their propensity to commit suicide and their preferred methods with them when they leave India. Chapter 15 presents a unique and detailed case study based on individual records of suicide in Pondicherry, which has the highest suicide rates in India. In about 40 per cent of cases, a conflict with a close relative was the immediately precipitating cause of suicide. The Pondicherry data also throw some light on the very much higher propensity of Hindus to take their own lives.

Chapter 16, the conclusion, argues that the complex patterns of suicide found in our study are best understood in terms of the major changes that are occurring in Indian family life and in economic expectations. Since these changes are most advanced in south India, we predict that similar patterns will emerge in the rest of

India as this pattern 'moves north'. In particular, India's youth suicide crisis, at present largely confined to the south, will become a national crisis in coming decades.

Notes

1 We are indebted to the Inter-university Consortium for Political Science for providing us with data from the World Values Surveys.
2 Krishnakumar received the 2002 Lorenzo Natali Prize for Journalism for the series of articles she wrote on weaver suicides in Andhra. See *Frontline*, 6 December, 2002, at http://www.flonnet.com/fl1924/stories/20021206007013400.htm, accessed 12 August 2005.
3 Each powerloom leaves a dozen handloom weavers unemployed while each jetloom does the work of 40 powerlooms, rendering hundreds out of work (Padma 2002).
4 Sainath has won many awards for his journalism, including the European Commission's Lorenzo Natali Prize and the Bharat Asmita national award.
5 It seems entirely plausible that similar cultural predispositions underlie the use by the Tamil Tigers in Sri Lanka of suicide bombing as a political tactic to further their demands for Tamileelam, a separate Tamil homeland in Sri Lanka (see for example, Pape 2003).
6 Sethi quotes a PUDR report, which states that most of those who attempted suicide were from poor or lower middle class families (Sethi 1991: 70).

2 Previous studies of suicide in India

Introduction

Although in absolute terms, Indian suicides constitute a significant portion of the worldwide burden of suicide deaths, there has been only limited study of the phenomenon at the national level, and almost no systematic examination of the problem from a sociological point of view. Much of the existing literature on suicide in India can be classified under four broad headings: the Indological tradition, which examines the evidence and ethical teachings found in Sanskrit texts; modern psychiatric evidence – largely drawn from hospital experience; sociological studies carried out at the state or union territory level; and anthropological studies of specific tribal groups.

Suicide in Indian culture

India is an ancient civilisation and an extremely complex one. Waves of migration, expansion and conquest have laid down layer after layer of cultural diversity, to the point that it is virtually impossible to make any uncontested social generalisation. In addition, when we seek to discover traditional Hindu attitudes toward suicide we must rely upon a narrow range of literary sources that may only reflect the views of a small, literate elite and tell us little about the views and practices of ordinary villagers. Any discussion of traditional attitudes toward suicide must acknowledge the significance of Hindu doctrines of reincarnation and rebirth, the belief that human beings are bound onto an endless and dreary wheel of births, deaths and rebirths and that the object of all classical religious teachings is the achievement of *moksha*, liberation from the cycle (de Bary, Hay *et al.* 1964, Chapter XIII).

The oldest evidence of Hindu attitudes towards suicide comes from fragmentary evidence found in the Vedas. These seem to indicate that, in an age when worship involved animal sacrifices to the gods, self-sacrifice was considered to be the highest and best form of worship (Venkoba Rao 1975: 231; see also Thakur 1963: 46–50).

These attitudes are said to have changed by the time the Upanishads were written, perhaps in the eighth to third centuries BCE. Professor Venkoba Rao cites a passage from the Iśa Upanishad that appears to condemn suicide: 'He who takes his self reaches after death the sunless regions covered by impenetrable darkness.' (Venkoba Rao 1975: 231; see also Thakur 1963: 51). Radhakrishna, however, suggests that what he translates as 'slayers of the self' may be interpreted as 'those who neglect the spirit' or 'those who do not know the Self' (Radhakrishnan 1953: 570). In a similar vein, Bhaktivedanta suggests that the phrase that he translates as 'the killer of the soul', refers to 'a person [who] does not fully utilize his human life for self-realization' (Bhaktivedanta 1969: 23). Varma also argues that 'this couplet does not actually indicate suicide' (1976: 138; see also Andriolo 1993, fn 20).

Thakur notes that the great Hindu epic, the *Ramayana*, recounts a remarkable mass suicide. At the end of the epic, after the deaths of Sita and Kausilya, Rama's own brother Lakshman kills himself by drowning:

> With the death of Laksmana, Rama also lost all interest in life. He then, together with Bharata and Satrughna, left this world by drowning in the Sarayu river near [Guptaraghata]. Aggrieved and depressed, thousands of inhabitants of Ayodhaya followed suit.
>
> (Thakur 1963: 52)[1]

A change of attitude towards suicide appears in the *smriti* (remembered) Sanskrit literature that emerged in the early centuries of the Common Era (for a general survey of this literature see Basham 1954: 112–121). Thakur cites a number of passages from these legal texts that condemn suicide as sinful (Thakur 1963: 54–59; see also Bilimoria 1995, fn 10: 176–177). Stietencron observes that, while:

> Most passages [of the Dharmashastra texts] condemned suicide as a mortal sin . . . Manu and the other Smr[i]tis were not equally strict in all cases of suicide. They admit of certain exceptions to the rule. According to Manu, for instance, a man who has committed a *mahapataka*, i.e. a sin so great that no other penance can be adequate, is allowed to atone for it by death.
>
> (Stietencron 1967: 12–13; see also Day 1982: 233–235)

Religious suicide

If the legal texts condemn suicide, medieval texts offer increasing support to those wishing to go down the *mahapatha* [great road], i.e. undertake an act of religious suicide. Thakur provides extensive evidence from this period of encouragement of suicide at sites of religious pilgrimage, such as falling from a cliff at Amarkantak, drowning at Kashi (Varanasi) or jumping from a sacred tree at Prayag (the convergence of the Ganges and the Jamuna at Allahabad) (Thakur 1963: 79–85).

> Prayaga is further noted for being the place where one is not only permitted but persuaded to commit suicide . . . [O]ne who jumps from the sacred banyan tree (*vata-vrksa*) into the river below and so ends his life goes to Rudraloka [the abode of Siva] . . . The number of suicides in Allahabad by jumping off this tree became so great from a belief that Akbar had committed such

a suicide in a past birth and been rewarded by becoming an emperor in the next that he had the tree cut down.

(Thakur 1963: 83–85)

Keith also offers a number of examples from Hindu sacred writings and from the epics which describe religiously meritorious self-sacrifice (Keith 1914: 34). Stietencron suggests that the growth in the influence of popular emotional religiosity in the form of *bhakti* movements in the first centuries CE was accompanied by the popularity of pilgrimage to holy places such as Prayag or Kashi (Stietencron 1967: 9–10; for an extended discussion of bhakti cults see Lannoy 1975, especially 205 ff.).

Over time, Stietencron argues, religious suicide at those places became increasingly accepted for those 'who wanted to gain *moks[h]a* quickly without much effort' (Stietencron 1967: 14). Benjamin Walker suggests that such religious suicides became relatively common at times in the past:

> ... suicide was once very commonly practised in India by all classes of people, and those who took their own lives were not regarded as having committed a sin, but on the contrary as having performed a meritorious act, and the record of their deed was often preserved in stone or metal. *Sati* stones commemorating the virtuous wives who voluntarily died on the pyres of their husbands are extant in large numbers. In the Deccan there are numerous inscriptions which commemorate the pious souls who in fulfilment of a vow leapt from pillars, starved to death or drowned themselves.
>
> (Walker 1983: 446)

Stietencron cites passages such as these from the *Puranas* written around the sixth century CE:

> a man who, knowingly or unknowingly, wilfully or unintentionally dies in the Ganges, secures on death heaven and *moksha* [release from the cycle of rebirths] (*Padma Purana* V: 60.55).
>
> (Stietencron 1967: 15)

> He who abandons his life in this *tirtha* [pilgrimage] (= Kasi) in some way or other does not incur the sin of suicide but secures his desired objects (*Skanda Purana, Kasikhanda* 22.76).
>
> (Stietencron 1967: 15)

In the medieval period, the acceptable means of religious suicide grew:

> the methods for permissible suicide were amended. One could cut one's throat, or throw oneself into the abyss, which meant jumping from a holy place atop a cliff or from a specially designated tree at Prayaga. If suicide was to facilitate quick release, perhaps one should compensate for the absence of

the renouncer's asceticism by adding an extra dash of pain. Roasting on top of slow-burning cow dung was considered to be the most meritorious form of cremation. Cutting off pieces of one's flesh and feeding it to the birds while bleeding to death demonstrated more courage and endurance than cutting one's throat.

(Andriolo 1993: 16; for an extended treatment see Thakur 1963: 77–96)

Religious suicides were also recorded occasionally at places such as the Jaganath Temple in Puri, Orissa. In the annual *rath* festival in June, the images of Jaganath, his brother Balabhadra and sister Subhadra are placed in immense *raths* or carriages – hence the English word *juggernaut*. The Jaganath *rath* is some 13.5 metres in height, 10.5 metres on a side and has wheels that are two metres in diameter. On some occasions in the past, devotees killed themselves by throwing themselves under the wheels as the *rath* was being pulled by thousands of devotees around the temple complex. Hunter cited with disapproval a lurid description of a fanciful engraving of the *rath* festival given in 1869 by the novelist William Makepeace Thackeray:

'It is called the Gin [djin?] Jagannath, and represents a hideous moving palace, with a reeking still at the roof, and vast gin-barrels for wheels, *under which unhappy millions are crushed to death.*' [Emphasis in original]

(Hunter 1872: 138)

Hunter observed tartly that his researches showed that such suicides have 'always been insignificant, and could at most occur but once a year' (Hunter 1872: 137). Nevertheless,

their fame made a deep impression upon early travellers . . . and I find that the travellers who have had the most terrible stories to tell are the very ones whose narratives prove that they went entirely by hearsay, and could not possibly have themselves seen the Car Festival.

(Hunter 1872: 137)

In another passage, Hunter observed:

[N]othing could be more opposed to the spirit of Vishnu-worship than self-immolation. Accidental death within the temple renders the whole place unclean. The ritual suddenly stops, and the polluted offerings are hurried away from the sight of the offended god.

(Hunter 1872: 38)

Walker and Keith give instances of other locations at which religious suicides occasionally occurred: at Girnar (by jumping from a high rock) or at the sacred conjunction of the Ganges and Jamuna at Allahabad (by drowning), or jumping into the sea at the mouth of the Ganges ('to be devoured by sharks'), or cutting one's throat before the image of Bhavani at the Vindhyavasini Temple at Mirzapur, or by starvation (Walker 1983; Keith 1914, p. 35; and see also Varma 1976, pp. 139–143).

Thakur provides an extensive citation from an 1822 manuscript of an eye-witness to a religious suicide by leaping into a steep ravine in the holy island of Omkarji at Mandhata (near Indore in Madhya Pradesh) in the Narmada River (Thakur 1963: xii–xiv).

Bishop Heber, travelling across north India in 1824, noted that:

> Suttees are less numerous in Benares than many parts of India, but self-immolation by drowning is very common. Many scores, every year, of pilgrims from all parts of India, come hither expressly to end their days to secure their salvation. They purchase two large kegeree pots between which they tie themselves, and when empty these support their weight in the water. Thus equipped, they paddle into the stream, then fill the pots with the water which surrounds them, and thus sink into eternity. Government have sometimes attempted to prevent this practice, but with no other effect than driving the voluntary victims a little further down the river; nor indeed when a man has come several hundred miles to die, is it likely that a police-officer can prevent him.
>
> (Heber 1828, vol. 1: 295)

Day argues that there is also abundant evidence in Hindu, Jain and Buddhist texts for broad approval of what he terms 'expiational suicide' (Day 1982: 231). Suicide could expiatate grave sins such as the murder of a Brahmin or adultery with the wife of one's guru, which could not be otherwise expunged in life (Day 1982: 232).

Sati and jauhar

As Walker mentions, memorials to *satis*, women who burned themselves on their husbands' funeral pyres, exist in a number of places, especially in central and western India. One of the most famous accounts we have of a voluntary *sati* is that witnessed by Sleeman near Jabalpur in 1829. Sleeman had sought to impede, if not completely ban, the practice in his jurisdiction. Accordingly he refused consent to a 65-year-old widow whose husband had been cremated that morning. After four days, in which the widow had commenced a fast unto death, Sleeman relented:

> Satisfied myself that it would be unavailing to attempt to save her life, I sent for all the principal members of the family, and consented that she should be suffered to burn herself if they would all enter into engagements that no other members of their family should ever do the same. This they agreed to . . .
>
> The ceremonies of bathing were gone through before three, while the wood and other combustible materials for a strong fire were collected, and put in the pit. After bathing, she called for a pawn [pan] (betel leaf) and ate it, then

rose up, and with one arm on the shoulder of her eldest son, and the other on that of her nephew, approached the fire. I had sentries placed all round, and no other person was allowed to approach within five paces. As she rose up, fire was set to the pile, and it was instantly in a blaze. The distance was about one hundred and fifty yards – she came on with a calm and cheerful countenance – stopped once, and casting her eyes upward said – 'Why have they kept me five days from thee, my husband!' On coming to the sentries her supporters stopped – she walked once round the pit, paused a moment; and while muttering a prayer threw some flowers into the fire. She then walked up deliberately and steadily to the brink, stepped into the centre of the flame, sat down, and leaning back in the midst as if reposing upon a couch, was consumed without uttering a shriek or betraying one sign of agony!

(Sleeman 1844, vol. 1: 29–30)[2]

Not all *satis* were voluntary suicides. The Abbé Dubois states his belief that 'these wretched victims' were often drugged and in his description of one *sati* notes that some of 'her relatives and friends . . . were armed with muskets, swords and other weapons . . . intended not only to intimidate the unhappy victim . . . but also to overawe any persons . . . tempted to prevent the accomplishment of the homicidal sacrifice' (Dubois 1906: 357–358, 363). Andriolo cites Nicolò dei Conti and others to the same effect (Andriolo 1993: 2–3 and 28–29).

There are also well-attested instances of mass suicides from the medieval and early modern period in India. The *jauhar*, the mass suicide by self-immolation of the wives of Rajput warriors faced with unavoidable defeat, occurred on a number of occasions. In 1533, for example, Chitorgarh was besieged by Bahadur Shah, Sultan of Gujarat. Having concluded that defeat was inevitable, the Rajput army went out for the last time to certain death.

The infant [king], Oody Sing [Udai Singh], was placed in safety with Soortan, Prince of Boondi, the garrison put on their saffron robes [symbolising their resolve to die in battle], while materials for the *johur* [*jauhar*] were preparing. There was little time for the pyre. The bravest had fallen in defending the breach, now completely exposed. Combustibles were quickly heaped up in reservoirs and magazines excavated in the rock, under which gunpowder was strewed. Kurnavati, mother of the prince, and sister of the gallant Arjoon Hara, led the procession of willing victims to their doom, and thirteen thousand females were thus swept at once from the record of life.

(Tod 1829: 249–250)

Sitting dharna

The *threat* of suicide is another relevant aspect of Indian custom.

As Chakrabarti reminds us, there is a religious form of *dharna* that is directed against the gods:

Dharna is a right of the Hindus seeking to establish a direct contact with the supernatural for receiving divine aid in the solution of their problems. It is an expression of the devotee's innate need to meet an emergency, by prostrating himself in front of the deity for days together without taking any food or drink, expecting the vision of the deity to appear in a trance and direct him to overcome his crisis.

(Chakrabarti 1979: 120)

Although it is not clear whether the origins of *dharna* are to be found in the religious form, it is more famous in its secular manifestation. Yule and Burnell define the practice as:

A mode of extorting payment or compliance with a demand, effected by the complainant or creditor sitting at the debtor's door, and there remaining without tasting food till his demand shall be complied with, or (sometimes) by threatening to do himself some mortal violence if it be not complied with.

(Yule and Burnell 1886: 315)

Thakur suggests that the efficacy of

the custom of *'sitting dharna'* – generally practised by creditors who sat down before the doors of their debtors 'threatening to starve themselves to death if their claims were not paid' [arose from] the sin attached to causing the death of a Brahmana [which] 'would further increase the efficacy of the creditors' threat.' It should be added that in India, as elsewhere, the souls of those who have killed themselves or met death by any other violent means are regarded as particularly malevolent and troublesome.

(Thakur 1963: 64–65 citing works by Stienmetz and Balfour; see also Shridharani 1972: 19–20 ff.)

Bishop Heber reported an instance in which the threat of collective *dharna* had been made by the Hindus of Benares in a dispute with Muslims, some time prior to his arrival there in 1824. He added:

[A]mong Hindoos it is very prevailing, not only from the apprehended dreadful consequences of the death of the petitioner, but because many are of opinion, that while a person sits dhurna at their door, they must not themselves presume to eat, or undertake any secular business. It is even said that some persons hire brahmins to sit dhurna for them, the thing being done by proxy, and the durna of a brahmin being naturally more aweful in its effects than that of a soodra could be.

(Heber 1828, vol. 1: 326)

William Crooke recounts the North Indian legend of the Brahmin Harshu Panre who sought to punish Raja Salivahana of Chayanpur, whom he served as family priest, for jealously destroying the priest's newly constructed house: 'The enraged Brahman did *dharna*, in other words fasted till he died at the palace gate' (Crooke 1896: 191). As a consequence of the Brahmin's curse, all of the Raja's descendants, except his daughter whose kindness secured her a blessing, were destroyed.

Yule and Burnell cite an extreme example published by Alexander Kinloch Forbes in his *Ras Mala, or Hindoo Annals of the Province of Goozerat* in 1856:

> A striking story is told in Forbes's *Ras Mala* ... of a farther proceeding following upon an unsuccessful *dharna*, put in practice by a company of Charans, or bards, in Kathiawar, to enforce payment of a debt by a chief of Jaila to one of their number. After fasting three days in vain, they proceeded from *dharna* to the further rite of *traga* ... Some hacked their own arms; others decapitated three old women of their party, and hung their heads up as a garland at the gate. Certain of the women cut off their own breasts. The bards also pierced the throats of four of the older men with spikes, and took two young girls and dashed their brains out against the town-gate. Finally the Charan creditor soaked his quilted clothes in oil, and set fire to himself. As he burned to death he cried out, 'I am now dying, but I will become a headless ghost (*Kavis*) in the Palace, and will take the chief's life, and cut off his posterity!' [Emphasis in original]
>
> (Yule and Burnell 1886: 317; see also the account of the
> Bhats in Russell and Lal 1916 [1969]: 259–263)

Spodek argues that the custom of 'sitting *dharna* or stationing oneself near the ruler's palace or in some other prominent place so as to call public attention to, and hopefully invoke public sympathy for one's cause' was an aspect of Kathiawadi tradition which Gandhi brought into the repertoire of modern Indian politics (Spodek 1970).[3]

Non-approved suicides

In opposition to the religiously and socially approved forms of suicide cited above, the weight of scholarly opinion holds that suicide for personal reasons was condemned and prohibited. A frequently cited passage comes from the famous Mauryan book of statecraft, the *Arthashastra* (*Treatise on Material Gain*) ascribed to Kautilya or Chanakya and written some time between 300 BCE and 400 CE (de Bary, Hay *et al.* 1964: 237).[4] The Fourth Book ('Removal of Thorns') of the *Arthashastra* deals with the maintenance of law and order in a kingdom. Chapter VII deals with the examination of the circumstances of sudden death to determine whether deliberate homicide is involved. The chapter concludes with these remarks:

> If a man or woman under the infatuation of love, anger or other sinful passions commits, or causes to commit, suicide by means of ropes, arms, or poison, he or she shall be dragged by means of a rope along the public road by the hands

of a Chandala [Untouchable]. For such murderers as the above, neither cremation rites nor any obsequies usually performed by relatives shall be observed.

(Shamasastry 1929: 247)

As with so much of the Sanskrit literature, it is impossible to know what influence Kautilya's strictures may have had on ordinary village life at any given period.

We have little direct evidence of the attitudes toward suicide held by ordinary Indians in earlier periods. The Abbé Dubois, writing of his experiences in south India at the turn of the nineteenth century, observed:

> . . . murder and suicide occur occasionally amongst the Hindus, though such crimes are regarded by them with greater horror than by other people . . . It is usually women who are guilty of suicide. Driven to despair by the ill-treatment of a brutal husband, or by the annoyances of a spiteful mother-in-law, or by any of those domestic worries which are so common in a Hindu household, they lay criminal hands on themselves and destroy the life which has become unbearable.
>
> (Dubois 1906: 315)

Bishop Heber reported in his journal the opinion of a British judicial official he met in 1824:

> 'The truth is, so very little value do these people set on their own lives, that we cannot wonder at their caring little for the life of another. The cases of suicide which come before me, double those of suttees; men and still more, women, throw themselves down wells, or drink poison, for apparently the slightest reasons, generally out of some quarrel, and in order that their blood may lie at their enemy's door . . .'
>
> (Heber 1828, vol 1: 269)

South India

Although many of the examples of traditional attitudes toward and examples of suicide come from north and central India, there is a small literature which focuses on south India, especially on the Tamil-speaking region. Somasundaram, Babu and Geethayan recount several suicides that are recorded in the *Sangam* literature composed between 100 BCE and 300 CE. Some of these are instances of voluntary starvation, others are *satis* by noble women (Somasundaram, Babu *et al.* 1989). Jagadeesan recounts a number of instances of suicide as a form of defence of temples threatened with invasion. Perhaps the most striking is the case of an unnamed devadasi (temple dancer) who defended Srirangam Temple in the middle ages:

> After the sack of Srirangam by Malik Kafur, a Muslim general was placed in the premises of that temple. Much danger was averted by the clever intercession

of that Devadasi who captivated the Muslim general by her wiles and finally succeeded in killing him by pushing him away from a tower and herself perishing with him. Her kinsmen still enjoy some privileges for the signal service she rendered to the cause of that temple.

(Jagadeesan 1983: 61)

Krishnan cites numerous examples from Tamil inscriptions on temples and hero stones. What is striking about these examples – though not surprising given the sources – is that these inscriptions do not record the religious suicides more common in the north. Instead, they usually record suicides undertaken for others: another individual – such as the recovery from ill health of a chief, protest against injustice – unjust taxes or the failure of priests to make daily offerings to a resident deity, or individuals fulfilling vows to serve their masters unto death (Krishnan 1983). Venkatraman provides epigraphic instances of an apparently uniquely Tamil form of suicide, the *navakhandam*, in which the subject offers their head to a deity in fulfilment of a vow after first cutting off flesh from nine parts of the body (Venkatraman 1983).

Traditional aspects of contemporary suicide

It is, perhaps, possible to recognise elements of traditional attitudes towards religious suicide in some contemporary suicides. Waters, for example, in her exploration of women's suicides in contemporary Maharashtra, draws our attention to the 'valorisation of suffering' in dowry deaths and 'suicidal household deaths':

The valorization of suffering by women in South Asia is explicit and has a specific discourse that is revealed in Marathi terms such as *sosane* (to endure suffering) and *sahan karne* (to suffer). This treatment of suffering operates on the level of ideology (e.g. the self-sacrificing, ideal wife of philosophical and legal texts) and mythology (e.g. the suffering of female figures in great epics) as well as within the daily social roles of the family. Suffering as a principle, an organizing theme, and a technology of the self is a subtle as fasting and as brutal as suicide . . . .

The valorization of suffering helps to explain burning as a dominant means of women's suicide in India: It is commonly known as the most painful (Waters 1999: 527).

Hinduism and suicide

Andriolo seeks to resolve the ambivalent attitudes to suicide found in Hindu tradition by arguing that they largely conform with two principal criteria:

Only a life which has reached completion may be terminated wilfully, and only a death whose meaning is invested beyond the self is meritorious. In contrast, a life abandoned before its completion, a death which is sought for self-centred reasons, effects the rejected suicide.

(Andriolo 1993: 45)

Perhaps the surest conclusion we can reach from the fragmentary evidence we have is that, for Hindus, suicide was not subject to the strong and unambiguous prohibitions found in Islam or Christianity. As Varma observes, 'there is no categorical denunciation of suicide in the Hindu Scriptures' (Varma 1976: 138).

Suicide in Jainism

The extreme respect for life in Jainism is apparently responsible for the early emergence in the religion of *sallekhanā* or fasting unto death, a religious ritual intended to end the cycle of death and rebirth. In a comprehensive review, Billimoria states:

The practice in question permits a member of the community, under certain circumstances, to terminate his or her own life, or more accurately, to actively welcome impending death in a non-violent manner.

(Bilimoria 1992: 333)

The practice goes back very far in the history of the religion. Krishnan cites epigraphic evidence of two south Indian cases. In the sixth century Chandiranandiasiriyar died after 57 days' abstinence; in the tenth century Ilaiyabhatarar died after 30 days (Krishnan 1983: 91; see also Venkatraman 1983: 98). Bilimoria cites a prominent instance of the practice in 1983 (Bilimoria 1992: 335–336). In a second article Bilimoria cites two cases of *sallekhanā* that have been reported in the press: one from 1987, the other from 1994 (Bilimoria 1995: 174, fn 2). In 2005, the *sallekhanā* of a 75-year-old Jain woman was prominently reported by the national press (2005). Around 100,000 pilgrims were reported to have come to her small village 120 km north of Bhopal in Madhya Pradesh:

'This was a way of ultimate purification of the soul', said Kiran Godre, a Jain nun who looked after Ms. Bai during her ritual. 'She became a saint in the eyes of the Jain community and hundreds of people visited her during her fasting days to pay their respect'.

(*The Hindu* 2005)

Traditional Buddhism

There are relatively few Buddhists in contemporary India. Traditional Buddhism, according to Becker, saw death as simply a stage in the cycle of birth and death: 'suicide is therefore no escape from anything' (Becker 1990: 547). While not condoning suicide, Buddhism accepted it where it was undertaken with a pure and serene mind.

Suicide in Islam, Sikhism and Christianity

The views of India's minority religions are more succinctly stated. Islam, the religion of over 11 per cent of India's population, is understood by believers to absolutely condemn suicide.[5] In a brief but frequently cited article, Patton notes:

> there is no specific text of the Qur'an which forbids suicide, though it would seem that the texts which bear upon the taking of human life in general are sufficiently clear as to their purpose to include any kind of wilful killing in private life.

> (Patton 1914: 38)

Hassan adds:

> Muslim societies, in general, have few suicides because of the nature of the Muslim's beliefs and the future life. The right attitude for the Muslim is *Islam*, an acceptance of life's events as settled by divine appointment. Suicide is an act of revolt against Allah, and the perpetrator of that act risks the wrath of Allah and the indescribable penalties of the Fire.

> (Hassan 1983: 49)

Christians constitute about 2.5 per cent of India's population. Like Islam, Christianity traditionally condemned suicide in the strongest terms. Although the Old Testament contains no explicit condemnation of suicide, the view of the Christian Church was settled by St Augustine who declared that suicide violated the Commandment 'Thou shalt not kill'. Until very recent times, this attitude was accepted by both Catholics and Protestants.

Sikhs constitute just under 2 per cent of the Indian population. According to Bhatia, the view of the Sikh Gurus was that 'suicide in the face of misery and misfortune implies lack of faith in the goodness and righteousness of God' (Bhatia 2002).

Studies of suicide in colonial India

The first comparative study of suicide in India was a relatively little known paper by Dr Kenneth McLeod 'On the Statistics and Causes of Suicide in India', which was read to the Bengal Social Science Society in Calcutta on 13 June 1878. McLeod's pioneering study reported suicide rates for virtually all of British India in the first half of the 1870s. He found suicide rates ranged from relatively low levels in some Indian provinces (1.27 per 100,000 in the Punjab) to much higher levels in others (6.65 in Madras; 7.05 in the Central Provinces) (McLeod 1878, Table 20). Although it was his opinion that the number of suicides recorded was 'considerably below the truth', he was nevertheless struck by the consistency in recorded rates by provinces and also by districts within provinces (McLeod 1878: 396). The districts with the highest rates of recorded suicide in 1872 were Puri (10.07), Cuttack (8.52), Nadia (7.1), Patna (5.67) and Gaya (4.95) (McLeod 1878: 397).

In 1917 Mayr published comparable figures for India in 1907 based on Sanitary Reports (Mayr 1917: 266–267, 299–300).[6] His figures are also reported in Tables 2.1 and 2.2. Mayr also provides figures for the Northwest Provinces (now the western portion of Uttar Pradesh), Agra and Oudh (now the eastern portion of Uttar Pradesh) and the Punjab (which then included west Punjab, now in Pakistan).

Nandi and his colleagues have utilised McLeod's data to attempt to assess changes in suicide rates over the 100 years since McLeod presented his findings. Although the exercise is not without some difficulties, the results, which are reproduced in Table 2.1, are interesting.[7] (We have added Mayr's figures, and roughly comparable data for 1972 to those provided by Nandi *et al.*) Because of the major changes in boundaries following Partition and States Reorganisation strict comparability is not possible. It is obvious nevertheless that rates appear to have increased in every area over the past 100 years. (The long-term trend in Indian suicide rates is discussed in detail in Chapter 6.)

Table 2.1 Incidence of suicide per 100,000 of population

	1872	1907	1972
Bengal (West Bengal)	2.36	6.2	15.96
Bombay Presidency (Maharashtra)	4.73	2.2	8.26
Madras Presidency (Tamil Nadu)	7.85	4.0	11.3
(Andira Pradesh)			[7.37]
Central Provinces (Madhya Pradesh)	6.10	8.1	7.83
Northwest Provinces (W. Uttar Pradesh)		0.8	4.49
Agra and Oudh (E. Uttar Pradesh)		6.4	4.49
Punjab		1.6	4.68

Source: Hegde 1980 table 1: 156; Miner 1922: 17; Mayr 1917: 267.

Table 2.2 Suicide rates by gender in the provinces of British India

Province	1872		1907	
	Male suicide rate	*Female suicide rate*	*Male suicide rate*	*Female suicide rate*
Bengal	6.42	10.44	4.47	7.93
N.W. Provinces	2.78	7.16	.57	1.04
Oudh	3.78	6.61	3.25	9.55
Punjab	1.07	1.52	1.41	1.79
Central Provinces	6.42	7.71	8.10	8.10
Madras	6.26	6.85	3.41	4.59
Bombay	4.17	5.69	2.11	2.29

Source: Adapted from McLeod 1878: table 20. figures for 1907 estimated from Mayr 1917: 267, 300.

McLeod noted strong regional differences in the means employed in suicide: in the Presidency towns of Bombay and Madras drowning was the most frequent means used while in Bengal, hanging was the most common means, while in the opium-growing areas of Bihar and the North-West Provinces, opium poisoning prevailed (McLeod 1878: 403–4). (We examine the means employed in contemporary India in Chapter 15.)

McLeod was struck by the fact that – unlike in England where there were three male suicides for every female – in India suicides by women exceeded those by men; his findings are summarised in Table 2.2.[8] He observed 'whatever the causes are which determine people to put an end to their own existence in this country, they press more strongly upon the female section of the population than the male' (McLeod 1878: 399). We have estimated comparable figures for 1907 from Mayr's data and included them in the table. We discuss gender and suicide in Chapter 7.

McLeod was unable to obtain data on the ages at which suicide occurred, though he observed, on the basis of his experience in Jessore, that the majority of female suicides were between 25 and 35 – or even younger, a surmise all too abundantly confirmed by later data (McLeod 1878: 398). (The age at which suicide occurs is discussed in detail in Chapter 8.)

McLeod was also unable to find information on caste or religion, though he found in Calcutta that the suicide rate amongst Muslims was 4.54 per 100,000, a little more than half the rate of Hindus (8.54) and those of other religions (8.64) (McLeod 1878: 405). Patel reported suicide rates in Bombay between 1883 and 1907. As in Calcutta, rates for Muslims (6.6) were lower than those for Hindus (10.4). The rate for Christians was slightly lower than that for Hindus (9.8), while that for Parsis was very much higher than for any other community (24.1) (Miner 1922: 27).

Patel also reported on the seasonal distribution of suicides in Bombay between 1895 and 1907. He found (Table 2.3) that suicide rates tended to reach a maximum during the months of the monsoon (i.e. June–September).

Post-Independence India

It is surprising to discover that the first post-Independence study to examine suicide in an all-India context, Paripurnanand Varma's *Suicide in India and Abroad* (1976) remains virtually alone in the field. Varma's pioneering study brings together many disparate materials relating to suicide in post-Independence India. Varma

Table 2.3 Distribution of suicides by month, Bombay, 1895–1907

Distribution by equalised months per 1,200 suicides in Bombay

January	90	April	94	July	110	October	108
February	59	May	95	August	105	November	95
March	102	June	121	September	121	December	100

Source: Miner 1922 p. 20, table XI.

presented a sensible and balanced assessment of the Indological evidence, summarised a number of unpublished papers by scholars working in a number of urban hospitals and summarised the results of official figures for the early 1970s.

Varma concluded from his examination of the Indological evidence that while 'there is no categorical denunciation of suicide in Hindu Scriptures' (Varma 1976: 138) nevertheless 'it should be clearly understood that suicide is permitted only for expiation of sins, otherwise it is strictly forbidden' (Varma 1976: 140). Varma followed in a long tradition and argued that modernity was tending to undermine religious adherence, resulting in rising suicide rates.

The psychological evidence that Varma presented came from a number of apparently unpublished studies carried out in Varanasi (Benares), Bhopal, Agra, Goa, Gujarat and Calcutta. These exploratory studies were on the whole fairly rudimentary. One exception was Dr Heeresh Chandra's report of post-mortem studies of all unnatural deaths ($N = 845$), which occurred in the Bhopal region in an undefined period before 1972. Chandra reported that 94 cases (11.1 per cent) were suicides (Varma 1976: 149). (By way of comparison, suicides comprised 51.9 per cent of the total – un-natural deaths plus suicides – reported for the city of Bhopal in official statistics in 1999.) Another study of interest was Sharma, Gopalakrishnan and Rao's study of police records of suicides that occurred in Goa between 1965 and 1970. They reported that 'by far, the largest single factor in the background of the suicides was mental illness. One-fourth of the suicides, i.e. 25.4 per cent, were suffering from mental illness' (Varma 1976: 160).

Although his was not a sociological investigation – indeed Varma repeatedly called for sociologists to undertake this work – he offered unsystematic assessments of the regional patterns he observed. He noted, for example, that the highest percentage of suicides occur in 'the most educated and industrially advanced states like West Bengal, Maharashtra, Kerala, Tamil Nadu and Haryana' (Varma 1976: 126–127). He also drew attention to the high percentage of suicides that occurs in India's southern states (Varma 1976: 132). Varma noted that 60 per cent of suicides in 1971 were committed by men and that just under half of all suicides (44.7 per cent) were by those aged between 18 and 30 years (Varma 1976: 132–133).

In his examination of official suicide statistics Varma repeatedly emphasised his view that suicides are grossly under-reported in India. In some cases, this arises from suicides being misclassified as accidental deaths (Varma 1976: 125).[9] He stated, without furnishing corroborative evidence, that:

> A good percentage of suicides or attempted suicides goes unreported and a certain percentage is suppressed by the police itself for considerations.
>
> (Varma 1976: 127)

Varma estimated that official figures report only half – or perhaps only one-third – of the actual number of suicides:

> We are quite convinced that no less than 100,000 persons commit suicide in this country every year, which must be nearly ten times more than murder in

the country . . . [and] on the analogy of Great Britain and the United States that at least five times more than the number of successful suicides must be attempting it.

(Varma 1976: 127)

In Chapter 3 we subject India's official suicide data to some eight tests that lead us to reject Varma's assertion of gross undercounting of suicides in India.

The sociology of Indian suicide

Although there have been no broadly-based sociological studies of suicide at the all-India level, a small number of interesting regional monographs appeared in the 1990s. Several of these, which deal specifically with farmer suicides, are considered in detail in Chapter 11.

Shamim Aleem, The Suicide

In 1994 Professor Shamim Aleem published a monograph that explored the causes of suicide in Pondicherry, the jurisdiction with the highest suicide rates in India. (Our own detailed analysis of suicides in Pondicherry appears in Chapter 16.)

Aleem based her study on 441 cases registered in Pondicherry and Karaikal in 1991, an intensive examination of 86 cases, and responses to a questionnaire sent to members of voluntary organisations. Aleem found that men constituted 65.9 per cent of the cases reported (Aleem 1994: 29). She found that those aged between 20 and 29 years constituted the largest number of suicides in 1991, 33 per cent, followed by those between aged 30 and 39 years (23.5 per cent) (Aleem 1994: 31). Virtually all of those studied were labourers, many of them migrant workers (Aleem 1994: 31).[10]

Aleem concluded on the basis of answers from upper and middle-class respondents to her questionnaire ($N = 50$, response rate 17 per cent) that excessive conumption of alcohol was the major contributing factor to suicide in Pondicherry (Aleem 1994: 33). A majority of her elite respondents (56.2 per cent) also expressed little confidence in the abilities of the police to properly investigate suicides (Aleem 1994: 40).

Aleem offered the hypothesis that high levels of literacy, especially female literacy (65.8 per cent in 1991), in Pondicherry were a contributing factor to the high rate of suicides (Aleem 1994: 49). Aleem also notes that Pondicherry has elevated suicide rates despite the remarkable density of social networks that exist there, observing that 'it is surprising that in such a small place there are more than 3,000 voluntary organisations of women.' (Aleem 1994: 49).

One of Aleem's most interesting conclusions is that the very high suicide rate in the Territory is largely an artefact of the 'fool proof system of recording all the cases of deaths whether natural or unnatural', itself an enduring legacy of the French administrative system (Aleem 1994: xi and 45). She concluded, on the basis of her intensive examination of the original files of 86 cases, that – contrary to the opinion expressed by her sample respondents – all had been 'handled very meticulously and no loop holes were found'; in addition, as required by law, every suicide of a woman married for less than seven years had been referred to the Executive Magistrate for investigation (Aleem 1994: x).[11]

Suicide in tribal India

Verrier Elwin, Maria Murder and Suicide

In addition to the regional monographs that have studied suicide in Pondicherry and the Punjab, we have also two tribal ethnographies, which include detailed material on suicide. In his pioneering *Maria Murder and Suicide* (1991 [1943]) Verrier Elwin devoted most of his attention to murder among the Maria of Bastar district in what is now Chhattisgarh State but reported also on cases of suicide.

Elwin reported that the suicide sex ratio among the tribal population of Bastar was very nearly even, unlike homicides, 96 per cent of which were committed by men (Elwin 1991 [1943]: 48).

Elwin notes that the Bison-horn Maria had 'long had a bad reputation for violence and drunkenness' (Elwin 1991 [1943]: 37), which was reflected in a homicide rate three times that of the more placid Ghotul Muria. The same differences are evident in the suicide data. Elwin's data show that the homicide:suicide ratio among the Maria was 1.3:1; for the Muria it was 0.95:1 (Elwin 1991 [1943], calculated from Table 1: 37 and Table 10: 47). Among the tribal population of Bastar, hanging was used in all but a single case of suicide (Elwin 1991 [1943]: 47).

Elwin's data, taken from a sample of 50 cases for which he had detailed information, displays a bi-modal distribution. Young adults comprised 42 per cent of the cases. Older adults were 32 per cent of Elwin's sample (Elwin 1991 [1943]: 49). If we infer that life expectancy in the Bastar in the 1930s was about the same as the rest of India, then the adult suicide rate was in all likelihood a relatively high one.

The most common precipitating reason for suicide among the Maria in Elwin's sample was what elsewhere in this study we call 'quarrel with kin'. In nearly half of the sample (46 per cent) 'antagonism between husband and wife', 'an intolerable home', resentment at a rebuke or 'regret for harsh behaviour to someone loved' were identified as the antecedent cause (Elwin 1991 [1943]: 58). Disease and fear of magic, insanity and a variety of other minor causes were responsible for the remainder of the cases. Elwin remarks that 'the majority [of suicides] seem to be have caused by a desire to escape from a physical or domestic situation that had become intolerable' (Elwin 1991 [1943]: 58).

A. B. Saran, Murder and Suicide among the Munda and the Oraon

Anirudha Behari Saran conducted a parallel study to that of Elwin in Ranchi District of what is now Jharkhand state in the second half of the 1950s, making a comparison of differences between the Munda and Oraon tribes. In both tribal societies, roughly equal proportions of men and women take their lives (Saran 1974: 166).

Suicide was relatively uncommon in tribal society in Ranchi, with rates among the Munda relatively higher than the Oraon. Saran attributes the difference to 'the Oraon's well-organized *Dhumkuria* [youth dormitory] and *Akhra* [dance ground] [which] provide socially accepted channels for the release of their aggressive impulses, [while] the Munda's Gitiora [dormitory] . . . is just a sleeping place for the unmarried youths and hardly fulfil[s] any other objective' (Saran 1974: 163). As in Bastar, hanging is the nearly universal means of suicide, with minor differences among both tribes in Ranchi (Saran 1974: 164).

The age distribution reported by Saran indicates that roughly one-third of suicides in Ranchi were committed by young adults (Saran 1974, adapted from Table XX: 166). The age distributions were quite similar in both tribal groups.

Saran's categories of causes of suicide are different from Elwin's. Nevertheless, in both Bastar and Ranchi, conflict with close relatives is the most commonly attributed cause of suicide (Saran 1974: 170). Disease (but apparently not witchcraft) is next most frequent, followed by mental illness.

Notes

1   Hari Prasad Shastri's translation of Valmiki's *Ramayana* is euphemistic in its depiction of the death of Rama: '. . . the supremely virtuous Rama formed his resolution and entered Vishnu's abode in his body with his younger brothers' (Valmiki 1959: 635).

2   The Abbé Dubois presents accounts of two *satis* that occurred when he was living in Thanjavur at the end of the eighteenth century. It is not entirely clear whether the Abbé actually witnessed the two events he describes in vivid detail (Dubois 1906, Chapter XIX), though Max Müller indicates in his preface to *Hindu Manners, Customs and Ceremonies* that these were eyewitness accounts (Dubois 1906: vii).

3   We wish to thank Tom Weber for drawing the work of Shirdharani and Spodek to our attention. Shridharani (1972: 22) argues that Gandhi came to see the practice as 'barbaric' and urged his followers not to use the practice. Bose (1962, Appendix) offers a discussion of fasting in the practice of *satyagraha*. And Ashe briefly traces the history of Gandhi's adoption of fasting as a political technique (Ashe 1968: 169 ff.).

4   We wish to acknowledge the kindness of the late C. L. Holden in making his copy of the *Arthashastra* available to us.

5   Dale (1988) reminds us that suicidal *jihad* has been utilized in anti-colonial struggles by a number of Muslim communities, including the Mappilas of Kerala.

6   Mayr's data are reproduced in Miner (1922: 17, 31).

7   In attempting to match colonial presidencies with post-Independence states, Nandi and his colleagues have, for example, equated Madras Presidency with present day Tamil Nadu. As McLeod's district-level data all refer to present day Andhra Pradesh, we have added the figures for that state in square brackets.

8   The data reported for 1872 in Tables 2.1 and 2.2 are not strictly comparable. Table 2.1 gives figures for West Bengal, while 2.2 reports the lower figure for undivided Bengal.

9   We discuss the reliability of official suicide data in India in Chapter 3.

10   Aleem is not specific, but one must assume that she is referring to male suicides here.

11   The requirement to investigate the death of every woman married for seven years or less is a measure adopted in India to detect and thus deter so-called 'dowry deaths'.

3 The reliability of Indian suicide data

This study attempts to achieve the inherently impossible: to understand an aspect of Indian society undergoing profound change. There are two principal causes of the difficulty of the exercise. The first – which at heart is irremediable – is the inherent complexity of Indian society. No single discipline, certainly no individual scholar, can pretend to grasp more than a small part of the infinitely complex whole. The second is inherent in any attempt to understand the present as history. Without the luxury of hindsight we attempt by giving meaning to fragments of evidence to discern the direction in which social change may be headed.

Our attempt to understand social change across India through the dark, sad lens of suicide rests unavoidably on the use of official statistics of suicide deaths. As we shall see, many Indian scholars believe these to be grossly inaccurate. If they are correct, it must place the reliability of this entire enterprise in grave doubt. Curiously, however, the confidant dismissal of the reliability of India's official suicide statistics is made in the absence of systematic published evidence. It is essential, therefore, at the outset that we do what has heretofore not been done and examine systematically and critically the evidence for the reliability of India's official suicide statistics as reported by the National Crime Records Bureau in their annual publication *Accidental Deaths and Suicides in India.*

Legal status of suicide and Attempted Suicide

Section 309 of the Indian Penal Code (IPC) defines 'Attempts to Commit Suicide' as criminal offences under the law, subject upon conviction to a term of imprisonment for up to a year, or a fine, or both (National Crime Records Bureau 1995: 2).

The Code defines suicide as the 'intentional ending of life'. There are three tests a death must meet to be classified as a suicide:

(i) it should be an un-natural death, (ii) the desire to die should originate within him/herself, (iii) there should be a cause to end life.

(National Crime Records Bureau 1995: 1)

A. K. Kaka notes that attempts to repeal Section 309 go back as far as 1971 when the Law Commission of India in its 42nd Report urged repeal of the provision, stating that 'this penal provision is harsh and unjustifiable ... It seems [a] monstrous procedure to inflict further suffering on even a single individual who has already found life so unbearable ...' (Kala 2001). Subsequently, a bill to amend the Indian Penal Code was introduced in 1972 into the Rajya Sabha, the upper house of the Indian Parliament, which subsequently passed the amendment in 1978. It was pending before the Lok Sabha, India's lower house, but lapsed after Parliament was dissolved in 1979. There have been no subsequent moves to amend the law (Kala 2001).

Bilimoria presents an extensive discussion of *Maruti Shripati Dubal v. State of Maharashtra* heard by the Bombay High Court in 1986 in which the learned judges ruled that the right to life established by Article 21 of the Indian Constitution logically implied a right to death. Affirming that positive rights, such as the right to free speech, implied the negative right to remain silent, their Honours stated:

> If this is so, logically it must follow that right to live as recognised by Article 21 will include also right not to live or not to be forced to live. To put it positively it would include *a right to die, or to terminate one's life*. [Emphasis in original]
>
> (Bilimoria 1995: 163)

Under the Indian Constitution, a judgement of the Bombay Court need not be followed by courts in other states nor by the Indian Supreme Court. On 27 April, 1994 in what was greeted at the time as a landmark judgement, Mr Justice B. L. Hansaria of the Indian Supreme Court ruled in *P. Rathnam v. Union of India* that Section 309 was unconstitutional and that attempted suicide could not be treated as a crime. Arguing on terms very similar to those advance by the Bombay High Court, Hansaria argued that the right to life implied the right not to live and that humans had a right to more than a mere animal existence. Going further, Mr Justice Hansaria argued that rather than punish an attempted suicide, the focus should be on offering psychological care:

> So what is needed to take care of suicide prone persons are soft words and wise counselling [of a psychiatrist] and not st[er]n dealing by a jailor following harsh treatment meted out by a heartless prosecutor ... Section 309 of IPC is void.
>
> (Kala 2001)

On 21 March 1996 a five-member panel of the Supreme Court headed by Mr Justice J. S. Verma reversed this judgement and declared that Section 309 was indeed valid law and that the attempt to take one's own life, or to assist another to do so – which is prohibited under Section 309 of the IPC – remained criminal acts (National Crime Records Bureau 1997: 2–3). The learned judges declared that the right to life, guaranteed by Article 21 of the Indian Constitution, did not imply a right to die, nor did the prohibition of suicide violate the guarantee of equal protection under the law guaranteed by Article 14 of the Constitution. Therefore, the provisions of Section 309 remain in force.

We should note that although the criminalisation of attempted suicide is the direct cause of the absence of any official statistics on attempted suicide in India, we could find no evidence that in recent years there have been any prosecutions or convictions for offences under Section 309 (National Crime Records Bureau 1997: 2). Kala presented evidence indicating that in Ludhiana District, Punjab between 1996 and 2001 there were eight prosecutions of cases under Section 306 (Kala 2001). He argued that the effect of the provision was to encourage the police to 'reconstruct' attempted suicides as accidents.

Suicide determination in India

The continued treatment of suicide and attempted suicide as criminal acts places responsibility for the determination for the classification of individual deaths on members of the state police force in each locality. We know almost nothing about how this local-level determination of suicides takes place. The only systematic investigation of the accuracy of police recording of suicides is Shamim Aleem's study of the Union Territory of Pondicherry (1994). As noted in Chapter 2, Aleem's opinion is that police procedures followed in Pondicherry, whose origins she traces to the period of French colonial rule, are particularly accurate, arising as they do from a requirement for an official determination of the cause of every death in the Territory.

Against this confidence we must set our own investigations in Pondicherry in 2000. With the very cordial cooperation of the Inspector General of Police (IG), Pondicherry, we sought to determine what criteria were invoked when the cause of suicides in an appendix to Aleem's book were listed as *thikkum* or others as 'stomach ache' or 'stomach pain' (Aleem 1994, e.g. 88). The consensus of the police officers at the meeting was that the first was really a case of 'overconsumption of alcohol and not really suicide'. Their opinion was that 'stomach pain' might refer to the consequences of inadequate post-operative care in the case of operations such as tubal ligation (meeting in Pondicherry, 3 February 2000). The IG's subordinates were unable to clarify these attributes of cause, and despite their searches, the IG subsequently reported that they had been unable to locate the First Information Reports on which the official statistics rested.

There are similar lacunae that need further investigation and clarification. Since 1995 national suicide statistics have reported the both the occupation and marital status of suicides at the national level. Those who compile the national data do not indicate from which states the data are drawn. A survey of suicide records for Reddi Chavri Police Station, Cuddalore in Tamil Nadu, which Sub-Inspector A. Sabibulla was kind enough to assist us to examine, did not consistently indicate either the occupation or marital status of the suicides for the years 1992–1993 and 1998.[1] As a brief example, of the first 20 cases recorded in 1993 in which the victim was an identifiable person (i.e. not a vagrant), occupations were reported for only eight; marital status was reported (or inferable in the case of a 13-year-old boy) for all but one. Since the total suicides listed under each category are the same as the overall national totals, it appears that the determination of profession, to take this one small example, must have been recorded or determined somewhere other than the entry in the register of suicides at the local police station or else included in the catch-all category of 'other'. In addition, there were quite a few cases listed in the register of suicides that appeared *prima facie* to be accidental deaths. Included in the register for 1993, for example, were a case of 'fire accident', three deadly snake bites, a deadly fly bite, goring by a bullock, a death occasioned by a house fire caused by faulty electrical wiring and a death by electric shock which might have been accidental. It is impossible to know whether at a later stage of data analysis these cases were properly accounted as accidental deaths, but to find nine apparent accidental deaths in a list of 31 suicides is cause for concern. Nevertheless we may note at this point that there was no evidence that possible suicides were being disguised as accidental deaths, quite the contrary.

Data collected from official police records in Pondicherry by Dr S. Vaidynathan and Mr S. Radjagopalane of Maitreyi, Befrienders India Centre, Pondicherry for the years 1995–1999, however, did not systematically record either marital status or profession, though Aleem records both in her appendix, so the difference in this case is likely to reflect choices made in transcribing the records. (Others have been less privileged in their access to official records. Dandekar *et al.* reported that they were unable to obtain official records of suicides in preparing their report for the Mumbai High Court and in consequence had to rely upon a list maintained by a Maharashtrian journalist (Dandekar, Narawade *et al.* 2005: 7).)

Although there is much we do not yet know about how police investigators reach their judgments in cases of apparent suicide, and how their findings are recorded and later aggregated at state and ultimately at national level, the records published by the National Crime Records Bureau are the only comprehensive, national data which are available for the study of the sociology of suicide in India. They are thus valuable and vitally important sources of basic information. Although we have no alternative but to base our study upon them, it is essential to subject the data to the most rigorous tests of reliability possible. If the basic data themselves are unreliable, any conclusions we draw from them will be doubly so.

Assessing the reliability of official suicide data

The 'severe under-reporting' thesis

In the previous chapter we noted that in his pioneering study *Suicide in India and Abroad* Paripurnanand Varma offered his opinion that official figures report only half – perhaps only a third – of the suicides which occur each year (Varma 1976). Comparable estimates to Varma's have been offered by subsequent commentators. For example, Dr Alexander Jacob estimated in 2001 that only one-fourth of suicides in Kerala were reported, implying an actual suicide rate of 136 per 100,000 (2001). On the basis of a detailed verbal autopsies on 38,836 deaths occurring between 1999 and 2000 in rural Villupuram District, Tamil Nadu, Gajalakshmi and Peto concluded that official statistics:

> . . . may not reflect the true suicide rates because of the possibility of non-reporting of deaths to police to avoid legal and social consequences. The estimated suicide mortality rates reported for India in the 2002 global burden of injuries are much lower than the rates observed in the present study in rural Tamil Nadu, South India. The number of suicide deaths estimated based on present study results for the year 2005 in India is 687,000 [vs 113,914 in official statistics].
>
> (Gajalakshmi and Peto 2007: 206)

If the reported data are indeed so seriously distorted, it might have major implications for any attempt to draw conclusions from those data. For example, are suicides actually fifty times more frequent in Pondicherry, which had an average rate of 66 per 100,000 between 1987 and 1996, than in Bihar, which had a rate of only 1.3 in the decade; or are suicides recorded fifty times more accurately in Pondicherry? If there is under-counting of suicides, are the errors random, uniform or systematic? If errors were random, there would be as many false positives (for example, accidental deaths erroneously classified as suicides) as false negatives (for example, actual suicides registered as accidental deaths). If there were uniform under-reporting, the reported rate would be a fraction of the true rate. If systematic factors are at work, social factors may lead to pressures to report suicides as accidental deaths (for a discussion of the different types of possible error, see Pescosolido and Mendelsohn 1986: 81). It is clearly important to attempt to discover if there is a pattern of consistent under-reporting in some or all states, whether any under-reporting that might occur seriously distorts the reported figures, and perhaps most importantly, whether it does so in a way that affects our ability to draw meaningful conclusions about the social causes of suicide in India. Surprisingly, despite the confidence with which some who study suicide in India declare published rates to be greatly below actual rates, there has been no systematic attempt to assess the reliability of the official data. In this chapter we consider the results of eight different methods of evaluating reliability.

i. International comparison

We may begin with a 'commonsense' test of the reliability of India's official suicide statistics by referring back to the international comparison presented in Table 1.3 in Chapter 1. As we saw there, some Indian states with high suicide rates rank with the highest reported for nations elsewhere. Suicide rates in other states place them very much in the centre of internationally reported rates. It is obvious that if real Indian suicide rates were twice the official rates then the population of many states would rank as among the most suicide-prone in the world. While such a conclusion cannot be ruled out, it does not appear *prima facie* to be plausible.

ii. Regional consistency

Next we can observe that geographically contiguous areas in India have comparable suicide rates. As we noted in Chapter 1 (Figure 1.4), we can discern a number of broad suicide regions in India. We can discern distinct differences in the mean suicide rates in five regions for the entire range of post-Independence data, 1967–1999 (Table 3.1). Lowest in the Hindi heartland and in the adjacent states in northwest India, they rise consistently as we move southwards and eastwards. Average suicide rates are highest in the four southern states. Analysis of variance shows that these differences are statistically significant ($p < 0.005$). Although these groupings are to some extent artificial, they correspond broadly to regions with long histories of common experiences (Dyson and Moore 1983). The fact that individual states in roughly homogeneous geographical clusters but with widely differing political systems and administrative cultures report broadly comparable suicide rates is another piece of evidence which adds to our confidence that we are observing real differences.

iii. The stability of suicide rates

One of the most straightforward tests of the reliability of Indian official data is to examine their consistency over time. Sainsbury and Barraclough (1968: 1252) employed this method to compare the consistency of suicide rates in forty countries between 1950 and 1960. They found a correlation of 0.95, indicating a high degree of consistency.

Lester (1987) examined the long-term consistency of suicide data in fourteen European countries between 1875 and 1975. The correlation was, unsurprisingly, lower, but still quite strong at 0.42.

A comparable examination of Indian suicide data for 21 Indian states over 40 years shows a very high rate of consistency. Table 3.2 indicates firstly that the correlations between decades are very high, with very high rates of statistical significance. Correlations between adjacent decades are, as we would expect, highest declining slowly but monotonically with separation in time. Thus the correlation between rates in 1967 and 1977 is 0.93; the correlation between 1967 rates and those in 1997 has fallen slightly to 0.89. The correlation between adjacent decades is nearly perfect: between 1977 and 1987 it is 0.98 and between 1987 and 1997 it is 0.97.

Table 3.1 Mean suicide rates 1967–1999

	Mean
Northern India	2.4
Northwest India	3.6
Western/Central India	7.1
Eastern India	12.2
Southern India	13.8

Table 3.2 Decadal suicide rate correlations

	1967	1977	1987	1997
1967	1.00			
1977	0.93	1.00		
1987	0.93	0.98	1.00	
1997	0.89	0.94	0.97	1.00

Note: All correlations are significant at 0.0001 level. States included in analysis: Andhra Pradesh, Assam, Bihar, Goa, Gujarat, Haryana, Himachal Pradesh, Jammu & Kashmir, Karnataka, Kerala, Madhya Pradesh, Maharashtra, Nagaland, Orissa, Pondicherry, Punjab, Rajasthan, Tamil Nadu, Tripura, Uttar Pradesh, West Bengal.

While it is possible to argue, as Douglas (1967) does, that the mere fact of consistency over time does not prove that the data accurately measure a real phenomenon, the principle of Ockham's razor would indicate that unless a variety of other factors can be shown to be interacting in a complex way to produce the consistency we observe in the data, then we should accept the most direct conclusion: that the data describe a real phenomenon.

iv. Internal consistency of the Indian data

We may combine regional clustering and changes over time in a further test of consistency. An examination of Table 3.3 demonstrates the detailed basis for our finding that there is a strong degree of regional homogeneity. As we have seen, the north Indian states Uttar Pradesh and Bihar have consistently low rates of reported suicide, while the southern states Andhra Pradesh, Karnataka, Tamil Nadu and Kerala have elevated rates (the small Union Territory of Pondicherry which has extremely high rates is included here for purposes of comparison only but is not included in the analysis of variance test).

The table also demonstrates that the data are not static. Suicide rates declined appreciably in the 1980s (the possible reasons for this decline will be examined in Chapter 6). What is striking is the consistency with which the declining incidence was reported from different jurisdictions. In a comparable way, a major increase in suicide rates in the 1990s was reported from many states.

An analysis of variance with repeated measures (Table 3.4) shows that both the regional effects and the changes over time make separate and statistically significant contributions to the pattern of rates we observe. The interaction term between the two is also statistically significant. The interaction effects are shown graphically in Figure 3.1.

The relative homogeneity of rates in geographically contiguous states and the general consistency in changes in patterns of incidence in successive decades is a further indication that official data record real phenomena with reasonable fidelity.

Table 3.3 Suicide rates: Decade means by region

	1967–1976	1977–1986	1987–1996
Northern India			
Bihar	2.2	0.9	1.3
U.P.	4.9	2.6	2.6
Northwest India			
H.P.	2.2	2.2	3.2
Haryana	7.1	4.3	7.0
Punjab	4.0	1.8	2.4
Rajasthan	1.9	2.4	4.6
Western/Central India			
Gujarat	5.9	5.1	7.5
M.P.	6.8	5.1	8.8
Maharashtra	7.7	5.9	10.9
Southern India			
Andhra Pradesh	8.1	6.0	9.3
Karnataka	11.7	13.1	17.9
Kerala	16.0	17.8	26.2
Tamil Nadu	12.3	11.5	15.7
Pondicherry	52.6	47.6	64.7
Eastern India			
West Bengal	15.5	13.4	17.2
Orissa	9.9	7.9	9.1

Table 3.4 Analysis of variance of regions and decades

	DF	Sum of squares	Mean square	F-Value	P-Value
Region	4	935.743	233.936	7.216	0.0053
Subject (Group)	10	324.206	32.421		
Category for Decades	2	65.075	32.538	18.671	< 0.0001
Category for Decades* Region	8	44.810	5.601	3.214	0.0162
Category for Decades* Subject (Group)	20	34.854	1.743		

v. Comparison of National Crime Records with Registrar General's cause of death statistics

An independent assessment of the relative incidence of suicide deaths is provided by sample survey data on causes of death of women of reproductive age (15–44) in rural India published by the Registrar General (2002, Statement 24: 34).[2] The correlation between NCRB data on the suicide rates for women (urban *and* rural, since no breakdown is available) aged between 15 and 44 (see Chapter 8

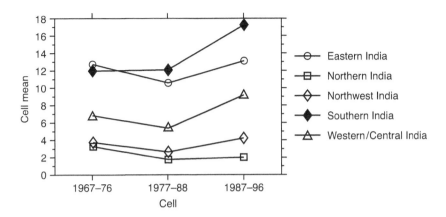

Figure 3.1 Interaction line plot for decades, interaction effect between decades and regions.

Table 8.2) and the Registrar General's estimates for the percentage of female deaths due to suicide is reasonably high ($r = 0.55$; $p = 0.05$). For Madhya Pradesh and Maharashtra, the Registrar General's sample appears to record many fewer suicide deaths than are included in the NCRB data. The opposite is the case for Kerala and Tamil Nadu, where the Registrar General's sample indicates a higher level of suicide deaths than are reported by the NCRB. The association is not as high as might appear desirable, but the differences may arise from sampling error in the Registrar General's data. For example, the Registrar General's data reports *no* suicide deaths for women of reproductive age in Bihar.

vi. The reliability of official Indian records: Are suicides hidden as accidents?

According to Durkheim's (1951) social integration theory, suicides increase when people feel less integrated into society. For example, modernisation can weaken traditional social ties, orthodox principles and values (Stack 2000). Indicators of modernisation include social correlates such as urbanisation, education, religion and divorce rate. Urbanisation with increased migration of people from rural to urban environments is considered to cause an erosion of social networks (Durkheim 1951).[3] Previous research has shown that urbanisation is associated with increased suicide risk (Pope, Danigelis *et al.* 1983; Simpson and Conklin 1989). Improved education or literacy is also a measure of modernisation and while this brings increased opportunities for people it may also increase their vulnerability to economic pressures (Stack and Danigelis 1985). In accord with this, previous research has shown a positive relationship between improved literacy and suicide (Gillis 1994; Kowalski, Faupel *et al.* 1987; Steen and Mayer 2003).

The relationship between religion and suicide has long been debated since Durkheim's (1951) tenet that religions with high integration should reduce suicidal behaviour. Most research has focussed on the Protestant–Catholic disparity (for a review see Stack 2000) and findings are mixed. Simpson and Conklin (1989) conducted one of the few studies investigating another religion, Islam, which does not traditionally condone suicide. They found in 71 countries that where the percentage of Muslims was higher there was an associated lower suicide rate. Marriage is another sign of high social integration and therefore divorce signals the weakening of the bonds of marriage and society and should therefore be associated with higher suicide risk (Durkheim 1951). Previous research has indeed demonstrated a strong positive link between divorce and suicide rates in many countries (Stack 2000), and particularly in India (Ziaian and Mayer 2002).[4]

Besides being related to social correlates, suicide rates are also partly a product of the social construction of the rates themselves (Pescosolido and Mendelsohn 1986). Different cultures have diverse attitudes towards suicide. While some societies are more relaxed and tolerant, in most the act of suicide is socially condemned and suicides may be misreported 'as accidents or other less socially stigmatised causes of death' (Stack 2000: 152). The actual recording of a death as a suicide may therefore be influenced by any number of factors such as attempts to disguise a suicide by family or officials and lack of objective evidence. Some have argued that this suspected underreporting invalidates the use of suicide statistics in research (Baechler 1975; Douglas 1967).

According to Pescosolido and Mendelsohn (1986), suicide statistics may be disguised or hidden due to systematic misreporting. This is most likely to occur as a result of the type of official system in charge of recording suspicious deaths. Characteristics such as the religious nature of a region or the kind of medico-legal system responsible for death classifications may bias the extent of true suicide reports. For example, a predominantly Catholic area may be more likely to discourage suicide and possibly encourage misreporting than an area with a less prohibitive religious stance toward suicide. Likewise, a medical examiner-based system is more likely to classify a death as a suicide, than a coroner-based system using the 'beyond reasonable doubt' standard to classify deaths. This observation may help to explain why hospital studies of suicide in India report higher rates than do those determined by official police machinery.

Pescosolido and Mendelsohn (1986) carried out a unique analysis to determine whether misreporting of suicide had occurred in 1970 mortality data from 404 county areas in the US. While their results were suggestive, they were not able to provide significant evidence that there were biases in the reporting of suicides. In this section we present a replication of their statistical technique[5] using data from India for 1991, although our data set was limited to 14 states.[6] Moreover, unlike the Pescosolido and Mendelsohn (1986) study, we did not have the data for gender- and age-specific analyses. The statistical analyses involve multiple regression techniques with total suicide rate as the dependent variable and social correlates and social construction factors as the independent variables. Total suicide rates for each state were provided by the Indian publication,

Accidental Deaths and Suicides in India, 1991. All other data were state-wise and provided by various official Indian sources.

Social correlates, which are generally linked to modernisation and for which we had specific data, included income, education, urbanisation, population density and divorce rate. Income was measured by the percentage of people living below the poverty line and education was measured by the literacy rate of all persons. Urbanisation was measured by the percentage of the state population living in urban areas and population density was measured by number of persons per square km. (in thousands). The divorce rate measure was percentage of divorced persons per state calculated from Census data, 1991.

Social construction factors suggested by Pescosolido and Mendelsohn (1986) included religion, type of medico-legal system and other causes of death rates. For the religion variable, we used the percentage of Muslims per state. While Muslims constitute a relatively small proportion of the population compared with Hindus, they are uniformly spread throughout India and, as mentioned, have a prohibitive stance toward suicide similar to the Catholics that Pescosolido and Mendelsohn (1986) included in their US study. As we noted in Chapter 2, suicide is not unambiguously prohibited by the Hindu religion.

Unlike the US, the types of medico-legal systems operating in India tend to be uniform across the country. However, there is little specific information available about the accuracy with which different police forces record suicides. Therefore, for this variable we used the Institutional Performance Index (Mayer 2001) as a 'proxy' for the quality of administration. This index measures the extent to which an administration provides effective services to the community. A high IPI indicates that an administration is relatively competent in delivering services to citizens, while a low IPI indicates a less capable administrative process.

The other causes of death we included were rates of deaths from accidental drowning, burning and unspecified accidents. These were included because it is frequently suggested that these categories are more likely to contain misclassified or hidden suicides than less ambiguous categories of death, such as multiple car crash deaths (Douglas 1967; Phillips and Ruth 1993; Wasserman and Värnik 1998).

We performed correlations on the data to determine which independent variables were suitable as core variables for the regression equations. Only education and divorce rates were significantly correlated to total suicide rates. Therefore, in the first equation, we regressed these social correlates onto the dependent variable. We then performed successive regression equations adding a single social construction variable to this basic group, one at a time. According to Pescosolido and Mendelsohn (1986), statistical differences between the first (control) equation and subsequent equations should reflect biases in misreporting.

Table 3.5 presents the results of the consecutive multiple regression equations for the 14 states. The statistics include the unstandardised regression coefficients (R^2), the standard errors (in parentheses) with asterisks to indicate significance (alpha = 0.05; 2-tailed). Column 1 represents the basic or 'naïve' model (Pescosolido and Mendelsohn 1986), with the relevant social correlates entered as independent

Table 3.5 Regression of social causation and social construction variables upon total suicide rate, 1991, India, 14 states

Independent variables	Col 1	2	3	4	5	6	7
Social causation							
Education	0.29*	0.28*	0.54	0.29*	0.31*	0.29*	0.29*
	(0.01)	(0.10)	(0.32)	(0.10)	(0.10)	(0.10)	(0.10)
Divorce rate	0.02*	0.02*	0.02*	0.02*	0.02*	0.02*	0.02*
	(0.01)	(0.01)	(0.01)	(0.01)	(0.01)	(0.01)	(0.01)
Social construction							
Religion (Muslims)		0.19					
		(0.17)					
Institutional Performance Index			−3.64				
			(4.41)				
Other causes of death							
Accidental drowning				−0.12			
				(0.63)			
Accidental burning					−0.46		
					(0.53)		
Unspecified accidents						−0.15	
						(0.28)	
Total accidents							−0.02
							(0.12)
R^2	0.77	0.80	0.79	0.77	0.80	0.78	0.77
Adjusted R^2	0.73	0.74	0.72	0.71	0.73	0.71	0.71
SEE	4.03	3.98	4.09	4.22	4.07	4.17	4.22
F	18.74	13.17	12.36	11.41	12.45	11.75	11.41

variables. Columns 2 to 7 of Table 3.5 show the results of subsequent attempts to control for misreporting. If there were any significant differences between the coefficients of social factors between columns 1 and 2, 3, 4, 5, 6 and 7, it could suggest systematic misreporting.

As can be seen, we found no appreciable difference between the coefficients for any combination of social causation and social construction variables. Coefficients for the core social causation variables, education and divorce rate, are both positive and significant across most of the equations indicating that more literate areas have higher suicide rates and also higher divorce rates. However, the coefficients barely change across the equations. It can be seen that this basic model accounts for about 77 per cent of the variance in total suicide rates [$F(2, 11) = 18.74, p < 0.001$] and there is little change in R^2 across the columns.

Adding the social construction variables, religion and institutional perform-ance, appears to have little impact. The negative sign of the latter indicates that areas of low institutional performance are associated with higher suicide areas, although this is not significant. This is contrary to what we would expect if ineffective administrations underreported suicides. There is, however, weak evidence to suggest that some suicides may be classified as accidental deaths: the sign of all categories of accidental death are negative indicating that where accidental deaths are higher, suicides are lower, but again the coefficients are not statistically significant. According to Pescosolido and Mendelsohn (1986), the fact that there is little change in the equations from column 1 to 7 suggests that this analysis fails to provide evidence of systematic misreporting or concealment of suicides in the Indian context.

vii. Evidence from clinical studies

A third major category of evidence regarding the accuracy of Indian statistics on suicides comes from clinical studies. These studies are illuminating because the investigators are trained psychiatrists who have investigated meaningful, if small, samples in great depth. There are clear problems, however, in extrapolating from the findings from these micro-level studies to an Indian state or the nation as a whole. For the most part, these studies were carried out in large public hospitals located in major urban centres. It is not clear that the populations that they have studied are representative of India's largely rural population. In addition, the investigators may have applied a less rigorous standard than that required of those administering the criminal law. It is possible, for example, that clinical studies commonly make decisions about suicides 'on the balance of probabilities' rather than requiring the evidence to be 'beyond reasonable doubt'. Different standards of proof may explain why clinical studies uniformly report higher levels of suicides than are officially recorded.

A clear illustration of this generalisation can be found in the study by Venkoba Rao and associates who studied 100 consecutive female patients admitted to the burns unit of the Government Rajaji Hospital, Madurai, Tamil Nadu, in 1988. Fifty-one cases were originally classified as accidental deaths. In 31 cases the classification was made on the basis of 'dying declarations' made by the women, which police are required to consider in determining the cause of death. In subsequent interviews with clinical staff, 26 of these women who did not imme-diately succumb to their injuries 'later confessed the[ir] suicidal intent to the project staff before death'. Thus Venkoba Rao and his colleagues concluded that over one-quarter of sample burns cases were wrongly classified as accidents in the first instance. In addition, the Madurai study found that one dying declaration of suicide was actually an attempted homicide and three dying declaration homi-cides were eventually discovered to be suicides. In all, of 48 dying declarations available to the Madurai researchers, 30 (62.5 per cent) were found to be inaccurate on further investigation. '[M]any women concealed [the] suicid[al] nature of their burns apprehending ill-treatment of their children by the family or/ and to avoid social stigma' (Venkoba Rao, Mahendran *et al.* 1989: 45). Most importantly though, Venkoba Rao's study indicates that the great majority of errors in recording suicide deaths arose, not from concealment or other failures on the part of the police or medical staff, but from deceptive depositions made by the burns victims about the circumstances in which they were burned and – crucial for a determination of suicide – about their intentions.

A study of 50 patients of both sexes admitted to King Edward VII Memorial Hospital in Mumbai between 1994 and 1995 for treatment of burns found that 20 (40 per cent) were the result of suicide attempts, while the rest were accidental burns (Wagle, Wagle *et al.* 1999: 159). Although Wagle *et al.* also found that conflict with close relations was a factor in a large proportion of cases (40 per cent), unemployment was a factor in another 32 per cent, these stressors not being exclusive. Fifty-five per cent of attempters came from joint families, as against 23 per cent of accidental burns victims (Wagle, Wagle *et al.* 1999: 159). In contrast to the study by Rao *et al.*, Wagle and colleagues did not report finding any inaccuracies in the cases they examined, suggesting that because in the period covered by their study, 'suicide or attempted suicide is no longer considered an offence in the court of law in India . . . more victims are likely to reveal and accept the true nature of burns injury' (Wagle, Wagle *et al.* 1999: 158). Later court rulings that we discussed in Chapter 2 may have altered this situation.

In a retrospective study of 25 years (1972–1997) of autopsies conducted on 375 acute poisoning deaths by the Postgraduate Institute of Medical Education and Research, Chandigarh, Singh *et al.* found that the number of poisonings rose sharply after 1982, primarily due to the wide availability of agrochemicals, an integral part of the 'Green Revolution' package. Despite the increasing availability of these commercial poisons, accidental deaths as a proportion of all acute poisonings have fallen steadily from 63 per cent in 1972–1977 to 17 per cent in 1992–1997. Suicides, by contrast, have risen from 33 per cent in 1972–1977 to 77 per cent in 1992–1997 (Singh, Jit *et al.* 1999: 205). Over the study period, the suicide sex ratio (male: female) fell from 3.5:1 in 1972–1977 to 1.64:1 in 1992–1977. Singh and his colleagues do not report finding any incorrectly classified deaths.

The evidence from clinical studies reinforces our earlier conclusions that Indian suicide data are unlikely to be seriously affected by systematic biases in the administrative procedures and processes by which they are recorded. Rao's study serves as a warning that in cases where suicide attempters deliberately misrepresent their intentions, it is difficult without employing extraordinary measures to detect the deception.

viii. Suicide rates of Indian migrants

Methodological considerations

A final means of testing the reliability of Indian suicide statistics is to compare the rates of suicides recorded for Indian migrants under different recording procedures with those in India itself. As there are many difficulties in making such comparisons, they serve at best as additional confirmation. We will consider the incidence of suicide among the Indian diaspora in detail in Chapter 14.

For the purposes of seeking to assess the validity of official Indian data on suicides, we may briefly examine a table, which we will consider in more detail later. The table compares average suicide rates for India between 1980 and 1990 with rates for Indian migrants in a few countries for which separate reports of the rates of suicide for Indian migrants are reported.

It can be seen that the Indian suicide rate is higher than that reported for Indians in the US, but lower than that reported for Indian migrants in either Australia or the United Kingdom.

It is very difficult to specify what relationship we should expect between the suicide rates of migrants and their country of origin. Migrants, almost by definition, are not typical of their populations of birth; they tend to be better educated and more ambitious. In addition, they are subject to many additional stresses in their country of migration and lack many of the social supports that they might have had in the land of their birth. All of these things would lead us to predict, *a priori*, that their suicide rates would be relatively high. The fact that the average suicide rate for India for the decade of the 1980s falls in between three rates we have is one further piece of evidence that the data are not deeply flawed. Indeed, the all-India rate for 1999 is virtually identical to that reported for Indian migrants living for more than ten years in Australia.

Conclusion

It is a commonplace of Indian scholars writing on suicide that official Indian statistics on suicide grossly understate the true rate of suicide in the country. If their claims are correct, it would constitute a major, possibly a fatal, weakness in the project to which this book is directed, relying as it does so heavily on those official figures. As we have seen, despite the frequent assertion that official figures report less than half the actual suicides that occur, those who make the claim have offered no systematic evidence to substantiate it. The most persuasive and significant evidence comes from a relative handful of clinical studies. While these *are* significant data, they are inadequate, in themselves, to refute the broader claim of systematic bias in the official figures. There are several reasons for this. First, because they are clinical studies, in most instances they reflect an unsystematic

Table 3.6 Suicide rates of Indian migrants in the USA, UK and Australia compared with the Indian population

Country	Suicide rate
India (average 1980–1990)	7.0
India (1999)	11.2
USA	4.0
UK	16.4
Australia (more than 10 years)	11.1

sample of largely urban populations. Second, in most instances the cases upon which they report are drawn from a single method of suicide such as burning or poisoning; none reports, for example, on hanging or drowning. Thirdly, most clinical studies have not been clear about the standard of proof they have applied; none seems to have applied the 'beyond reasonable doubt' test of the criminal law. Finally, with the exception of Vijayakumar and Rajkumar's unique series of psychological autopsies conducted in Chennai, none of the clinical studies has compared their cases with official statistics of which they are generally critical. In a personal communication, Dr Vijayakumar has informed us that in Chennai, at least, the police records were generally quite accurate.

Appendix

As the discussion in this chapter has indicated, the core data on which the book relies are those compiled each year by the National Crime Records Bureau (NCRB) in New Delhi. We have used differing base years for different investigations. In some cases the year was chosen because it was closest to the date of collection of other variables. In some cases, it was necessary to use data from a single year because it was only in that year that a particular breakdown of the data was presented. For many analyses we rely on data from 1997, which the NCRB were gracious enough to generate for us.

The statistical analyses presented in this and subsequent chapters are standard ones and were generated using SPSS for Windows 10.0 (SPSS Inc, 2000). The statistical tests used in the book are also conventional ones.

At a few points in the book we also utilise the less familiar power tests, which rely on 'effect size' (ES). At the core of the logic of effect size is the observation that with a sufficiently large sample, even quite minor and 'sociologically insignificant' correlations can be statistically significant. Cohen suggests that for correlation coefficients, we may take $r = 0.1$ as a small effect, $r = 0.3$ as a medium effect and $r = 0.5$ as a large effect:

> 'My intention was that medium [effect size] represent[s] an effect likely to be visible to the naked eye of a careful observer . . . I set small ES to be noticeably smaller than medium but not so small as to be trivial, and I set large ES to be the same distance above medium as small was below it.'
>
> (Cohen 1992: 156)

Given the limited number of states for which we have data, only large effect sizes are likely to also be statistically significant.

Notes

1 We wish to express our deep thanks to Sri S. C. Sharma, IPS, Inspector General of Police for Tamil Nadu, and Sri J.P. Singh, IPS Inspector General of Police for Pondicherry for their kindness in assisting us in our study of suicide records in Tamil Nadu and Pondicherry.

2 The Registrar General's data omit the figure for West Bengal.
3 The differences in urban and rural rates will be examined in Chapter 9.
4 We discuss the relationship between marital status and suicide in Chapter 12.
5 For full details about the statistical technique see Pescosolido & Mendelsohn (1986).
6 Data for 1991 were used to be coincident with Census and other data used in the analysis.

4   The aetiology of suicide in India

The motives for suicide

The motives of suicide were among the first aspects of suicide to be investigated by nineteenth-century sociologists and to be reported as part of official recording of suicide in Europe.[1] As the collection of records became more systematic, the lists of possible motivations used by different jurisdictions and investigators grew and changed enormously. The great Italian sociologist Dr Enrico Morselli, reviewing what he sardonically termed 'the so much despised tables of . . . "determining cause"' (Morselli 1881: 267) which were available to him in 1881, noted that:

> The French statistics of suicides, for example, enumerate about 60 causes, the Italian 25, Des-Étanges 15, De Boismont 20, Lisle 50, whilst Wagner reduces them to 14, Oettingen to 10, the Bavarian statistics to two or three groups of 4.
> (Morselli 1881: 266)

Morselli[1]

Morselli's own work utilised 10 broad categories to classify the causes of suicides. He was struck by the consistency of the patterns that he found, both over time and across nations, in Europe. Year after year very similar proportions of cases appeared in each category of causes, leading him to speculate that he was observing something approaching a sociological 'law'.[2] Morselli, like investigators in our own time, was struck by the high proportion of cases in which psychological disorders such as melancolia and *toedium vitae* – forms that would now be termed depression – prevailed (Morselli 1881: 280–286). Morselli also noted a theme that has been repeated by innumerable subsequent investigations: the importance of alcohol (and other drugs) as a causal factor in suicide (Morselli 1881: 288–291).

Durkheim

The best-known and most influential approach to the aetiology of suicide is that developed by Émile Durkheim in his classic study *Le Suicide*, published in 1897.

Durkheim's four causes of suicide – egoism, altruism, anomie and fatalism – have been subject to many subsequent analyses and referred to in innumerable studies.[3] Douglas argues that Durkheim did not himself create these categories; rather they were already well established in nineteenth century European sociology (Douglas 1967: 16–20). Durkheim believed that each of these causes had specific social forces that were responsible for them.

Scholars have offered widely differing interpretations of Durkheim's aetological cal scheme. Douglas argues that we best understand Durkheim as having conceived of two pairs of opposing or balancing social forces – egoism restrained by altruism, and anomie opposed by fatalism – each pair corresponding to two overarching social mechanisms: *social integration* for the first pair and *social regulation* for the second (Douglas 1967: 56). Egoism referred to individuals directed by self-interest, over whom social controls are weak; altruism, by contrast, referred to the subservience of the individual to the general good. Anomie referred to the unbounded, emotional desire for experience and wealth while its balancing force, fatalism, referred to an unquestioning acceptance of the prevailing social order. When egoism and altruism are in balance, individuals are 'integrated'. When anomie and fatalism are in balance, then an appropriate degree of social regulation has been achieved. When either pair is unbalanced, suicidogenetic [suicide-causing] currents are set in motion (Douglas 1967: 57).

Johnson, by contrast, has argued that Durkheim's different categories really represent a single dimension (Johnson 1965). He argues that Durkheim locates altruism only in preliterate traditional societies and in the armed forces. Similarly, fatalism is found only in exceptional and narrow groups, such as slaves and others subjected to despotism. For these reasons, Johnson argues that neither altruism nor fatalism is applicable to contemporary societies (Johnson 1965: 879–881). Johnson also presents evidence for understanding anomie as a subset of egoism (Johnson 1965: 881–886; see also Gibbs and Martin 1964; Pope and Danigelis 1981).

Durkheim's broad argument that suicide rates are inversely related to social integration has been the aspect of his theory most frequently utilised by subsequent investigators. Thus, Henry and Short in their study of suicide and homicide used the rate of marriage as a proxy for Durkheim's 'involvement of an individual in relationships with other persons'. They found that, as predicted, the suicide rate of married individuals was lower than for single, widowed or divorced persons (Henry and Short 1954: 73). In a similar replication, Stack utilised female labour participation rates as a measure of social disintegration in a study of 45 nations. He found that suicide rates were positively correlated with women's labour force participation (Stack 1978). Lester utilised measures of political and civil rights to estimate degrees of social regulation and marriage and birth rates as proxies for social integration in a cross-cultural study of 53 countries. He found that nations with high scores on both dimensions or low scores on both had the highest suicide rates. Nations with moderate scores on both dimensions had low suicide rates. Lester also found, unexpectedly, that countries with low social regulation and high social integration had the highest suicide rates (Lester 1989: 38–39).

Despite the entrenched tradition of referring to Durkeim's aetiological categories, contemporary scholarly analyses rarely use them in studying the causes of individual suicides. As Hassan notes, typologies such as Durkheim's are not 'very useful in analysing . . . individual cases and the specific circumstances leading the individual to commit suicide' (Hassan 1995: 133).

More recent psychological autopsies

The most prominent contemporary technique based on the analysis of the causes of suicide is the Psychological Autopsy Method.[4] Pioneered by the Los Angeles Suicide Prevention Center, psychological autopsy was developed to assist medical examiners determine the cause of death in ambiguous cases. At the core of the method is a process of extended, usually structured, interviews by trained psychiatrists or psychologists within a few months of death with a number of informants such as close relatives or friends. These are supplemented by interviews with ancillary informants such as health or social workers and police. The interviews elicit information on the personality, mental health, family relations, drug dependence, and so forth of the deceased. The objective is to construct as accurately as possible, after the fact, the mental state of the deceased so as to inform the classification of death.

The method has been extended to the specific investigation of the causes of suicide. One of the consistent findings of psychological autopsy studies is that psychiatric disorder is found in over 90 per cent of cases (Brent 1989: 48; Isometsä, Heikkinen *et al.* 1997: 382) with major affective disorder or alcoholism in 60–90 per cent of all suicides (Clark and Horton-Deustch 1992: 147). About two-thirds of suicides communicated their intention in broad terms in the period preceding their deaths, with over a third doing so in very explicit terms (see Clark and Horton-Deustch 1992: 148–149, 153).

The psychological autopsy has its critics. They note that it is reliant upon indirect evidence about the mental state of a deceased person gathered from emotionally involved individuals, often at a considerable period after a suicide has occurred (see for example, Hawton, Appleby *et al.* 1998; Selkin 1994). In addition, it seems likely that the explicitly psychological focus of the method may predispose those using it to privilege psychological over other social or economic causal factors.

The causes identified in psychological autopsy may also be used to inform suicide prevention strategies. Thus, the finding of a number of studies that 'two-thirds of the suicide victims communicated their suicidal intent over a period of weeks prior to their death, usually to several different persons, and 40 per cent communicated their suicidal intent in very clear and specific terms' (Clark and Horton-Deustch 1992: 149; see also, Isometsä 2001: 382) provides the evidential basis for youth suicide prevention programmes that inform parents, teachers, peers and medical personnel of the importance of taking such warnings with the utmost seriousness. Befrienders International reflects these findings in their succinct list of warning signs of suicide:

- Suicide is rarely a spur of the moment decision. In the days and hours before people kill themselves, there are usually clues and warning signs.
- The strongest and most disturbing signs are verbal – 'I can't go on,' 'Nothing matters any more' or even 'I'm thinking of ending it all.' Such remarks should always be taken seriously.[5]

Studies of the motives for suicide in India

Virtually every study of suicide in India includes a brief examination of its causes, based in most instances on official determinations. McLeod examined the fragmentary evidence available for a number of causes of suicide in his path-breaking 1878 study of suicide in British India. Evidence from Madras Presidency indicated that during the famine year of 1877 suicides rose by one-third above their average level. He reported that physical pain, especially abdominal pain, 'is the common cause of suicide in Bengal, more particularly, among women' (McLeod 1878: 407). McLeod cited post-mortem findings of Assistant Surgeon Guru Dayal Das Gupta in Tangail District that two-thirds of suicides by hanging suffered from roundworm infection (McLeod 1878: 408). McLeod also noted that, as in Europe, mental illness and drug addiction were also significant factors in Indian suicide, though he could cite nothing by way of firm evidence. Lastly, McLeod offered the impressionistic conclusion that 'the immediate motive to suicide is no doubt in most cases of a domestic kind of quarrel, slight, some petty annoyance, grief, shame, jealousy or the like' (McLeod 1878: 412).

A representative post-Independence presentation of the causes of suicide is provided in Varma's *Suicide in India and Abroad*. Varma offers a brief table drawn from the official figures for 1971, noting that dreadful diseases and quarrels with family members were the most frequent causes. Varma is sceptical at the extremely low rate of suicide due to unemployment found in the official figures (less than 0.8 per cent of all cases), given the large numbers of educated unemployed alone: 'obviously [these] data [are] not to be relied upon' (Varma 1976: 130).

Another typical survey of the causes of suicide is Gehlot and Nathawat's 1983 investigation of suicide in the family context, which begins with a brief summary of the official national figures published in 1976. These showed that just under 20 per cent were prompted by despair over incurable diseases, another 16 per cent arose from quarrels with relatives or spouses, 5 per cent from disappointment in love, 4 per cent from disputes over property and 4 per cent from poverty (Gehlot and Nathawat 1983: 274–275).

Pandey's extended examination of 'The Aetiology of Suicide in India Today' arranged the official classifications of suicide from 1979 under four major headings (physical causes, social causes, psychological causes and miscellaneous). The largest group (50 per cent) were those for which no cause was established. Physical causes (dreaded diseases) were the cause of 15 per cent of deaths, familial causes, including quarrels with close relatives, were implicated in 20 per cent of cases, questions of social status (including failure in examinations) for 3 per cent, economic causes for 8 per cent, and psychological causes for 3 per cent (Pandey 1985: 434). Pandey concluded his paper by noting the significance of social causes of suicide, arguing that 'this speaks of deteriorating family relations in India' (Pandey 1985: 438).

A number of Indian studies have reported the causes of suicide for smaller, local-level populations. Venkoba Rao *et al.* in their study of 100 female burns cases in Madurai, found that of the 69 cases for which causes could be established, 96 per cent had a social cause. Marital conflict precipitated 51 per cent of cases, other stressful relationships or events 37 per cent and conflicts over dowry a further 8 per cent (Venkoba Rao, Mahendran *et al.* 1989: 45–46).

Banerjee *et al.* studied all suicides recorded at Deganga Police Station, North 24 Parganas District, West Bengal, in 1979. They found that conflict with one's spouse (18 per cent), relatives (10 per cent) and parents (23 per cent) were the most frequently recorded causes of suicide. Women were more likely to have quarrelled with a spouse (33 per cent vs 25 per cent) or in-laws (13 per cent vs nil) than men, who were more likely to quarrel with parents (33 per cent vs 20 per cent for women) (Banerjee, Nandi *et al.* 1990: 307). Illness was the other major cause of suicide (14 per cent; 7 per cent for males, 13 per cent for females).

Stomach pain or other physical illness was the most common cause of suicide (about 22 per cent in Hyderabad and 24 per cent in surrounding rural districts) recorded for 2,181 suicides by poisoning examined at the Andhra Pradesh State Forensic Laboratory between 1994 and 1998. About 10 per cent of cases involved conflicts with close relatives. Economic difficulties or conflicts were listed as causes in about 7 per cent of cases. Mental illness was a cause in about 2 per cent of cases (Gautami, Sudershan *et al.* 2001: 169).

Bhalla *et al.*'s 1998 study of 14 Punjab villages with above average suicide rates was unique in looking for both psychological and socio-economic antecedents of suicides. Nearly 55 per cent of suicides studied had shown signs of depression and over 90 per cent had some form of psychological disorder (Bhalla, Sharma *et al.* 1998: 57). If psychological factors may be considered as predisposing factors, a combination of social and economic factors were important in precipitating suicides. A conflict with close relatives was the proximate cause in 77 per cent of cases (Bhalla, Sharma *et al.* 1998: 66). Alcohol and drugs were implicated in 18 per cent of cases. Indebtedness and poverty were stated as causes in 24 per cent of cases and a loss of status in 16 per cent (Bhalla, Sharma *et al.* 1998: 64). The Punjab study is particularly valuable in illustrating the importance of sociological *and* psychological factors.

Psychological autopsy in India

Vijayakumar and Rajkumar's 1999 study in Chennai is unique in the Indian literature for undertaking a psychological autopsy study using case controls. As noted in Chapter 2, the Chennai study found 88 per cent of the 100 suicides had clinical disorders at some point in their lives. Seventeen per cent of suicides suffered from major depression. Alcoholism was a factor in 34 per cent and adjustment disorder in a further 12 per cent (Vijayakumar and Rajkumar 1999: 409).[6]

'Stomach pain'

Gautami's finding, noted above, that stomach pain or stomach ache was the immediate aetiology for just under a quarter of suicides by poisoning in the region around Hyderabad in Andhra Pradesh raises an important issue but one that is relatively neglected in the Indian context. It is entirely understandable that journalists treat such cases with righteous anger and ironic humour. Sainath in a two-part report on farmer suicides in Anantapur district, Andhra Pradesh stated that 1,016 cases – 58 per cent of the total – which he believed arose from the economic distress of farmers, were recorded by the police as due to 'stomach pain'.

> Why did these numbers never come into the debate on distress suicides among farmers? Simple. Hundreds of them went into the police registers with these lines: 'the man (or woman) had severe stomach-ache. Unable to bear the pain, he (or she) swallowed pesticide in despair'.
> The despair, then, did not arise from the economic distress of the farmer. It came from an epidemic of stomach-aches. A number of farmers ended their tummy pain with the pesticide, Monocrotophos. An item provided free by the State.
>
> (Sainath 2001a)

Nevertheless, as we shall see in our detailed study of suicides in Pondicherry in Chapter 15, there, too, stomach pain – or more rarely 'chest pain' – is given as the cause of nearly a quarter of suicides. Is this, too, evidence of, at best, weak police investigation, or, at worst, of attempts to cover up the 'real' causes of suicides? We suggest that it is neither but rather that in many instances the police aetiologies actually point to unrecognised evidence of depression. Evidence for this conclusion comes from a number of studies both from India and elsewhere.

Raguram *et al.* reported finding an inverse relationship between stigma and somatisation (physical symptoms such as stomach pain) and a positive correlation between stigma and depression (Raguram, Weiss *et al.* 1996). Although patients had high scores on the Hamilton depression scale, 60 per cent identified somatic symptoms as most troubling (Raguram, Weiss *et al.* 1996: 1046). In other words, patients manifesting signs of depression tended to describe their symptoms in terms of physical pain. Raguram *et al.* comment:

> the social meaning of somatic symptoms is less distressing because they closely approximate experiences that everyone has from time to time. Depressive symptoms, on the other hand, are considered to be private and even dangerous. They are experienced as socially disadvantageous; they might interfere with marriage, diminish social status, and compromise the self-esteem required to perform effectively in society.
>
> (Raguram, Weiss *et al.* 1996: 1048)

Chandra *et al.* report that pain symptoms explained 32 per cent of the variance in depressive and anxiety symptoms in a study of 51 HIV-positive subjects studied in Bangalore (Chandra, Ravi *et al.* 1998). Venkoba Rao also notes that many female burns patients studied in Madurai offered somatic pain as the precipitating circumstance of attempted and completed suicide. He suggests that 'the link between abdominal pain and suicide behaviour needs further study especially from the physicians to ascertain the quantum of high risk patients proceeding to suicide behaviour.' (Venkoba Rao, Mahendran *et al.* 1989: 47). He emphasises, however, that although some instances of pain may be depressive manifestations, others may have physical causes such as ulcer or appendicitis.

It is possible that the frequent appearance of somatic pain as an antecedent circumstance of completed suicide reflects the difficulties that individuals in a largely pre-psychological society such as India have in verbalising their emotional distress. The presentation of a constellation of somatic symptoms is utilised to diagnose depression in the Out-Patient Department of the Jawaharlal Institute of Postgraduate Medical Education & Research (JIPMER) in Pondicherry.

It is equally possible, however, that somatic pain is offered by survivors as an antecedent cause of suicide because it is perceived as a culturally less stigmatised reason. In a careful case–control psychological autopsy of 100 cases in Chennai, Vijayakumar and Rajkumar found 88 per cent had a lifetime diagnosis of clinical disorders. Major depression was found in 17 per cent of cases, alcoholism – which may itself be a form of self-medication for depression – in 34 per cent and somato-form disorder in only 1 per cent.

The failure to recognise the significance of stomach pain as a marker of possible psychological disorder is not confined to India. Chynoweth *et al.* in their study of 135 suicides in Brisbane, Australia, found that 52 per cent of their sample showed evidence of physical ill health; in 25 per cent of these cases the illness affected the gastrointestinal tract.

> ... disorders of the gastrointestinal tract occurred more frequently among the physically ill suicides than would be expected from their distribution within an adult population attending a medical practitioner with physical illness.
>
> (Chynoweth, Tonge *et al.* 1980: 40)

They conclude:

> The recurrence of abdominal pain in the absence of clear cut pathology such as alcoholic gastritis or peptic ulcer suggests the need for a fuller psychiatric and social assessment ... The importance of the gastrointestinal symptoms as a sign of emotional stress is reflected in the high proportion of 'functional' disorders in this system and also in the reported high referral rate to a psychiatric department that occurs from physicians within a general hospital.
>
> (Chynoweth, Tonge *et al.* 1980: 43–4)

Official determination of causes of suicide in India

The causes of suicides in India are determined in most cases by police officials at the local level. There are strengths and weaknesses inherent in this process of determination. The procedure has the virtue of being an official investigation conducted immediately after a case has been reported, in most cases with the body of the suicide *in situ*. Those undertaking the investigation are trained in the observation of crime scenes including homicides and accidental deaths. The investigating officers are legally authorised to interview all persons who may be in a position to assist them to establish whether the death was unnatural and above all, whether the individual took their own life. In only a relatively limited number of urban areas are the determinations of suicide and its causes made by hospital-based medical officers. And there is no evidence that trained psychologists or psychiatrists assist in the determination of the nature of more than a small percentage of ambiguous cases.

Changing categories of causes of suicide in India

Official statistics on the causes of suicide in India have shown a tendency, somewhat akin to that noticed by Morselli in nineteenth-century Europe to change and expand over time to include finer and more precise categories. They have also exhibited a remarkable consistency in pattern over the years.

As can be seen in Table 4.1, what were ten basic categories in 1967 have grown over the decades to 22 major categories and five sub-categories for illnesses in 1997. At the same time, a few significant older categories such as quarrel with spouse and quarrel with parents have disappeared, to be replaced by more inclusive if less informative categories such as 'family problems'.

Patterns of suicide causes 1967–1997

The patterns of causes reported for suicide in India have shown a robust consistency over the past 30 years. Until recently the most important aspect of that consistency was actually a deficiency, in that until the mid-1980s about half the cases were either attributed to causes other than those listed or to unknown causes (Figure 4.1). The separate listing of suicides for which causes were not determined in 1984 marked the first significant reduction in the size of this residual category. The subsequent inclusion of 11 additional categories of cause in 1995 reduced the remaining numbers attributed to 'other causes' by about half.

The broad consistency of patterns of suicide causes over the years can best be appreciated if they are amalgamated into fewer, more inclusive, categories. Figure 4.2 compares causes of suicide between 1967 and 2007, consolidated under seven broad headings. Two major causes, each accounting for between 15 and 25 per cent of cases, predominate over the years: suicides attributed to diseases and suicides attributed to antagonistic relations with close kin such as a spouse, parents or in-laws. Loss of reputation, which includes failure in examinations, regularly accounts for between 5 and 10 per cent of suicides. About the same percentage of

Table 4.1 Causes of suicide, 1967–2007 (percentage)

	1967	1977	1987	1997	2007
Failure in examination	3.9	1.8	1.7	2.7	1.6
Quarrel with parents-in-law	9.0	10.1	8.1	•	
Quarrel with spouse	7.2	6.5	5.9	•	
Family problems	•	•	•	18.4	23.8
Poverty	5.4	0.03	2.2	3.4	2.3
Frustration	3.6	•	•	•	
Love affairs	3.4	5.8	4.4	3.7	2.8
Insanity/mental illness	3.5	2.9	3.3	5.0	7.0
Disputes over property	1.2	3.0	1.8	1.8	1.2
Despair over dreadful diseases/illness	17.2	16.7	13.8	15.2	
AIDS/STD	•	•	•	0.2	0.8
Cancer	•	•	•	0.6	0.6
Paralysis	•	•	•	0.4	0.4
Other illness	•	•	•	14.0	13.4
Unemployment	•	1.4	1.5	2.0	2.0
Bankruptcy	•	0.8	1.0	1.7	2.7
Death of dear person	•	0.9	0.7	0.7	0.6
Fall in social reputation	•	0.9	0.8	1.0	0.9
Dowry disputes	•	•	1.6	2.6	2.6
Illegitimate pregnancy	•	•	0.4	0.4	0.1
Suspected/illicit relationship	•	•	•	1.3	1.1
Cancellation/non-settlement of marriage	•	•	•	0.9	0.8
Barrenness	•	•	•	0.6	0.7
Divorce	•	•	•	0.4	0.3
Drug abuse	•	•	•	1.0	1.9
Hero worship/ideology	•	•	•	0.1	0.2
Physical abuse/rape	•	•	•	0.4	0.2
Professional/career problem	•	•	•	0.6	1.0
Causes not known	•	•	15.2	18.9	16.6
Other causes	45.6	46.2	37.6	17.3	14.4

cases are attributed to economic causes such as bankruptcy or poverty and to bereavement at the loss of 'a dear person' or tragic love affairs. Mental illness is reported as the cause of around 4 per cent of the cases over the long term.

Aetiological interrelationships

To determine the relationships between different causes of suicide in the Indian states and their relationship to major socio-economic factors a factor analysis was undertaken which included eight major antecedent causes of suicide and six socio-economic variables. The causes included in the model were the suicide rates for: unemployment, bankruptcy, family problems, insanity, exam failure,

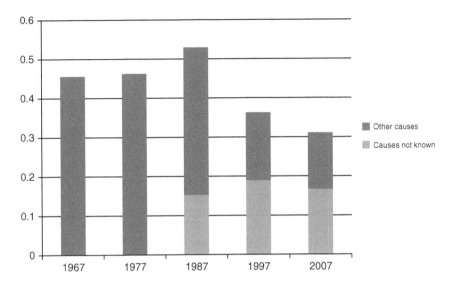

Figure 4.1 Unclassified suicides, 1967–1997.

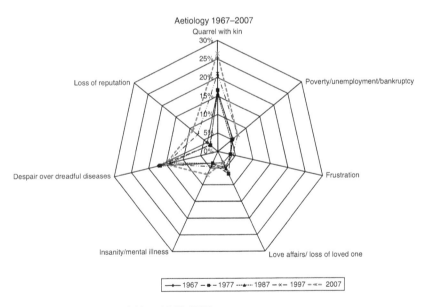

Figure 4.2 Causes of suicides, 1967–2007.

suspected/illicit relationship, love affair, cancelled/non-settled marriage.[7] The socio-economic variables utilised were chosen to measure the effect of integration into traditional society, urbanisation, industrialisation, political engagement and human capital accumulation: average household size, percentage urban, factory employment, the Civic Community Index and percentage female literacy in 1991.[8]

The results of the factor analysis are very interesting but somewhat unexpected. As can be seen in Table 4.2, three factors emerged.[9] The suicide causes that loaded on the first factor were unemployment, bankruptcy, family problems and insanity. The socio-economic variables highly associated with the factor were female literacy and the Civic Community Index; family size, a measure of integration into traditional social structures, had a negative loading on the factor. The association of female literacy and the Civic Community Index with this factor indicates that it measures a dimension of personal empowerment associated with modernisation.

Although it is possible to assimilate this first factor with Durkheim's observations concerning the destructive effects on traditional beliefs that arise from education and the moral individualism that results from knowledge and to see this factor as representing Egoistic suicides[10] (Durkheim 1951: 168), we prefer an interpretation that sees human development as unambiguously positive. This interpretation recognises that for small numbers of individuals, the social and cultural changes that accompany expanded human capability and empowerment create conflicts and crises that they are unable to endure. It is for this reason we have chosen to label this as a Human Development Crisis Factor. It accounts for 46 per cent of the variance in the model.

Table 4.2 Suicide causes, factor scores

Causes of suicide	Crises of human development	Crises of personal relationships	Economic development
Unemployment	0.96	−0.05	0.001
Bankruptcy	0.96	−0.08	−0.02
Family problems	0.90	0.31	0.11
Insanity	0.89	0.27	0.02
Exam failure	0.08	0.97	−0.07
Suspected/ illicit relationship	−0.10	0.95	−0.13
Love affair	0.21	0.97	0.02
Cancelled marriage	0.28	0.91	0.05
Socio-economic variables			
% Female literacy 1991	0.82	0.12	0.48
Civic Community Index	0.81	0.16	0.51
Average household size	−0.55	−0.20	−0.58
NDP per capita 1997	0.06	−0.10	0.92
Factory employment per capita	0.06	−0.02	0.99

The second factor brings together a number of causes that reflect crises in personal relationships: failed love affairs, suspected or actual illicit relationships and cancelled or non-settled marriages. The apparently odd association with this factor is 'failure in examinations'. What is striking is that none of the socio-economic variables load on this second factor. We have labelled this as a Crisis of Personal Relationships Factor. It is possible to identify the characteristics of this cluster of causes with Durkheim's Anomic Suicides. This factor accounts for 33 per cent of the variance in the model.

The third factor brings together the socio-economic variables related to economic development: urbanisation, industrialisation and per capita income. We have here the apparent mirror reflection of the second factor: none of the aetiological variables load on this factor. We have labelled this as an Economic Development Factor. This factor accounts for 21 per cent of the variance in the model.

We may conclude our examination of the aetiology of suicide in India by noting that there are important regional and gender aspects to the two broad factors we have identified. First we may note that there are two unmistakable outliers: Kerala and West Bengal. Kerala has a very high score on the Human Development Crisis Factor but a relatively low score on the second factor. The other conspicuous outlier is West Bengal, which has a very high score on the Personal Relationship Crisis Factor and a low score on the Human Development Crisis Factor.

We next used the Human Development Crisis Factor to generate individual 'factor scores' for each state. When we do this, we can see that the two regional extremes of Kerala and West Bengal are part of a broader regional pattern. Looking at Table 4.3 we can observe that scores on the Human Development Crisis Factor are highest in the South, moderate in the West, moderate to low in the East and consistently low in the North. These differences are statistically significant.

In Table 4.4 we see the distribution for the Personal Relationship Crisis Factor

Table 4.3 Human development crisis factor score vs region (no. of states)

	South	West	North	East	Totals
High	1	0	0	0	1
Medium	3	2	0	1	6
Low	0	0	6	1	7
Totals	4	2	6	2	14

Note: Significant at 0.03.

Table 4.4 Personal relationship crisis factor score vs region (no. of states)

	South	West	North	East	Totals
High	0	0	0	1	1
Medium	3	1	1	1	6
Low	1	1	5	0	7
Totals	4	2	6	2	14

Table 4.5 Suicide causes – factors and gender

	Human development crisis factor	Personal relationship crisis factor
Male suicide rate	0.91[†††]	0.29
Female suicide rate	0.67[††]	0.64[††]

Note: †† = significant at 0.01; ††† = significant at 0.001.

scores. Here the East is high to medium, the North and West are medium and low and the South is medium and low. Though striking, these differences are not statistically significant.

It can be seen that the South and East have exchanged relative positions between the two factors. Taken together the two tables suggest that the traumatic effects resulting from changes in human development are greatest in the South, which as we have already seen has the highest suicide rates in the country. The higher impact of Personal Relationships crises in the East, especially West Bengal, is particularly noticeable when we examine suicide rates attributed to individual causes. The suicide rates in West Bengal for failure in examinations, tragic love affairs and cancelled marriages are many times higher than the rates for those causes in other states.

In addition to the regional patterns there is also an important gender dimension as well, which can be seen in Table 4.5. Indian male suicide rates are highly and statistically significantly correlated with the Human Development Crisis Factor; there is only a weak and statistically insignificant association with the Personal Relationship Crisis Factor. This suggests that Human Development crises have a disproportionately high impact upon men.

Female suicide rates are strongly and statistically significantly correlated with both aetiological factors. The implication of this finding is that while women are very much affected by the same conflicts and crises of modernisation as men, they are disproportionately affected by the causes associated with the Personal Relationship Crisis Factor.

The aetiology of suicide in Pondicherry

In Chapter 15 we present a detailed case study of suicide in Pondicherry using individual case records compiled by the suicide-prevention association Maitreyi in Pondicherry between 1995 and 1999. Without repeating the detail given there, it is appropriate to note here that we found nearly 40 per cent of suicides in Pondicherry had a 'quarrel with kin' as the immediately precipitating factor.

Notes

1 For a review of nineteenth-century writing on suicide, see Goldney and Schioldann 2000.

Appendix

Table 4.6 Suicide rates due to various causes in the Indian states, 1997

	Bankruptcy	Suspected/ illicit relationship	Cancelled marriage	No child	Insanity	Other illness	Dowry dispute	Failed examination	Family problem	Love affair	Poverty	Unemployment
Andhra Pradesh	0.17	0.10	0.08	0.10	0.82	3.80	0.37	0.22	2.12	0.24	1.20	0.09
Bihar	0.01	0.02	0.01	0.01	0.07	0.07	0.03	0.03	0.23	0.05	0.05	0.02
Goa	0.27	0.00	0.14	0.21	2.19	1.03	0.21	0.34	2.53	1.10	0.07	0.55
Gujarat	0.23	0.08	0.14	0.13	0.76	1.53	0.16	0.13	2.13	0.32	0.25	0.36
Haryana	0.04	0.11	0.01	0.02	0.35	0.42	0.22	0.16	1.17	0.20	0.13	0.12
Himachal Pradesh	0.00	0.00	0.02	0.00	0.32	0.77	0.05	0.21	0.64	0.19	0.05	0.40
Karnataka	0.31	0.11	0.18	0.13	1.02	5.49	0.20	0.37	3.11	0.40	1.05	0.54
Kerala	1.70	0.07	0.12	0.04	1.89	3.98	0.12	0.28	5.91	0.56	0.04	0.95
Madhya Pradesh	0.11	0.18	0.05	0.07	0.36	1.10	0.61	0.15	1.55	0.28	0.19	0.14
Maharashtra	0.28	0.09	0.07	0.07	0.63	1.83	0.43	0.28	2.48	0.30	0.43	0.26
Orissa	0.02	0.31	0.09	0.07	0.31	0.42	0.22	0.15	2.64	0.54	0.05	0.29
Punjab	0.01	0.03	0.01	0.01	0.15	0.38	0.21	0.03	0.31	0.07	0.07	0.04
Rajasthan	0.10	0.11	0.03	0.05	0.53	0.45	0.15	0.13	1.18	0.16	0.09	0.14
Tamil Nadu	0.19	0.09	0.09	0.05	0.27	2.24	0.15	0.33	3.85	0.48	1.23	0.30
Uttar Pradesh	0.05	0.04	0.01	0.02	0.11	0.20	0.30	0.04	0.51	0.09	0.07	0.07
West Bengal	0.07	0.59	0.35	0.12	0.89	0.91	0.33	1.43	2.78	1.60	0.05	0.07

2 'these motives or "causes" are regularly and constantly the same for men or women, for young or old, for Italian or English, for the physician or the peasant; each one of the individual states has also a specificness in its own determination, since ... given a certain condition of a social society, a determinate number of individuals must put an end to their own existence' (Morselli 1881: 271).

3 See for example (Douglas 1967; Henry and Short 1954; Lester 1989; Pope 1976; Johnson 1965).

4 For a review of studies utilising the psychological autopsy method, see (Clark and Horton-Deustch 1992; Isometsä 2001). For a critical assessment of the method, see (Selkin 1994).

5 http://www.befrienders.org/suicide/warning.htm (accessed 29 August 2002). Other warning signs listed by Befrienders are: i) becoming depressed or withdrawn; ii) behaving recklessly; iii) getting affairs in order and giving away valued possessions; iv) showing a marked change in behaviour, attitudes or appearance; v) abusing drugs or alcohol; vi) Suffering a major loss or life change.

6 We discuss the impact of alcohol consumption on suicide in India in Chapter 13.

7 Four other causes were initially examined but then excluded from further investigation because of their weak relationship to the other major causes: other illness, childlessness/impotence, dowry dispute, poverty.

8 Other variables suggested by Chauhan (1984) were also investigated, but dropped from subsequent analysis as they added little to explanatory power: homicide rate, percentage Scheduled Castes, electoral participation. Other variables tested but subsequently rejected were: son preference, population per hospital bed, females with no exposure to media and the headcount poverty rate. The degree of urbanisation was also utilised initially but because it was highly correlated with other modernisation variables it created a singularity in the correlation matrix and had to be excluded from subsequent analysis. The Civic Community Index is described in Mayer (2001).

9 The analysis used the Principal Components method to extract the factors and then Varimax rotation.

10 Hassan's linkage of causes for Australian suicides to Durkheim's broad types is largely consistent with this interpretation (Hassan 1995: 139).

5   The methods of suicide

In his classic work, *Suicide*, Durkheim considered the study of the *methods* of suicide to make little contribution to the understanding of the social meanings of suicide:

> The social causes on which suicides in general depend, however, differ from those which determine the way they are committed; for no relation can be discovered between the types of suicides which we have distinguished and the most common methods of performance.
>
> (Durkheim 1951: 291)

Because he believed that the methods chosen in suicides merely reflected familiarity and opportunity, the study of methods 'has nothing to teach us' about the social causes of suicides themselves (Durkheim 1951: 293). Durkheim's position is not that taken by other early suicidologists such as Morselli and Halbwachs. Halbwachs, for example, asked pointedly whether 'since every suicide results from the collaboration of decision and means, has one the right to neglect the latter?' (Halbwachs 1978: 28).

Using similar data from nineteenth century Europe, Morselli and Halbwachs both emphasised the remarkably consistent national patterns in choice of method of suicide. Even when suicide rates were rapidly increasing, the methods by which these suicides were completed remained constant over time. Different nationalities preferred different methods of suicide, tied both to logistical concerns (the accessibility of a particular method) and the social factors mentioned by Durkheim. For example, Scandinavians committed suicide by drowning far less frequently than all others in Europe and it is suggested that this was because of the extreme coldness of their waterways for most of the year. Also, the English hanged themselves far less frequently than all others in Europe and for this it was suggested that the social injunction against hanging was due to its use as a method of punishment for criminals. Further, Halbwachs suggested that national 'temperament' may play a part in method preference, that the 'chivalrous spirit' of the Spanish and Italians might have contributed to their national preference for dramatic and aesthetic forms of suicide – firearms and poison (Halbwachs 1978: 40). To emphasise this consistency even more, Morselli demonstrated that even when persons emigrated to another country, in this case the US, the choice of method of suicide remained remarkably similar to that of the home nation (Morselli 1881: 327).

This is not to say that there are not variations in choice of method of suicide both within nations themselves and between national groups. Morselli demonstrated that there were distinct differences between city and country areas in regards to method of suicide. Cities had peculiar patterns of their own, in part an avoidance of 'ignoble' forms of suicide by the sophisticated classes. In country areas, however, away from the influence of urban society, hanging and drowning were much more common. Also, Morselli reported distinct variations in preferred mode of suicide between the regions of Italy, with more violent methods being employed in the southern provinces (Morselli 1881: 334). There was also a common pattern whereby women, though committing suicide less frequently than men, chose different methods to do so. Commonly, women drowned themselves far more frequently than men and used violent methods, such as firearms, far less.

These patterns in method of suicide have changed somewhat over the last century however, for reasons of both availability and acceptance. The historically low rates of hanging in England and Wales have dramatically increased since the prohibition of capital punishment in 1965 (Pounder 1993). Removing the stigma appears to have made hanging more socially acceptable. Similarly, making a form of suicide more available, such as in the case of firearms in the US, also dramatically increases the number of suicides utilising this method. Since the early 1960s firearms have been increasingly easier to obtain in the US and the increase in the number of suicides using firearms accounted for almost all increases in suicide rates to at least 1975 (Boor 1981). The increase in high-density housing has also been accompanied by an increase in the rates of 'jumping' deaths, particularly in Asia (Cheng and Lee 2000).

Making a form of suicide less available or less lethal is an effective way of reducing the suicide rate. When Britain reduced the carbon monoxide content of the domestic gas supply, the suicide rate fell sharply though the number of attempted suicides increased (Boor 1981). Similar findings were reported after Vienna reduced the lethality of its gas supply. Similarly changes to the packaging of paracetamol in the UK led to changes in the use of the drug in suicide attempts. Thus some changes are noted in the methods of suicide over time, but it nonetheless remains one of the most stable characteristics of suicidal behaviour nonetheless.

Examining the Indian data regarding method of suicide shows this largely consistent character. McLeod reported very similar patterns of method of suicide in 1878 as are found in India today (McLeod 1878). Working principally in Bengal, McLeod reported that hanging and poisoning were the two dominant methods of suicide in this region, poisoning usually taking the form of opium overdose (McLeod 1878: 402). There were important regional differences, however, like those described by Morselli. Hanging was customary in the Bengal (now West Bengal and the independent nation Bangladesh) and Orissa while poisoning was dominant in Bihar. Unlike the urban–rural differences noted by Morselli however, McLeod reported that the pattern of method of suicide for Calcutta, the largest city in the region, was the same as the region at large (McLeod 1878: 402).

Modern literature discussing the methods of suicide chosen in India reveals a fairly consistent preference for hanging, poisoning and drowning. Hegde (1980) reported that in northern Karnataka, drowning, poisoning and hanging accounted for 39.21 per cent, 33.33 per cent and 25.50 per cent of the total number of suicides respectively. This is a similar result to that found by Ganapathi and Venkoba Rao (1966) in the city of Madurai in the adjoining state of Tamil Nadu. Of the 912 suicides on which autopsies were performed in the Department of Forensic Medicine, Madurai Medical College between the years 1958 and 1962, 45.5 per cent of these were by organophosphate (insecticide) poisoning. The authors comment that since their introduction in late 1958, organophosphoric compounds were increasingly used as a method of suicide, with their easy availability thought to promote this as a method of suicide. Incidences of hanging and drowning are reported to have slightly decreased in 'popularity' since the introduction of organophosphoric compounds (Ganapathi and Venkoba Rao 1966: 21). Further research in the south of India supports the pre-eminence of hanging and poisoning as methods of suicide in this region (Latha, Bhat *et al.* 1996; Ponnudurai and Jeyakar 1980).

Studies incorporating data collected India-wide report similar patterns to those noted in the southern regions. Having collected hundreds of reports of suicides from newspapers across India, Varma's (1972) analysis indicated that drowning was the most 'popular' method (33.5 per cent of the sample) followed by hanging (25.25 per cent) and poisoning (15.35 per cent). Although Varma's data collection method leaves the sample open to bias and the period over which these reports were collected is unstated, similar results are reported by other authors around this time. Pandey (1968) reported that in 1965 drowning, hanging and poisoning together accounted for over 66 per cent of suicides nationally. Seven years later, the figures remained virtually the same; Chauhan (1984) reported that the 1972 statistics showed that poisoning, drowning and hanging accounted for over 65 per cent of the total number of suicides for that year. The only difference here is that poisoning has become the method of choice, overtaking drowning and hanging as preferred methods.

In the remaining regions of India, the patterns of method of suicide can be quite different to those observed in the south. A study by Shah using early 1950s data from Saurashtra, in the west of the nation, reported that close to 58 per cent of suicides were by drowning at this time. Self-immolation accounted for a further 19.13 per cent of suicides and hangings another 15.06 per cent (Shah 1960). Phal's (1978) work in Panaji, the capital of Goa, also in the west, reported a similar pattern to that of Shah (1960). There 56.45 per cent of suicides were by drowning, while hanging and self-immolation accounted for a further 16.13 per cent and 9.68 per cent respectively (Phal 1978). Bhatia, Aggarwal *et al.* (2000) reported that of the completed suicides brought to a teaching hospital in Uttar Pradesh, 43.6 per cent of the sample were hangings, 38.3 per cent were burns and 12.7 per cent were poisonings. A comprehensive study of suicides in rural areas of the Punjab, in the northwest, observed that the large number of sui-cides by pesticide ingestion show 'the impact of the green revolution on the mode of suicide in the state' (Bhalla, Sharma *et al.* 1998: 28). Here 58.5 per cent of suicides sampled were by poisoning while all other methods accounted for less than 10 per cent each. The introduction of organophosphate insecticides in the late 1950s appears to have had an extreme impact upon chosen methods of suicides, reflected in the findings of Bhalla, Sharma *et al.* (1998), Ganapathi and Venkoba Rao (1966) and Banerjee *et al.* (1990). The study by Banerjee, Nandi *et al.* (1990) was conducted in a rural area of West Bengal, and so allows comparison with the nineteenth century study by McLeod (1878) already discussed. Banerjee, Nandi *et al.* (1990) reported that 7 per cent of suicides were by hanging (*n* = 4) while 93 per cent of suicides were by ingestion of organophosphate insecticide, which is a marked change to the finding by McLeod that the most common form of suicide in this area in the nineteenth century was hanging. Banerjee *et al.* contend that 'the almost exclusive use of an insecticide was obviously a function of its easy availability in the locality' (Banerjee, Nandi *et al.* 1990: 307).

From the data presented above, we can surmise that even though there are consistent patterns of methods of suicides selected, there are distinct differences between regional areas and changes in method over time. To analyse both regional differences and changes over time we have analysed data collected by the National Crime Records Bureau over a four-decade period using data from the years 1967, 1977, 1987 and 1997.

Indian suicides most commonly take the form of drowning, hanging, poisoning and burns (self-immolation). In the east (West Bengal and Orissa), the area in which McLeod was working, poisoning predominates accounting for 44.02 per cent of the region's suicides in 1997. While most of the earlier literature concerning other regions of India reported drowning as the most common method of suicide, poisoning had become the predominant form of suicide in most regions by 1997. It can be seen in Table 5.1 that in the south, 40.56 per cent of the 1997 suicides were poisonings and in the west, 37.20 per cent, while poisoning accounted for 31.48 per cent of the 1997 suicides in the northwest. In the north, hanging was as frequent a choice of method as poisoning in 1997, accounting for 29.12 per cent and 29.67 per cent respectively. Only in the northeastern states does the supremacy

Table 5.1 Regional percentages for methods of suicides, 1997

	East	North	Northeast	Northwest	South	West
Poisoning	44.02	29.67	19.76	31.48	40.56	37.20
Hanging	31.28	29.12	40.64	17.43	25.73	20.00
Fire/self-immolation	5.64	12.38	3.01	9.44	8.87	19.93
Drowning	3.02	8.31	7.77	13.64	11.00	11.89
Railways/roads	4.56	4.57	4.18	6.37	2.71	2.54
Jumping	1.56	0.80	0.50	2.89	1.57	0.83
Firearms	0.17	1.87	1.64	0.60	0.66	0.07
Machine	0.26	0.25	0.02	0.14	0.03	0.12
Other methods	9.50	13.04	22.47	18.01	8.88	7.43

of poisoning as a method of suicide falter, hanging being the most frequent form of suicide in 1997 accounting for 40.64 per cent of the suicides as opposed to 19.76 per cent for poisoning.

As we can see from the table, in most regions poisoning and hanging account for the majority of all suicides with most other forms of suicide accounting for less than 10 per cent of the annual figure. In the west however, and to a lesser degree the north, self-immolation accounts for a large percentage of the 1997 suicides and drowning ranks a poor third in all other regions.

The predominance of drowning as a method of suicide as suggested by the earlier literature is not seen in the 1997 data. Although accounting for around 10 per cent of the annual suicides in most regions, this is nothing like the 58 per cent mentioned by Shah (1960). As we have seen, a number of authors have suggested that the advent of organophosophate poisons and their easy availability in this predominantly rural nation has altered the pattern of method choice since their introduction in the late 1950s (Ganapathi and Venkoba Rao 1966; Gautami, Sudershan *et al.* 2001). What changes over time, then, can be seen in the regional Indian data?

Taking the method of suicide data from 1967 (the earliest year available), 1977, 1987 and 1997, we calculated all-India and regional rates per 100,000 of population as well as the percentage proportions for each method of suicide (Figure 5.1). At the all-India level, drowning, the dominant form of suicide in 1967 declined by about half over the four-decade period as did the category including suicides involving vehicles (on railways and roads). A similar pattern of decline over time is evident for the miscellaneous category of 'other methods'. Whether or not this is an artefact of improved reporting and categorisation cannot be determined, except to say that new categories appearing in statistics published after 1967 appear to be

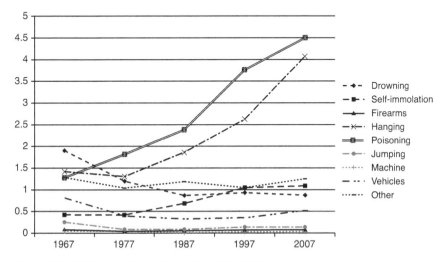

Figure 5.1 All-India methods of suicides, 1967–2007.

expansions from existing specific categories. For example, the 1967 category 'poisoning' equates with three categories in 1997: 'poisoning (consuming insecticides)', 'consuming other poison' and 'overdose of sleeping pills'.[1]

Counter-balancing these declines are notable increases in the percentages of suicides by poisoning, hanging and self-immolation. Even by 1977, the predominance of poisoning as a method of suicide is clear and this is consistent with the theory that the availability of organophosphates as part of the Green Revolution 'package' has facilitated these changes.

Changes in regional areas show a similar trend although not a uniform one. In the eastern states, the two most 'popular' forms of suicide, hanging and poisoning, increased at a similar rate from 1967 to 1997 with concomitant decreases in drowning and 'other methods'. (In the interest of clarity, only the trend by decade for poisoning is shown in Figure 5.2.) The southern states show a very similar trend. The western region shows a similar pattern of change to that of the east and south; poisoning and hanging increased while drowning and other methods decreased, but with the singular difference of a marked increase in the rate of self-immolations. The northern and northwestern regions show marked change in actual suicide rates, declining sharply after 1967 and increasing again after 1987.[2] But here too poisoning became the predominant form of suicide by 1987. The lack of uniformity in these statistics is probably due to the low rate of suicide overall in these areas. Finally, the northeastern region shows a distinct difference from the other Indian regions in that while suicides by poisoning increased in rate from 1967, hanging remained by far the most frequent form of suicide in this region.

Despite overall increases in suicide rates across the country, and small differences in preferred methodologies between regions, a multiple analysis of variance

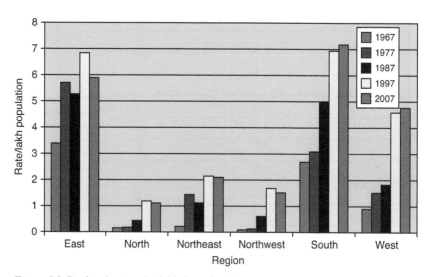

Figure 5.2 Regional rates of suicide by poisoning.

reveals that there is not a significant interaction between sampled years and regional suicide but that the interaction between sample year and method of suicide *is* significant. We can conclude from this that over the four decades sampled there have been some significant changes in the methodologies chosen to complete suicides.

In the absence of other evidence, we can posit that the changes in suicide methodologies observed over time in the Indian data can be attributed to the increasing availability of highly lethal organophosphate poisons. Supporting the ideas of Morselli and others, it appears that the most readily available suicidal agent is being utilised by Indian suicides. In direct contrast to the patterns observed in the United States (Boor 1981), firearms deaths in India, where it is comparatively difficult to access such weapons, are extremely rare. Likewise, where Singapore has a high rate of jumping deaths (Peng and Choo 1990), India, with its relative absence of high-rise buildings, has a comparatively low rate of suicides by jumping.

We can also examine long-term changes in methods utilised in urban areas by comparing McLeod's (1878) data for Calcutta, Madras and Bombay with the 1997 data for these cities (Table 5.2).

Unlike our all-India and regional trends, poisonings have actually decreased in proportion to other methods in these three urban areas, as have drowning, wounding and firearm deaths. Many of the categories now recorded for these cities were not listed by McLeod (1878), but his near-100 per cent tallies for the categories he does include indicates that large proportionate increases have also occurred for self-immolation and jumping deaths. The fact that deaths by poisoning have not greatly increased is in all probability due to the difficulty of obtaining agricultural chemicals, the poisons most frequently used in such suicides outside cities. The increase in jumping deaths can also be inferred to be due to the increase in high-rise architecture in these huge cities. It is not known what has provoked the large increase in portion of suicides by self-immolation, except to attribute this increase

Table 5.2 Comparison of city methodologies (percentages)

McLeod (1878)				*NCRB 1997*			
	Calcutta	*Madras*	*Bombay*		*Calcutta*	*Madras*	*Bombay*
Drowning	5	78.1	48.5	Drowning	1.03	6.83	2.45
Poisoning	44.2	5.3	31.5	Poison	16.92	14.12	21.38
Hanging	41.3	10	7.1	Hanging	52.31	31.37	33.33
Self-immolation				Self-immolation	17.95	16.61	35.79
Firearms	3.5			Firearms	0.51	0	0.16
Jumping				Jumping	10.25	6.09	5.07
Wounding	5	4.8		Wounding	0	0	0.48
				Other methods	1.03	24.98	1.34
Total	99	98.2	87.1	Total	100	100	100

to social causes. Waters' (1999) observations on the 'valorization of suffering' mentioned in Chapter 2 are clearly relevant to the choice of self-immolation. As suggested by various authors, Morselli included, both the availability and the social acceptability of a particular method of suicide are influential in determining its use, so social and technical changes in urban India over the last century may largely explain these increases.

We may conclude that the methods of suicide chosen by Indians are reasonably stable over relatively short periods of time, as has been observed in other nations (Morselli 1881; Halbwachs 1978). However, as has also been demonstrated in other nations (Peng and Choo 1990; Pounder 1993), changes in availability of a certain method of suicide or in the social mores surrounding a method's use can cause significant changes in the methods chosen irrespective of the actual rates of suicides observed.

Notes

1 For our analysis we have combined sub-categories in order to be able to compare these methods.
2 See also Chapters 3 and 6 for additional discussion of the decline that occurred in the 1970s.

6   Trends in suicide in India

Suicide rates are not constant but vary considerably over time, both at the scale of a few years and over the range of many decades. Suicide rates in Finland, for example, rose slowly but steadily throughout the nineteenth century, rising from around 2 per 100,000 to around 5. In the next thirty years they shot up suddenly to nearly 23. They fell slightly during the Great Depression and the Second World War and resumed their upward tendency, reaching 25 per 100,000 by 1975 (Stack 1993: 142). Stack concluded from his analysis that Finland's experience of urbanisation over a century and three-quarters explained much of the change in suicide rates. A 1 per cent increase in urbanisation was associated with just under a 0.2 per cent rise in the suicide rate. (Stack 1993: 145).

By contrast, Hassan reports that male suicide rates in Australia declined from a high of around 20 at the beginning of the twentieth century to a low of 10 at the end of World War II. In between they reached a momentary peak of 24 in 1930 at the height of the Depression. Male suicide rates increased rapidly after 1945 reaching 20 again in 1963 (Hassan and Tan 1989: 377–379). They dipped down to 15 in 1975, then rose again above 20 in the late 1980s (Hassan 1995: 35). Female rates in Australia, by contrast, were virtually constant at about 4 between 1901 and 1952 (Hassan and Tan 1989: 377–379). They peaked suddenly to 11 in 1967 and declined back to their historical level after the mid-1980s (Hassan 1995: 35). Hassan and Tan concluded that modernisation variables including urbanisation, industrialisation, education and female workforce employment, explained 84 per cent of the variance in the male–female suicide rates (Hassan and Tan 1989: 369).

Trend of suicides in British India

The colonial Government of India began to publish consolidated data on the causes of death early in the 1860s. Since their primary concern was with deaths from cholera, smallpox, fevers, dysentery, plague and so on, these reports were prepared by the government's Sanitary Commissioner. After 1870 the Sanitary Reports also included the numbers of suicides for most provinces. These reports were published on a consolidated all-India basis until 1898, after which all-India figures for suicides were no longer included. However, suicide figures *were* reported in annual Public Health Reports published at the Presidency and provincial level until Independence in 1947. In the years after Independence, especially following States Reorganisation in 1956, these reports were truncated in a number of states and increasingly only numbers of deaths from major diseases were reported. The modern suicide data series dates to 1967. The transfer of responsibility for recording accidental deaths and suicides to the police appears to have been the consequence both of the institution of a national cause of death sample survey under the Registrar General, and of the recognition that under the Indian Penal Code suicide was a punishable offence and hence was more appropriately a police than a public health responsibility.

The break in the continuity of consistent reporting after Independence, coupled with the drastic redrawing of administrative boundaries after 1954 means that, with the exception of Bengal (to be considered in detail below), it is not possible to trace suicide trends for the entire 120 years for which data have been collected.

The broad trend for the nearly 80 years from the 1870s to the 1950s can be seen in Figure 6.1. At the broadest level of generalisation, we may say that suicide rates on the eve of Independence were at roughly the same levels they were in the 1870s. There were also consistent differences in rates between provinces. The overall level of suicides was relatively high in the Central Provinces & Berar and in the Madras Presidency. Suicide rates were consistently low in the Punjab. The trend in Bihar and Orissa from 1910, following their separation from Bengal, is one of general increase up until 1940.

In several provinces we can see relatively sudden peaks in suicide rates. In the United Provinces (previously the Northwest Province and the United Provinces of Agra and Oudh), for example, we can see a peak in suicides around 1898, which may be associated with a major famine. There is a major peak in suicide rates in Bengal, which appears to coincide with the Great Influenza Pandemic of 1918, though as we will see, the actual peak in suicide rates was reached in 1925.[1]

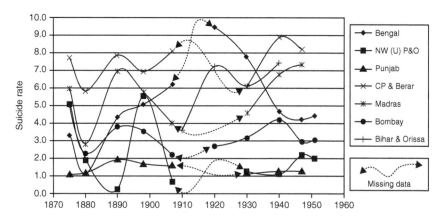

Figure 6.1 Trend of suicides 1872–1950.

Source: (McLeod 1878), Annual Reports of the Sanitary Commissioner with the Government of India 1875–1898, and thereafter, Provincial Annual Public Health Reports.

A unique series: Bengal, 1872–1999

Although it is not possible to link the provincial data presented in Figure 6.1 with post-1967 data, there is one partial exception: Bengal and after 1905 West Bengal. McLeod reported a rate of 2.36 for undivided Bengal in 1872 (McLeod 1878: 156). Mayr reported a rate of 6.2 for Bengal in 1907 (cited in Miner 1922: 17). Thereafter we have two ten-year suicide series that were reported in the *Census of India*. The first covers undivided Bengal between 1921 and 1930 (Porter 1933). This is followed by a decade gap, occasioned by the Second World War, which reduced the Census for 1941 to a bare minimum. We then have a series for West Bengal for the decade 1941 to 1950, which was reported in the *Census of India, 1951* (Mitra 1952: 37).[2] Finally, after a 17-year gap, we have the uniform national series that commenced in 1967, which will be discussed in greater detail later in the chapter.

This incomplete 135-year series presents a history of suicide trends with many apparent resemblances to what Stack found in Finland. Suicide rates in Bengal rose from around 2 per 100,000 in undivided Bengal in the late nineteenth century to over 6 early in the twentieth century and reached a peak in the first half of the century around 1925. Suicide rates appear to have begun to fall just before the beginning of the Great Depression and to reach a low around 5 per 100,000 during and after World War II. While it is difficult to explain why rates fell during the Depression, in Bengal as elsewhere in the world, suicide rates fell during wartime. What is perhaps surprising, however, is that there is no evidence of an increase in suicides following the Great Bengal Famine of 1943. In the first two decades of Independence, suicide rates shot up rapidly to around 16 per 100,000. Here again Bengal followed a post-war pattern seen elsewhere. After a minor decline in the 1970s suicide rates rose to their current level, around 18 per 100,000.

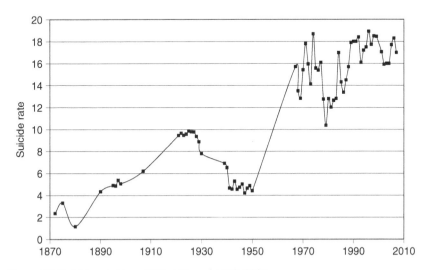

Figure 6.2 Suicide rate Bengal/West Bengal 1872–2007.

The trend of suicides in India, 1965–2007

There has been little study of the trend of suicides in India (an exception is Lester and Natarajan 1995). As can be seen in Figure 6.3, between 1967 and 2007 the all-India suicide rate has risen in an approximately linear fashion from around 8 per 100,000 in 1967 to nearly 11 in 2007.[3] This represents a linear increase of 1.27 per cent per year or a compound annual growth rate of 0.86 per cent. If the linear trend of the past 40 years were to continue for another decade, India's suicide rate would reach 12.05 per 100,000 in 2020.

Trends in suicide rates in the states[4]

South

Southern suicide rates have consistently been the highest in India.[5] The tiny Union Territory of Pondicherry has exceptionally high suicide rates in both national and international terms. Over the long-term it has had an average rate of 54.5. Like the rest of the Southern states, rates in Pondicherry have risen consistently since 1980. Because of its small population (0.81 m in 1991) there is greater year-to-year variability in Pondicherry's suicide rates than is found in larger states.

Of the larger states, Kerala has the highest suicide rates in India. Its long-term average is 22.3. Suicide rates in Kerala reached a peak of 30.4 in 2002, since when they have declined slightly.

The trend of rates in Karnataka and Tamil Nadu is quite similar, though in recent years rates in Karnataka have been slightly higher. The long-term average rate in Karnataka is 16.5, in Tamil Nadu 14.7. Rates in both states reached a peak around 2002.

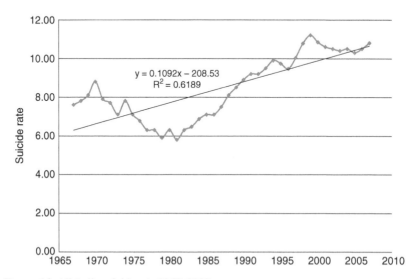

Figure 6.3 All-India suicide rate 1967–2008.

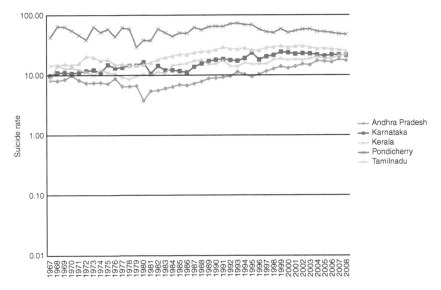

Figure 6.4 Trend of suicides in South India, 1967–2008.

Andhra Pradesh has had the lowest suicide rates in the South. The long-term average rate in Andhra has been 9.7 and here too rates have increased steadily since 1980.

West–Central

The West–Central states are tightly clustered together. Goa, with a long-term average suicide rate of 13.6, has the highest suicide rates in this region. It too exhibits a rising trend after 1980. There is also one exceptional year in Goa's recent history. In 1996 suicide rates shot up to 42.2, falling immediately to more normal levels in following years.

Over the long term, Maharashtra has had an average rate of 8.8; Madhya Pradesh of 7.3 and Gujarat of 6.5. Like the other states considered so far, these three states have also experienced increasing suicide rates since 1980.

Northwest

Suicide rates in northwest India are generally low. Regional rates are highest in most years in Haryana, which has a long-term average rate of 6.4. Rajasthan, Himachal Pradesh and the Punjab have had very similar historical experiences and their trend lines are bunched closely together. The historical average rate for Rajasthan is 3.5, for Punjab 2.9 and for Himachal Pradesh 2.7. The manifest outlier in this grouping is Jammu and Kashmir, which has the lowest suicide rates in India (the historical average is only 0.6). Suicide rates in Jammu & Kashmir

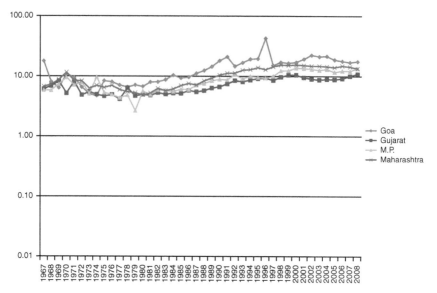

Figure 6.5 Trend of suicides in West India, 1967–2008.

fell to zero in 1971. Suicide rates in the state have also been highly variable over the years. While the other states in this region have experienced a general, if modest, increase in suicide rates since 1980, rates in Jammu & Kashmir show no evident trend.

East

The historical rates of suicides in the two eastern states are relatively high. The long-term rate since 1967 in West Bengal has been 15.9. For Orissa the average has been 9.5. Unlike the experience of the regions so far examined, no increasing trend of rates is evident in the eastern states, both of which experience constant rates year after year.

Northeast

We have not plotted 1967–2007 time series data for all the small, mountainous and largely tribal states of eastern India. Those that we include here show a greater diversity of rates than in India's other regions. Tripura has one of India's highest average rates – 20.6 – while Nagaland has one of the lowest – 1.7. Assam has a reasonably high rate at 9.3. Like the eastern states, no rising trend of suicides is evident in the Northeast.

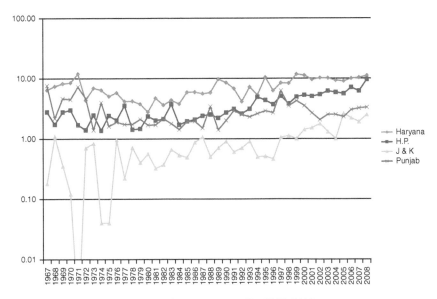

Figure 6.6 Trend of suicide rates in Northwest India, 1967–2008.

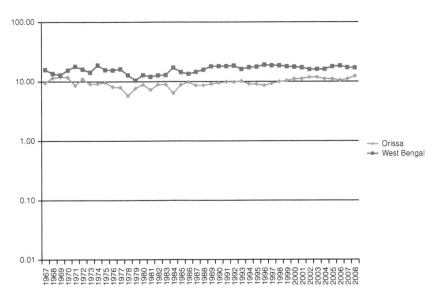

Figure 6.7 Trend of suicides in East India, 1967–2008.

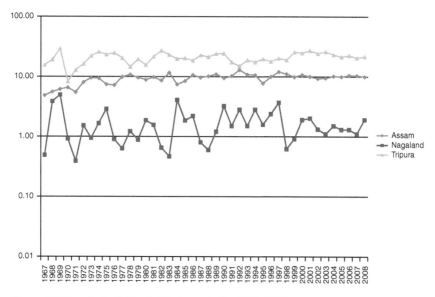

Figure 6.8 Trend of suicides in Northeast India, 1967–2008.

North

There are a number of features that emerge from an examination of the trend of suicides in North India. On the whole, suicide levels in both states are quite low. The historical average for Bihar is only 1.4, for Uttar Pradesh, 3.1.[6] One remarkable feature of the trend in both states is the extended decline in suicide rates between 1967 and the late 1980s to early 1990s. Unlike the south and west, we find no period of consistent increase in suicide rates after 1980. It is possible that rates began to increase in these two states around 1990, but it is too soon to be certain that this is so.

The great 1970s decline in Indian suicide rates

One of the most puzzling questions surrounding the trend of suicides in India is the significant decline in suicide rates that occurred in the 1970s. If we examine again the full range of national data for suicides from 1967 to 2007 shown in Figure 6.3 we see that suicides rose to a peak in 1970 and then fell sharply to a trough in 1981. From 1982 to 1994 suicide rates then entered the period of rapid and consistent increase we have already noted. In 1995 and 1996 suicide rates appeared to have turned onto a downward path, turning however upwards again in the following years. What explanation is there for this remarkable ten-year period of declining rates of suicide?

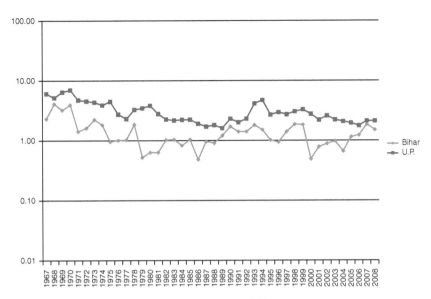

Figure 6.9 Trend of suicides in North India, 1967–2008.

Modernisation and suicide

One powerful causal factor that is often linked to suicide trends in other countries is modernisation. Can the great 1970s suicide decline in India be linked to the impact of urbanisation and industrialisation, two major indicators of structural transformation in society that are often seen as the sources of social dislocation? There is, for example, an established literature that has its roots in the studies of Maine, Tönnies and Durkheim, which finds a strong relationship between increasing urbanisation and industrialisation and rising crime rates.

Clinard and Abbott, who made of one of the first studies of crime in the newly independent Third World, exemplify this approach. They argued that Third World crime was caused largely because the expectations of better employment and education of the new migrants were not met in the rapidly growing cities. In this variant of the 'revolution of rising expectations' argument, high crime rates are understood to be the inevitable outcome of the growing gap between material desires and urban reality (Clinard and Abbott 1973). Most deeply affected by these forces, and hence most drawn into criminal activities, are unemployed young male slum dwellers.

We must note immediately that almost all detailed historical studies of nineteenth century Europe have rejected both the proposition that homicides increased during periods of rapid urbanisation and industrialisation, and that the hypothesised linkage is valid. Howard Zehr found that during the formative period of industrialisation in the nineteenth century overall homicide rates tended to fall in both France and Germany (Zehr 1976). Ted Robert Gurr cites several studies that have traced declining homicide rates over the long term in Europe, the United States and Australia (Gurr 1980: 44). And Lane reports, 'Every single study of nineteenth century Britain, the most rapidly urbanising society in the world, shows that "serious" crime was declining, whatever the methods or definitions used and whatever the period or area covered'. Lane's data for nineteenth-century Philadelphia show a similar trend (Lane 1980: 92–93).

Durkheim maintained that suicides would increase with modernisation. This would occur because modernisation processes, such as urbanisation and the emancipation (i.e. education) of females, are thought to encourage the erosion of traditional values and movement away from the family. This may then isolate the individual from social integration or 'the collective', making them more vulnerable to suicide.

We can readily test the validity of the linkage between urbanisation and industrialisation for suicides in India.

It is hard to discern an overall relationship between the possible cyclical trend in suicides in India and the constant growth of either industrial production (Figure 6.10) or urbanisation (Figure 6.11). Neither indicator experienced a decline between 1970 and 1980, which might explain the significant decrease in suicide rates during that period.

We have examined literally dozens of social and economic series for India in the search for a possible factor that might shed light on the 'Great 1970s Decline in Suicide Rates'. Most, like urbanisation and industrialisation, exhibit a constant rising trend with no discernible dip in the 1970s. Only one series that we have examined exhibits a similar pattern and its possible association with national suicide trends raises as many questions as it answers.

Table 6.12 shows a very strong similarity in pattern between the post-Independence trend in Indian suicide rates and the percentage of the vote received in national elections by minor parties and independents since 1965.[7] (The correlation between the two series is very strong: $r = 0.91$.) The percentage of the vote received by minor parties and independents is a reasonable proxy for the fragmentation of major opposition parties and thus appears to measure the fragmentation of the political system.

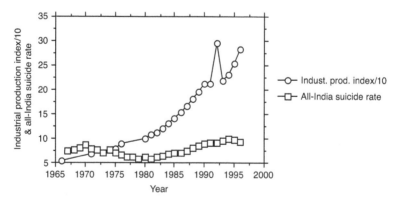

Figure 6.10 Trend in suicides and industrial production, 1965–1996.

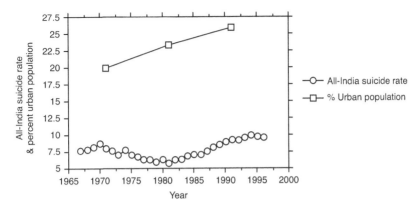

Figure 6.11 Trends in suicides and urbanisation 1965–1996.

Overall, as the commanding majority received by the Congress Party and its major party opponents has declined, and as the overall coherence of the political system has fragmented, there appears to have been a corresponding rise in the suicide rate. During the 1970s, the period of political domination by Indira Gandhi and in the period following the 'Emergency' (1975–1978), partisanship and the coherence of the Indian political system rose and the vote for minor parties and independents fell, and we observe a corresponding dip in the suicide rate during this period.

Although the correspondence between the political series and the trend in Indian suicide rates is striking, there is no well-accepted theoretical explanation that would help us see this relationship as *prima facie* plausible.

The idea that there can be a relationship between changes in suicide rates and political crises is not new. Durkheim noted a tendency for suicides to increase as societies passed maturity and began to disintegrate (Durkheim 1951: 203). Nevertheless, he concluded that the general rule to emerge from European experience of the nineteenth century is that suicide rates decline during periods of political crisis, much as they do during wartime (Durkheim 1951: 203–204).

Watt found a sharp increase in the number of suicides in early modern Geneva in the years of the French revolution, though few of these deaths seem to have had a directly political cause (Watt 2001: 196–203).

More recent investigations have found a relationship between the parties in power and increases and decreases in suicide rate. Page *et al.* have reported that suicide rates in New South Wales, Australia in the twentieth century tended to rise when there were conservative (Liberal Party) governments in power at either the state or federal levels (Page, Morrell *et al.* 2002). The increased relative risk of suicide under conservative governments at both levels was for 17 per cent for males and a remarkable 40 per cent for females (Page, Morrell *et al.* 2002: 767). Correspondingly, suicide rates tended to be lower when Labor party governments were formed at either level of government. They conclude:

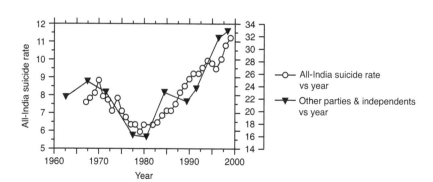

Figure 6.12 Trends in suicide vs non-congress percentage of vote, 1963–1999.

government programmes or perceived prospects under particular governments may be influential [in affecting population suicide rates] . . . Conservative ideology traditionally is less interventionist and more market orientated
than that of a social democratic ideology. . . . [I]f hopelessness is a necessary
but not sufficient condition for suicide, the regimes that offer less hope to the
bulk of the population will also increase the probability of suicide in groups
that have pre-existing or newly acquired risk factors for suicide.

(Page, Morrell *et al.* 2002: 770–771)

The findings of Page and his colleagues were replicated for the United Kingdom
by Shaw and her associates (Shaw, Dorling *et al.* 2002). As in New South Wales,
when Conservative governments were in power in Westminster, suicide rates
were higher. The rates tended to fall in periods when Labour formed government.
Shaw *et al.* found that between 1921 and 1940 the suicide rate under Conservative
governments was 17 per cent above the average. It was equally elevated between
1950 and 1965, and was 16 per cent greater during the Thatcher years 1981–1990
(Shaw, Dorling *et al.* 2002: 724). Overall, they conclude, 'roughly 35,000 of
[those who killed themselves in the 45 years the Conservatives were in govern-
ment] would not have died had these Conservative governments not been in government' (Shaw, Dorling *et al.* 2002: 725). They note that there is an important
regional dimension to their findings. Suicide rates fall in firm Conservative electorates when the Tories are in power and rise in Labour electorates (Shaw, Dorling
et al. 2002: 725).

If there is a political connection with trends in suicide rates in India, it appears
to be different to that found in Australia and the UK. Rather than a possible correlation between concerns about personal welfare under governments of left or
right persuasions, the connection in India appears to be associated with concern
about political stability at the national level. Importantly, there does not appear to
be a corresponding state-level relationship (Figure 6.13). On the contrary, there is

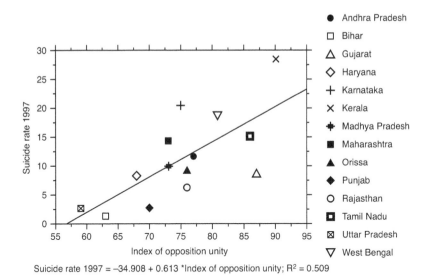

Suicide rate 1997 = −34.908 + 0.613 *Index of opposition unity; R² = 0.509

Figure 6.13 Suicide rates and opposition unity in the Indian states.

a strong positive relationship between state suicide rates and a measure of opposition unity, developed by David Butler and his colleagues.[8] The contradictory nature of these findings must make us cautious about forming a firm conclusion regarding the relationship between political fragmentation and the suicide rate in India.

Notes

1 We are indebted to Professor Lance Brennan for his interpretation of the data.
2 In computing the rates for the series, we have used the comparative population figures for the districts of West Bengal in 1941 and 1951 given in Statement I.10: 138 of Volume 1 of the 1951 Census. We have computed the rates on the basis of equal growth over the decade, necessarily ignoring major demographic catastrophes such as the Great Bengal Famine of 1943 and Partition in 1947.
3 We will consider the pre-1980 period later in the chapter.
4 All rates in this section are shown using a logarithmic scale.
5 To aid comparison of suicide rates in different regions, the vertical axes in this and the following figures use a logarithmic scale.
6 The series for Bihar includes Jharkhand, which was separated in 2000. The Uttar Pradesh series incorporates Uttaranchal, also separated in 2000.
7 The data come from Brass (1994), p. 101.
8 Butler, Lahiri *et al.* 1995.

Part II

7   Gender and suicide

One of the most consistent findings in suicide research emerged from the earliest studies in Europe: males are more likely than females to take their own lives. Enrico Morselli, the great Italian psychologist of the late nineteenth century observed:

> It was evident from the first attempt at comparative statistics that suicide is much more frequent amongst men than amongst women. In every country the proportion is 1 woman to 3 or 4 men, as in crime it is also 1 to 4 or 5. [Emphasis in original]
>
> (Morselli 1881)

Durkheim, following in the same tradition, declared suicide to be 'an essentially male phenomenon' (1951: 72).[1]

Let us now consider the overall national differences in Indian male and female suicides. Over the period 1967–2007 the average suicide rate for females was 7.0; for males it was 9.9. In general, suicide rates for men and women have tended to fall and rise in tandem, as shown by the nearly invariant suicide sex ratio line (average = 1.40) in Figure 7.1. The first signs of divergence have appeared since 2000 when female suicide rates have fallen slightly while male rates have continued to increase.

Over this period, the average male suicide rate was just under 9 per 100,000 (Table 7.3) and the female rate was 6.6. Over approximately the same period (1965–1995), the average global suicide rate for males was 21.6. Thus the average male rate in India was about 40 per cent of the international average rate for men. By contrast, the Indian female rate was nearly 90 per cent of the global average rate for females (7.4). These differences are summarised in differences in the male–female suicide ratios (the suicide sex ratio). At the global level, men were almost three times more likely to take their own lives as females. In India the differences are much narrower, with 1.4 male to every female suicide.

The distinctiveness of the gender pattern of Indian suicides is highlighted when we compare it with that found in a number of other nations (Table 7.4). In industrialised Anglophone countries such as Australia, Canada, the UK and the US, suicide sex ratios range from 3.4 to 4.4. In the countries of the Russian Federation,

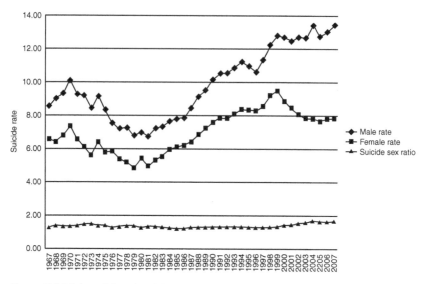

Figure 7.1 Male and female suicide rates, suicide sex ratios, all India, 1967–2007.

Table 7.1 Average male, female suicide rates and suicide sex ratios, 1967–1997

	Male suicide rate	*Female suicide rate*	*M/F suicide ratio*
India	8.9	6.6	1.4
Global	21.6	7.4	2.9

where male suicide rates are extremely high, the suicide sex ratio is over five to one. In Sri Lanka, the only other south Asian country for which the WHO provides data, male suicides exceed those for females by nearly three to one. Singapore, which has a sizeable minority of Indian descent, and Fiji, a major part of whose population is also of Indian descent, have suicide sex ratios quite similar to that found in India itself. Only in China, as already noted, do female suicides exceed those for males. These results support Lester's claim that females in Asian countries tend to kill themselves at a proportionately higher rate (Lester 1982). This phenomenon may well be related to the awareness of women's rights, women's dependency on men and women's social status. As a result of their subordinate position, women may experience high levels of stress that are intensified by family structures in Asian societies such as India. It may also be due to the use of more lethal methods such as the ingestion of highly toxic pesticides in Asia. The Indian pattern of near parity in suicide rates between males and females appears to be relatively distinctive in the global context.

Table 7.2 Suicide sex ratios in selected countries

	M/F suicide ratio
Russian Federation 1995	5.3
USA 1996	4.4
Canada 1995	4.0
Australia 1995	3.7
Finland 1996	3.6
UK 1997	3.4
Hungary 1997	3.2
Sri Lanka 1991	2.7
Singapore 1994	1.5
India 1997	**1.3**
Fiji 1998	1.1
China 1994	0.8

Contemporary international suicide rates vary tremendously, from very high levels for males in the Russian Federation (72.9 per 100,000) and for females in China (17.9 per 100,000), to what are reported to be zero rates for males and females in Jordan, the Dominican Republic, Honduras, and Saint Kitts and Nevis (World Health Organisation 1999, Tables 1 and 2).

If we now place the Indian states in this international context, a number of important observations can be made. First, it becomes immediately apparent how very high are the rates of female suicide in a number of Indian states. In Table 7.3, female suicide rates are ranked among a selected list of countries. The five highest ranks in this hybrid list are all occupied by south Asia states or countries: Tripura, West Bengal, Kerala, Sri Lanka and Karnataka. Of the 15 countries and states with the world's highest suicide rates, seven are Indian states.

Though a number of Indian states have very high male suicide rates, Kerala, which has the highest male suicide rate in India, ranks only eleventh in the hybrid world list. There are seven Indian states in the first 50 countries in the complete list and nine states in the bottom 50. As can be seen from the list of selected countries in Table 7.4, male suicide rates are relatively broadly dispersed when compared internationally.

The World Health Organisation (WHO) (World Health Organisation 1999) reported that global male suicide rates and total suicide rates in 1995 were the highest rates recorded in the entire 1950–1995 period (24.7 and 16 per 100,000 respectively). Conversely, the global female suicide rate had decreased from 8 in the 1975–1980 period to 6.9 per 100,000 in 1995 (World Health Organisation 1999). Thus, as noted in other literature, while male and total suicide rates seem to be rising worldwide, female rates do not (Lester 1997).

The impact of modernisation on the male–female suicide ratio in India, 1967–1997[2]

Let us now consider whether modernisation itself alters the risk of suicides in India. The classical viewpoint was offered by Durkheim (1951), who implied that

Table 7.3 Indian female suicide rates in an international context

Country/state	Female rate	Year
Tripura	**19.9**	1997
West Bengal	**18.1**	1997
Kerala	**17.2**	1997
Sri Lanka	16.8	1991
Karnataka	**15.7**	1997
Hungary	14.8	1999
China (selected areas)	14.8	1998
Tamil Nadu	**13.1**	1997
Maharashtra	**12.5**	1997
Estonia	12.1	1999
Cuba	12.0	1996
Sikkim	**11.9**	1997
Japan	11.9	1997
Russian Federation	11.6	1998
France	10.1	1997
Andhra Pradesh	**10.0**	1997
Singapore	9.5	1998
Madhya Pradesh	**9.0**	1997
Gujarat	**8.9**	1997
Sweden	8.5	1996
Orissa	**8.4**	1997
Republic of Korea	8.0	1997
Assam	**7.7**	1997
Australia	6.0	1997
Haryana	**6.0**	1997
Zimbabwe	6.0	1990
Arunachal Pradesh	**5.2**	1997
Italy	3.7	1997
Himachal Pradesh	**3.7**	1997
Israel	2.6	1997
Uttar Pradesh	**2.6**	1997
Kuwait	1.6	1999
Punjab	**1.6**	1997
Chile	1.4	1994
Meghalaya	**1.4**	1997
Bihar	**1.3**	1997
Nagaland	**1.3**	1997
Bahrain	0.5	1988
Manipur	**0.5**	1997
Iran	0.1	1991

Source: World Health Organisation, Geneva, October 2001 and National Crime Records Bureau 1997.

male and female suicides should diverge with modernisation. He believed that male suicides would increase with modernisation, but because women remained better integrated with family life and thus society, female suicides would tend to remain static (Durkheim 1964: 60, 247). If, on relatively infrequent occasions,

Table 7.4 Indian male suicide rates in an international context

Country/state	Male rate	Year
Lithuania	73.8	1999
Russian Federation	62.6	1998
Sri Lanka	44.6	1991
Kerala	**40.4**	1997
Japan	26.0	1997
Karnataka	**25.0**	1997
Australia	22.7	1997
Tripura	**20.4**	1997
Canada	19.6	1997
West Bengal	**19.0**	1007
United States of America	18.6	1998
Goa	**18.2**	1997
Tamil Nadu	**17.4**	1997
Maharashtra	**16.1**	1997
Assam	**15.9**	1997
China (selected areas)	13.4	1998
Andhra Pradesh	**13.2**	1997
Sikkim	**12.7**	1997
Italy	12.7	1997
United Kingdom	11.7	1998
Madhya Pradesh	**10.9**	1997
Haryana	**10.5**	1997
Portugal	8.7	1998
Gujarat	**8.4**	1997
Arunachal Pradesh	**7.6**	1997
Rajasthan	**6.9**	1997
Himachal Pradesh	**6.5**	1997
Greece	6.1	1998
Nagaland	**5.9**	1997
Mexico	5.4	1995
Meghalaya	**5.2**	1997
Punjab	**3.6**	1997
Uttar Pradesh	**2.8**	1997
Kuwait	2.7	1999
Bihar	**1.5**	1997
Manipur	**0.6**	1997
Peru	0.6	1989

Source: World Health Organisation, Geneva, October 2001 and National Crime Records Bureau 1997.

women did commit suicide it was because those individuals had deviated from their traditional roles and entered the modernisation process, which was, historically, the realm of males. By doing this they were taking on the male role with its inherent responsibilities, thus increasing their vulnerability to suicide (for example, in education, Durkheim 1951: 166).

More recent research has provided contradictory findings for the theory that male–female suicide rates diverge with modernisation. Stack and Danigelis (1985) found that modernisation in 17 industrialised nations from 1919 to 1972 was related to a rise in female suicide rates relative to male rates. This resulted in a decrease in the suicide sex ratio. By contrast, Hassan and Tan (1989) found that female suicide rates in Australia increased from 1901 but then decreased after the mid-60s, producing a divergence of rates. Steffensmeier (1984) also found that during the late 1970s, emancipation appeared to have curtailed the rise of suicide among White American females, relative to White males. Krull and Trovato (1994) reported that modernisation had a more detrimental effect on males than on females in Quebec during the years 1931 to 1986, again suggesting that rates diverge.

In a contrasting study, Trovato and Vos (1992) found that between 1971 and 1981 the risks of suicide associated with change in traditional roles for Canadian women initially reversed for both sexes. As women's participation in the work-force became more accepted, the risk of suicidal deaths fell for both males and females. Trovato and Lalu (2001) reported that the survival probabilities from suicide for Canadian males have improved more than for females.

A possible explanation of the contradictory results can be found in Stack's (1987) suggestion that there is a curvilinear relationship: as more women enter the work force, female suicides first rise, then plateau and finally decline as people adjust to urban life. Stack suggests that there should be a convergence of rates followed by a divergence (Stack, 2000). Pampel (1998) used 1953 to 1992 data from 18 industrialised countries and found that the ratio generally converged and then later diverged, due to a fall followed by a rise in male suicide rates, although this varied depending upon age group.

In an important argument Kushner (1993) stated that neither a convergence nor a divergence theory could be supported because there is no persuasive historical evidence that women were immune to suicidal behaviour in the early stages of modernisation in Europe, Britain or North America. Any differences observed by Durkheim are due to the fact that early theorists looked only at completed suicides. If they had also studied attempted suicides, the most common form and one in which women outnumber men, the gender differences would have largely disappeared.

Because suicide in India is still unlawful, reliable data about attempted suicides are not available. As we saw in Chapter 5, very lethal methods including poisoning, hanging and self-immolation are the means employed in nearly 75 per cent of suicides in India (National Crime Records Bureau, 2001: 123). For this reason, the number of attempted suicides in India is probably far lower than in economically developed countries.

In a previously published paper (Steen and Mayer 2004), we investigated whether increasing modernisation in India had affected the suicide sex ratio. Our measure of modernisation was an equally weighted index that aggregated all-India data on the urbanisation rate, the female literacy rate and female workforce participation from 1967 to 1997.

It was evident from our earlier consideration of Figure 7.1 that there has been relatively little variation in the suicide sex ratio. Hence it was not surprising that we found once the impact of time was included in a multiple regression analysis, there was no positive correlation between our measure of modernity and the ratio of male to female suicide rates. When we repeated the analysis for the individual components of the modernity index, only urbanisation initially appeared to be positively correlated with the male–female sex ratio. Once we found that there was multicollinearity between the individual variables we had to conclude that this result was spurious and that there was no evidence to support the theory that modernisation would bring convergence in the suicide sex ratio.

Female equality and suicide in the Indian states

A second strand of the literature suggests that rather than modernity per se, the achievement of greater female equality is responsible for rising female suicide rates. Several studies have shown that as the status of women and men becomes more equal, suicide rates in women tend to rise. Lester (1996: 88) has shown using cross-national data for the 1960s and 1970s that as gender equality in education and economics rise, suicide rates also increase. In a comparison that we conducted of 37 nations, a component of the United Nations Development Programme Human Development Index – the Life Expectancy Index – was found to have a significant negative correlation with male suicide rates (Mayer 2000: 369). The Gender Empowerment Measure was found to be significantly correlated with both male and female suicide rates for a subset of 26 nations (Mayer 2000: 371).

In a second published study,[3] we replicated the international comparison using data for the Indian states based on a second UN measure, the UNDP's Gender-Related Development Index. This Index summarises the achievement of gender equality in three dimensions: per capita income, life expectancy at birth and the literacy rate. As gender differences are reduced, the Index score is also reduced.

We utilized the Gender-Related Index for the Indian states computed by Siva Kumar (1996) to test the relationship between gender equality and female and male suicide rates for 1994. We found only a weak, positive correlation between the Gender-Related Index and female suicide rates, one that was not statistically significant.

When we tested the individual components of the Index, we found a moderate ($r = 0.52$, $p < 0.05$) correlation between the male suicide rate and the Equally Distributed Life-Expectancy Index. The strongest associations were with greater equality in education. Male suicide rates were strongly associated with greater equality in literacy ($r = 0.79$, $p < 0.01$) as were female suicide rates ($r = 0.54$, $p < 0.05$). Our analysis showed that male suicide rates increased more rapidly than female rates as attainments in literacy became more equal. Since both literacy and suicide rates are highest in southern India, we suggested that as education attainment for girls and boys rises and becomes more equal in northern India, we might expect a substantial increase in suicides in that region.

Notes

1 Kushner provides an excellent critical examination of nineteenth-century discourse on gender and suicide (Kushner 1985).
2 The material in this section is summarised from Steen and Mayer 2004.
3 The material in this section is summarised from Mayer 2003.

8   Age and suicide

In most countries suicide rates increase with age (Lester 1982). Schmidtke (1997) reported that globally most correlation coefficients between suicide rates and age are positive and significant for both males and females. However, he noted that the co-variation in males in most countries is more pronounced. Lester (1982) found that for females the suicide rate distribution by age varied with the level of economic development of the country. He reported that for the wealthiest countries, female suicide rates peak in middle age; for poorer countries the peak shifts to elderly women; in the poorest nations, young adult women are at greatest risk of suicide (Lester 1982). Pritchard (1996) also found that there were increases in young male (aged under 35) and female suicides (25 to 34 year olds) as well as an excess of elderly female suicides in the majority of Western countries between 1974 and 1992.

Data on the age composition of suicides in India have been become available only relatively recently. McLeod, for example, complained as early as 1878: 'I have found it impossible to obtain any information regarding the age at which suicides are most common' (McLeod 1878, 398). State-wise breakdowns by age and gender were first reported in 1994; the information was then omitted for six years, being resumed in *Accidental Deaths and Suicides in India* from 2001 onwards.[1]

It is striking that in 1997 the suicide sex ratio increased monotonically with age, becoming more masculine with each increase (Table 8.1). By 2007, there was a discernible decline in the rate of over-60 female suicides leading to a fall in the suicide sex ratio. It can be seen that in 1997, in the 'up to 14' and '15 to 29' age categories the suicide sex ratio was under one, indicating a higher female suicide rate in these categories; by 2007, this held only for the under 14 age group. Nonetheless, it is suggestive that male and female youth suicide rates in the 'up to 14 years' and '15 to 29' groups have come down (Table 8.1). If this trend is sustained in future years, it may point to common factors at work in India as overseas where data indicate that a majority of nations experienced a decrease in female youth suicide rates in the 1980s (Lester 1997).

Table 8.1 indicates that although for age categories 15-plus, the M/F ratio in 2007 was over 1, it was not especially high (2.96 was the highest, for the 45 to 59 age category).[2] For males the peak ages for suicide are the 30 to 44 and 45 to 59

Table 8.1 Suicide rate in India classified by sex and age group, census years 1997 and 2007

Year	Male						Female						M/f ratio
	Up to 14 yrs	15–29 yrs	30–44 yrs	45–59 yrs	60+ yrs	All ages	Up to 14 yrs	15–29 yrs	30–44 yrs	45–59 yrs	60+ yrs	All ages	All ages
1997	0.8	13.9	21.8	22.4	14.2	11.4	0.9	14.5	14.9	11.5	7.1	8.6	1.33
M/F Ratio 1997	0.9	0.95	1.5	1.9	2.0	1.32							
2007	0.6	14.9	24.9	29.5	16.7	13.5	0.7	13.5	12.3	10.9	10.9	7.9	1.82
M/F Ratio, 2007	0.9	1.19	2.15	2.96	2.70	1.82							

categories, whereas for females the peak ages are the 15 to 29 and 30 to 44 categories. Ponnudurai and Jeyakar (1980 cited in Banerjee, Nandi *et al.* 1990) in their study of suicide in Madras also found women between 15 and 20 years of age to be at greatest risk. The age distribution of suicide in India is in contrast with the typical age distribution for industrialised nations, which is highest among the elderly.

Of particular note is that in every country, the male suicide rate is higher, and most of the time is considerably higher, than that for females (Diekstra 1989).

A comparison of the average suicide rates[3] in the eight developed countries that constitute the G-8 (Canada, France, West Germany, Italy, Japan, Russia, the UK and the US) with data for India is presented in Figure 8.1. It can be seen that the suicide pattern for India is quite different from these developed countries. In the developed countries the suicide rate increases with age for both sexes, reaching a peak in old age, whereas, as we have seen, in India the peak for male suicides is in the 30 to 59 age group and for women is in the 15 to 44 age group.

Interpreting patterns of suicide[5]

Different interpretations have been advanced in the literature to explain both why suicide rates tend to increase with modernization and why there are distinctive age patterns for each gender. A frequent finding in the literature is that suicide rates increase with modernization and social change.

The theorising behind these findings suggests that modernisation affects men and women differently. As women gain greater equality and enter new sectors of the workforce it may have an adverse impact on men who feel a loss of status (Hassan, 1995). Those same changes, however, may also subject women to the same competitive economic pressures and thus increase their risk of suicide (Stack and Danigelis 1985).

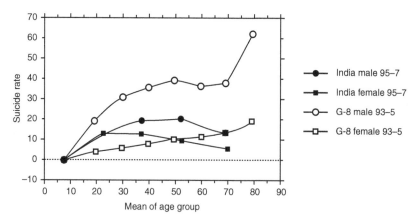

Figure 8.1   A comparison of male and female suicide rates per 100,000 in India and in eight developed countries (G-8)[4].

The effects of modernisation on gender role identity and suicide

Girard (1993) suggests that the observed patterns of suicide are better explained by considering changes in gender role identity as well as stages of economic development. Girard argues that the psychological foundation of an individual's self-image is derived from the 'carer' role with which they identify. Traditional male identities have been formed by their roles as 'breadwinners', while women's roles have emerged from their traditional roles as mothers and housewives. Each of these traditional carer roles has distinct ages at which vulnerability to suicide is greatest. For women traditionally, the shocks may arise from failure to marry or inability to have children. Once any children have grown up and left home, suicide risks tend to fall. For men, the loss of employment at any point may threaten their breadwinner role. Other shocks may come with failure to achieve promotion. Retirement, the severing of the connection with the world of work, is the period when men are most at risk.

Girard (1993) suggests that there are distinct age-related patterns of peak suicide risk that correspond to different stages of national economic development. In less developed countries where the ties of kinship are stronger for both women and men, most suicides occur in young adulthood, resulting in what he terms a 'downward sloping' pattern (Figure 8.2). When countries have reached an intermediate stage of industrialisation, one tends to find a bimodal pattern with peaks in youth and again at old age. Industrialised countries are characterised by convex and upward sloping patterns because most suicides occur in middle or old age. Girard speculated that the shift from a downward-sloping to a convex pattern occurs sooner for men than women, at any particular stage of economic development (Girard 1993: 559).

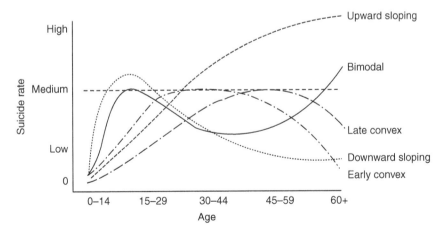

Figure 8.2 Schematic representation of differing ideal typologies representing suicide rates across the life-span.

Source: Steen and Mayer (2003: 250) adapted from Girard (1993: 558).

Examination of Table 8.1 and Figure 8.1 shows that India, taken as a whole, does not have the downward-sloping pattern that one might expect in light of its relatively low level of economic development. The pattern is convex, one more characteristic of an industrialised nation.

Age and suicide in the Indian states

There is a very wide range of age patterns at the state level in India. Table 8.2 presents the state-level suicide rates for all age groups and for each gender in 1997.[6]

The highest suicide rate, an extraordinary 146.01 per 100,000, occurs in the Union Territory of Pondicherry for middle-aged males (45 to 59 years); the rate for males in Pondicherry between 30 to 44 years is also very high: 95.75. The next highest, at 94.3, occurs in Kerala for males (45 to 59 years). Pondicherry, with an overall male suicide rate of 66.09 has a far higher incidence of suicide than either Kerala, with a total state male rate of 40.36 or the next highest state, Karnataka, at 24.97. At the other end of the range, the male suicide rate is lowest in Manipur at 0.60. The suicide rates in some Indian states for middle-aged males are high on a world scale. By way of comparison, the rate for males 30 to 59 in Denmark in 1985–1986 was 47.1; for France 41.5 and for Japan, 40.3 (World Health Organisation 2004). In a few states Indian suicide rates for older males are also quite high in comparative terms (for example, Pondicherry 66.09, Kerala 59.71), even though this is the category with the highest suicide rates in industrialised nations. By way of comparison, the rates for those over 60 in Singapore were 99.4; for France, 93.7; for Belgium, 85.8, and for Japan, 64.7.

The suicide rates for females are generally lower than for males in most age categories. However, in both of the under-30 age groups, female suicide rates are greater than male suicide rates in up to 50 per cent of the states for which data are reported. For females, the highest rate occurs once again in Pondicherry, where the rate among young women aged between 15 and 29 years was 68.78. The state with the next highest rate was Tripura at 57.43 among those aged between 30 and 44 years. Pondicherry also had the highest overall female suicide rate, 38.53, followed by Tripura at 19.87 and West Bengal at 18.06. The most at-risk ages for males are between 45 and 59 years, closely followed by those aged between 30 and 44 years. Females are also most at risk between 30 and 44 years, but the next most vulnerable group is much younger than the males and aged between 15 and 29 years. As with the males, the lowest recorded suicide rate for women also occurs in Manipur at 0.546. In comparison with industrialised nations, suicides among women over 60 are relatively low; the rate in Singapore (1985–1986) was 69.4; for Japan, 45.5 and for Denmark, 29.5. Suicide rates for middle-aged Indian women, by contrast, are relatively high in comparison with industrialised countries. The rate for women aged 30 to 59 in Denmark was 30.4, in Belgium, 21.3, and for France, 16.2.

Although the total female suicide rates in both the under-30 age groups are higher than the respective male suicide rates, they are not significantly so. However, older males do commit suicide at significantly greater rates than do older females. For the 30 to 44 year age group, male suicides were significantly

Table 8.2 Indian states and suicide rates classified by gender and age group for 1997; all rates per 100,000

States	Male suicide rates per age group						Female suicide rates per age group						All
	Up to 14	15–29	30–44	45–59	60+	Total	Up to 14	15–29	30–44	45–59	60+	Total	Total All
Andhra Pradesh	0.54	14.00	22.67	25.50	30.30	13.24	0.82	15.51	15.48	15.28	12.84	10.04	11.60
Arunachal Pradesh	0.45	7.64	16.98	18.56	0.00	7.55	0.47	14.02	6.90	0.00	0.00	5.19	6.46
Assam	0.27	24.37	32.33	26.90	12.75	15.91	0.32	11.20	16.14	17.07	5.29	7.69	11.96
Bihar	0.22	1.81	2.78	3.30	2.28	1.51	0.22	1.98	2.36	2.13	1.89	1.33	1.43
Goa	0.94	21.16	33.71	17.70	31.34	18.21	1.46	18.38	16.54	12.88	6.84	11.58	14.95
Gujarat	0.53	11.10	15.60	13.83	9.26	8.35	0.79	16.11	14.26	7.62	7.85	8.86	8.59
Haryana	0.55	18.35	17.02	20.89	6.31	10.47	0.49	10.35	11.47	9.10	2.82	5.95	8.38
Himachal Pradesh	0.27	9.20	12.83	12.12	4.12	6.49	0.00	7.70	6.11	3.64	0.84	3.73	5.13
Karnataka	1.02	27.74	47.33	54.82	29.69	24.97	1.26	25.77	26.15	22.25	13.55	15.66	20.41
Kerala	1.08	33.13	72.59	94.30	59.71	40.36	0.85	20.06	26.42	29.42	24.15	17.21	28.58
Madhya Pradesh	0.91	16.51	18.47	19.47	14.51	10.93	0.72	18.45	14.89	10.06	4.27	9.01	10.00
Maharashtra	1.20	18.56	32.32	29.81	15.37	16.11	1.46	21.04	21.95	14.06	8.13	12.47	14.35
Manipur	0.00	1.17	0.92	0.85	0.00	0.60	0.00	1.76	0.00	0.00	0.00	0.54	0.57
Megalaya	0.21	6.51	8.97	9.56	18.44	5.17	0.00	2.95	1.73	3.54	0.00	1.40	3.32
Mizoram	0.59	9.65	12.34	4.81	0.00	5.82	0.00	2.45	1.46	0.00	0.00	0.97	3.49
Nagaland	0.35	9.60	12.15	6.11	2.12	5.90	0.00	2.34	3.36	0.00	0.00	1.27	3.72
Orissa	1.05	13.86	18.93	15.54	9.62	10.11	1.01	15.46	14.71	6.08	6.61	8.42	9.28
Pondicherry	1.25	82.73	95.75	146.01	71.12	66.09	1.93	68.78	67.93	21.70	15.83	38.53	52.45
Punjab	0.17	4.55	7.15	7.49	2.26	3.62	0.05	3.36	2.63	1.26	0.37	1.62	2.69
Rajasthan	0.59	10.03	13.98	13.22	5.54	6.88	0.64	9.44	11.05	7.47	4.10	5.58	6.26
Sikkim	3.96	14.24	22.54	26.25	7.54	12.74	3.05	21.30	10.52	27.70	10.13	11.94	12.36
Tamil Nadu	0.80	18.15	35.14	30.30	13.61	17.43	0.78	19.43	23.78	15.00	6.90	13.10	15.30
Tripura	2.83	22.67	49.75	30.64	13.89	20.42	1.08	17.63	57.43	47.78	8.39	19.87	20.15
Uttar Pradesh	0.26	4.34	5.31	5.09	2.89	2.83	0.37	5.95	3.63	2.28	1.44	2.60	2.72
West Bengal	3.33	20.93	32.30	36.24	29.50	19.03	3.36	25.68	32.33	29.51	13.33	18.06	18.57
Total	0.8	13.9	22	22.7	14.4	11.5	0.9	14.5	15.1	11.7	7.2	8.7	10.14
Average	0.92	14.14	22.67	21.80	13.38	11.86	0.80	12.85	14.22	11.84	5.82	8.09	10.01

Source: Steen and Mayer 2003: 254.

higher than females ($t = 4.05$, $df = 23$, $p < 0.01$) as were male suicides in the 45 to 59 age group ($t = 3.35$, $df = 23$, $p < 0.05$). Finally, males aged over 60 were more suicidal than were females of the same age ($t = 3.97$, $df = 23$, $p < 0.05$).

Age patterns of suicide

In addition to having a national age pattern of suicides that is quite different from that of economically developed economies, there are also striking regional differences within India. Two major aspects are evident even in the dense mass of data in Table 8.2. The first is the great range in incidence of suicide for different age categories. Rates are very low at all ages for some northern states such as Bihar, Uttar Pradesh, the Punjab and the small northeast state of Manipur. At the other extreme, rates are very high for all but minors in a number of southern and eastern states such as the Union Territory of Pondicherry, Kerala, Karnataka, Tamilnadu, West Bengal and the northeast state of Tripura.

The second immediately evident feature is that the pattern in most states is convex, as we would expect, given the same pattern of the all-India curve in Figure 8.2. Nevertheless, closer inspection reveals a wider range of patterns. Five examples of different patterns have been selected in Figure 8.3. The pattern for Goa is an example of a downward-sloping pattern indicating that more suicides occur between the ages of 15 and 29 years. The pattern for West Bengal is an example of 'early' convex with more suicides occurring between the ages of 30 and 44 years. The pattern for Kerala, on the other hand, is an example of 'late' convex with suicides peaking around the age of 52 or within the 45 to 59 age group. The pattern for Meghalaya is clearly upward-sloping with most suicides being completed by those aged 60 years and over; this is the pattern which Girard suggests is characteristic of industrialised societies. This last pattern was only found for males in two states, Andhra Pradesh and Meghalaya, and was not found for females at all. Sikkim is an example of bimodal, a pattern that only showed up in two states for females and in one for males.

For male suicides, while most of the states demonstrated some type of convex pattern, there were two other exceptions besides Andhra Pradesh and Meghalaya. Haryana demonstrated a bimodal pattern with peaks around 22 and again around 52 years of age, while Manipur showed a downward-sloping pattern. According to Girard's theory, states with convex patterns should be economically advanced. This appeared to be true for the Punjab and yet we identified convex patterns (early and late) for six of the northeastern states. We have little socio-economic data on these states and while some are reported to have high literacy levels, they are still generally considered to be economically poor.

Many of the states reflected different patterns for female suicide rates. For example, more states demonstrated downward-sloping patterns for females than they did for males. These patterns for women are consistent with Girard's (1993: 558) theory that in less developed countries females are more likely to attempt suicide more at 'the usual age of marriage' than are males. However, patterns for female suicide in the northeastern states were mixed, which does not support the notion that less advanced places should show predominantly downward sloping patterns.

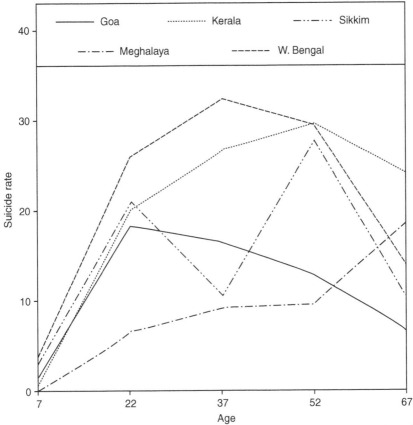

Figure 8.3 Examples of suicide patterns: convex (early and late), downward- and upward-sloping and bimodal.

Source: Steen and Mayer (2003: 258).

We examined economic and human development indices to obtain a clearer picture of the most and least advanced states based on predicted patterns. Overall, the most advanced states economically were Maharashtra and Gujarat. Maharashtra demonstrated early convex patterns of age-related suicide for both males and females while Gujarat demonstrated early convex for males and a downward-sloping pattern for females. This is consistent with Girard's theory.

The most advanced states, from a human development perspective, were Kerala and Tamil Nadu. For both males and females, Kerala showed late convex patterns, which are consistent with the notion that high development is associated with more suicides. However, because Kerala is an economically poor Indian state, this finding indicates that economics alone are not enough to explain suicide rates. Kerala had the lowest birth rates and maternal mortality rates and the highest female literacy levels in India for 1997. Women in Kerala also received the most exposure to the media during that time. However, it had one of the lowest levels of electricity use for industry indicating its relative economic poverty. Tamil Nadu demonstrated early convex patterns for both males and females, which is consistent with Girard's theory.

The least advanced states, both from an economic and social development perspective, were Bihar and Uttar Pradesh. Bihar showed convex patterns of suicide for both males (late convex) and females (early convex). Uttar Pradesh showed early convex for males and downward-sloping for females. Only the latter pattern is consistent with Girard's theory about relationship of pattern to development.

In a published study we tested the probability that these state-level patterns were associated with variables related to either human development or economic development, as suggested by Girard. We found that at low levels of either aspect of development, the most probable pattern for males was a convex one while at higher levels a bimodal pattern was most probable (Steen and Mayer 2003). For females, contrary to Girard's proposal, the probability of a downward-sloping pattern increased with either aspect of development (Steen and Mayer 2003).

When we assessed the impact of specific indicators of development on the most 'at risk' age groups, we found that for males between 30 and 59, the suicide rate was positively correlated with female literacy ($r = 0.56$, $p < 0.05$) and negatively with the birth rate ($r = -0.71$, $p < 0.01$), infant mortality rate ($r = -0.72$, $p < 0.05$) and females with no regular exposure to the media ($r = -0.63$, $p < 0.05$). For females suicide rates were negatively correlated with birth rate ($r = -0.65$, $p < 0.05$) and the size of the household ($r = -0.58$, $p < 0.05$). Lack of media exposure had a negative impact on women aged 30 to 44 ($r = -0.54$, $p < 0.05$).

Changes in age rates between 1981 and 1994

We have a limited ability to trace the changes in the incidence of suicide in different age categories. In 1981 and in 1994, however, comparable age categories were reported by the National Crime Records Bureau.[7]

To evaluate the changes that occurred between 1981 and 1994, we have used the 'reference with self' method developed by Pritchard (1996). Prichard's approach compares suicide rates per state against themselves and national rates over time and also contrasts changes found between the various states. In this method, a ratio of change is calculated between a 'base' year and an 'index' year to form an 'index of change'. The base year is indexed as 100 and compared to the latest year for which comparable data are available. We tested whether there were significant changes among different age brackets over time, using chi-square statistics.[8]

It can be seen in Table 8.3 that the general male suicide rate rose in all states, from 13 per cent in Haryana to more than double in Rajasthan (140 per cent), Maharashtra (134 per cent) and Bihar (116 per cent). More specifically, 50-plus-year-old males in the Punjab show the greatest increase in suicide rates for males of all the states (219 per cent). Males aged 30 to 49 years in Rajasthan showed the next greatest change in suicide rate (201 per cent). Proportionally greater increases can be seen in

Table 8.3 Summary of indices of change for male and female suicide by age, 1981–1994

States	All ages, male	0–17 yrs	18–29 yrs	30–49 yrs	50+ yrs	All ages, female	0–17 yrs	18–29 yrs	30–49 yrs	50+ yrs
Northern										
Bihar	216	206	246	231	114	304	395	403	213	139
Gujarat	189	137	164	227	184	175	187	190	139	140
Haryana	113	82	121	119	72	114	95	123	119	55
Madhya Pradesh	195	175	195	201	160	224	288	278	154	108
Orissa	121	103	106	129	128	133	154	132	124	76
Punjab	183	108	128	293	319	99	109	95	113	49
Rajasthan	240	261	186	301	294	226	317	194	215	242
Uttar Pradesh	163	152	169	156	138	187	208	239	148	101
West Bengal	152	99	141	180	213	137	103	150	130	129
Southern										
Andhra Pradesh	195	69	208	282	142	183	121	224	204	97
Karnataka	192	89	151	258	266	166	152	171	148	136
Kerala	189	113	107	221	282	147	243	114	135	157
Maharashtra	234	229	208	246	231	268	491	275	207	175
Tamil Nadu	156	80	135	208	180	169	132	187	157	121
All India	163	100	141	200	191	165	159	176	149	122

the 30 to 49 year age group in most states. A chi-square test showed that the index of change for this age group was significantly above the national average more often compared to the other age groups ($X^2 = 16.12$, $df = 1$, $p < 0.001$). The suicide rate also fell in some states for different groups. For example, the suicide rate among males aged up to 17 years fell by about 40 per cent in Andhra Pradesh and for males aged over 50 years in Haryana, the rate fell by nearly 30 per cent.

Table 8.3 shows the changes that have occurred across the states and all India for females. The only state to show generally no change over the time period is the Punjab. All the others show an overall increase from 14 per cent in Haryana to more than double in Bihar (204 per cent). As with the males, a closer inspection of the age groups demonstrates discrepancies among female suicide rates over time. Among all the states, the most striking change for young women aged less than 18 years occurred in Maharashtra. The suicide rate for this group increased by a massive 391 per cent. The next greatest change occurred for females aged 18 to 29 years in Bihar (303 per cent). Moreover, overall the greatest change in rates occurred for this age group. A chi-square test showed that the index of change for 18 to 29 year olds was significantly above the national average more often compared to the other age groups ($X^2 = 6.22$, $df = 1$, $p < 0.05$). As with the males, suicide rates fell in some places. For example, the rates for over-50s in both the Punjab and Haryana fell by about 50 per cent. Of the southern states, only Andhra Pradesh showed a slight decrease in the suicide rate for females aged over 50 years.

The shaded cells in Table 8.3 highlight the age group by gender by state with the greater change over time; those with equal or nearly equal changes are indicated by a lighter shading. It can be seen that overall there is a striking pattern. In almost all states, females aged below 30 years saw considerably greater changes in suicide rates over time than did males of similar age. Moreover, in almost all states the index of change in suicide rates for males aged over 30 years is greater than that for females in the same age category.

There are clear differences between gender and age groups. Apparently paradoxically, more states demonstrated rates above the national average than below for both sexes; this result is largely an artefact of the low suicide rates in northern states that have large populations such as Uttar Pradesh. However, these differences between males and females of all ages were not statistically significant. Moreover, chi-square tests to compare indices of change between northern and southern states also showed no significant difference between locations for either females or males or between the genders.

Youth and young adult suicide in India

The most striking and concerning aspect of India's suicide patterns is that which arises from an examination in detail of youth and young adult suicides.

In the 1980s and 1990s many developed countries experienced rapid increases in the suicide rates of young people and young adults. For example, Pritchard (1996) reports that in most industrialised economies between 1974 and 1992, there was a disproportionate rise in suicide rates among males aged under 35 and among females aged 25 to 34 years and over 75. In the US, for example, young male suicide rates rose by more than three times from 6.3 per 100,000 suicides in 1955 to 21.3 in 1977 and 21.9 in 1991–1993. In the same period, suicide rates for young women more than doubled, rising from 2.0 to 5.2. Although overall youth suicide rates fell in the 1990s from 6.2 to 4.6 in 2001, suicide was the third leading cause of death for teenaged Americans (Lubell, Swahn *et al.* 2004: 471). Suicide rates for young males remained at over 17 per 100,000 between 2000 and 2002.[9]

In Australia, suicide rates for young men aged 15 to 19 rose by three times, from 5.8 in 1964 to 17.8 in 1990; in the same period for males aged 20 to 24, rates more than doubled, rising from 16.3 to 36.1 (Hassan 1995: 50.). In 1991–1993, the rate for the 15 to 29 age group was 27.3. Comparable figures for young women in Australia were: 15 to 19 (1964): 7.7–5.0 (1990); 20 to 24 (1964): 7.7–3.9 (1990). The rate for the combined 15 to 29 year age group in 1991–1993 was 5.6.

The rapid increase in suicide among young males in industrialised countries was rapidly recognised as a public health crisis and numerous suicide prevention and counselling programmes were initiated in most jurisdictions in attempts to reduce the tragic waste of young lives.

There is, of course, no generally accepted level of youth suicide above which a crisis situation may be said to exist. It is the perception of a rapid rise in rates that most frequently leads to the perception of a crisis. Nevertheless, we suggest as a 'rule of thumb' that when youth suicide rates have risen above 15 per 100,000, nations have frequently perceived a public health crisis to exist.

In that context, it is striking – and most concerning – to see that youth suicide rates in a number of Indian states are as high – or in many cases *higher* – than those in a number of industrialised countries that have experienced youth suicide crises (Figures 8.4 and 8.5). The Union Territory of Pondicherry has far higher youth suicide rates for both males and females than *any* of the countries listed by UNICEF in its *The Progress of Nations 1996*.

Suicides by young females in India tend to be the highest in the world. Of the 18 nations and states in Figure 8.4 that have female suicide rates over 10 per 100,000, 17 are Indian states. Of the 32 nations for which UNICEF figures for young women are reported by age, only one, Estonia, exceeds 10. Of the 15 states and nations in which suicide rates for young women exceed our crisis level of 15 per 100,000, *all* are Indian states: Pondicherry (68.8), Karnataka (25.8), West Bengal (25.7), Sikkim (21.3), Maharashtra (21.0), Kerala (20.1), Tamil Nadu (19.4), Madhya Pradesh (21.0), Goa (18.4), Tripura (17.6), Gujarat (16.1), Andhra Pradesh (15.5) and Orissa (15.5).

Around the world, suicide rates for males are generally several times higher than those for females. It is, therefore, to be expected that relatively more nations will have youth suicide rates above our suggested threshold level. While this is certainly the case, of the 31 nations and states in Figure 8.5 with youth/young male suicide rates above 15, 11 are Indian states: Pondicherry (82.7), Kerala (33.1), Karnataka (27.7), Assam (24.4), Tripura (22.7), Goa (21.2), West Bengal (20.9), Maharashtra (18.6), Haryana (18.4), Tamil Nadu (18.2) and Madhya Pradesh (16.5).

Suicide is the leading cause of death among young people in India. In rural India, young people aged 15 to 24 are almost five times more likely to take their

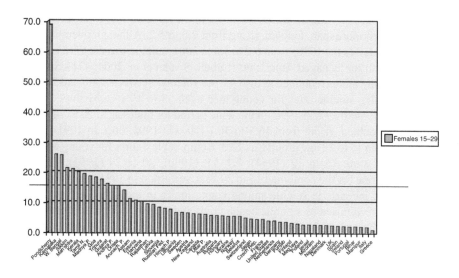

Figure 8.4 Female (15 to 19) – suicides, India and international comparisons.

Source: UNICEF: *The Progress of Nations*, 1996 (http://www.unicef.org/pon96/insuicid.htm).

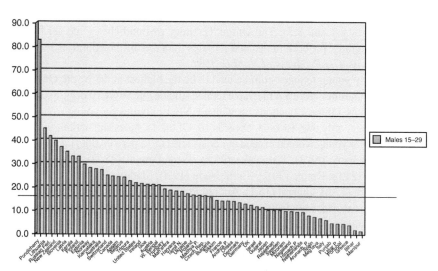

Figure 8.5 Male (15 to 19) – suicides, India and international comparisons.

Source: UNICEF 1996.

own lives than to die from the next leading cause, tuberculosis (Registrar General 2002, Statement 7; see also Ramanakumar 2004, Table 4).[10] Suicide is also the leading cause of death for rural Indians aged between 25 and 34, who are twice as likely to take their own lives as die from TB (Registrar General 2002, Statement 7). The Registrar General observes that for rural women aged between 15 and 44, suicide 'has been reported as the top killer in India' (Registrar General 2002: 35). Data from the sample registration system (Table 8.4) confirm that women between 15 and 29 are at greatest risk of suicide.

The state-wise significance of suicide as a leading cause of death in females of reproductive age can be seen in Table 8.5, which reports the rank of suicide among the top ten causes of death. In eight of 13 states for which data are given, suicide was the leading cause of death. In Bihar, the sample survey of the Registrar General did not report any suicides. For Rajasthan, suicides ranked behind tuberculosis. In Maharashtra, suicide ranked behind burns, TB, cancer, bronchitis, asthma, and drowning. In Madhya Pradesh, the leading causes were TB, burns, heart attack and acute abdominal diseases followed by suicide.

Another way of illustrating the significance of suicide as a cause of death among young Indians is to compare suicide deaths with accidental deaths. In a number of states with very high youth/young adult suicide rates, suicide deaths are a major cause of death (Figure 8.6). This is especially true of young women.

Table 8.4 Suicides as a percentage of deaths of rural females of reproductive age, 1998

Age	15–19	20–24	25–29	30–34	35–39	40–44
Percentage	23.5	27.7	22.9	11.9	11.6	2.4

Source: Registrar General 2002: 35.

Table 8.5 Rank of suicide as leading cause of death in rural females of reproductive age, 1998

State	Rank of suicide as cause of death
Andhra Pradesh	1
Bihar	10
Gujarat	1
Haryana	=1
Karnataka	1
Kerala	1
Maharashtra	5
Madhya Pradesh	6
Orissa	1
Punjab	1
Rajasthan	2
Tamil Nadu	1
Uttar Pradesh	3

Source: Registrar General 2002: 34. Note that no data were given for West Bengal.

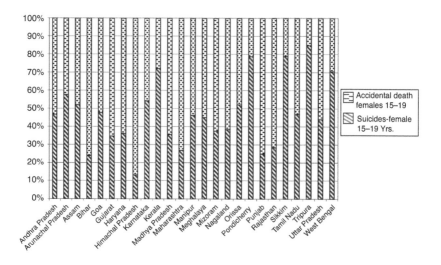

Figure 8.6 Accidental vs suicide deaths, females (15 to 29 years).

Female suicide deaths exceed accidental deaths in Tripura, Sikkim, Pondicherry, West Bengal, Arunachal Pradesh, Karnataka, Orissa and Assam.

Young men, for reasons that arise jointly from culture and heredity, are more likely to be exposed to both occupational and other risks of accidental death, as a consequence of which their accidental death rates tend to be considerably higher than those of young women. Despite the fact that accidental deaths are generally a cause of more young male deaths than suicides, in five states suicide deaths exceed accidental deaths (Figure 8.7): Tripura, Pondicherry, Nagaland, Kerala, West Bengal, while deaths from the two causes are virtually equal in Assam.

Conclusion

The evidence considered in this chapter sheds light on the impact that the broad social changes which are occurring in India are having on small but significant numbers of vulnerable individuals.

We have seen in terms of suicide rates alone that young-middle age (15 to 44 years) is the most precarious stage of life for both genders in the Indian states. This finding for India is consistent with studies of some other developed nations. Furthermore, and in contrast to findings for economically developed nations (Pritchard 1996), the evidence on changes over the medium-term presented in the chapter shows that both male and female suicide rates increased dramatically in a majority of the Indian states between 1981 and 1994.

In terms of male suicide, the suicide rate increased the most for those aged 30 to 49 years. This is a much older age group than predicted by Girard (1993),

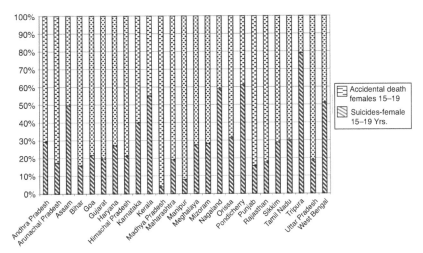

Figure 8.7 Accidental vs suicide deaths, males (15 to 29 years).

who argued that males in developing countries are more at risk during the usual years of marriage and childbearing, i.e. 15 to 34 years. Moreover, the age group is a slightly older one than predicted by Pritchard (1993) and slightly younger than we found from looking at 1997 alone. Looking at the trend suggests that 30- to 49-year-old males have been the most vulnerable group over time in terms of financial hardship and family conflict, typical antecedents of suicide in Indian society. This is an important finding as this group may have been overlooked in terms of risk of death by suicide.

Perhaps an even more striking finding is that female suicide rates increased the most rapidly for those aged under 30 years, while the major changes in male rates occurred for those aged over 30 years. More specifically, the greatest change for females occurred in the 18 to 29 year age group while the greatest change for males occurred among 30 to 49 year age group.

Although the suicide rates for young males and young male adults are relatively lower than those who are somewhat older, young people in some Indian states are taking their own lives at levels which are among the highest in the world – levels which elsewhere are treated as constituting a public health crisis. The apparent invisibility of India's youth and young adult suicide crisis may in part explain why there is so little sense of urgency in providing adequate levels of counselling and prevention services (a rare exception is Ahmed 2010).

Young females are particularly vulnerable in Indian society. With modernisation, young women in India are likely to become increasingly conscious of their powerlessness in a patriarchal society. Despite the social progress that has seen a rise in female literacy and a fall in birth rates, young women are still at the mercy of India's patriarchal culture. For example, violence against young women by young males, in particular, increased dramatically in Maharashtra during the early 1990s (Rai 1993). The sense of powerlessness appears to be especially acute at those ages when there are intense social expectations that they will make suitable marriages and have children, especially sons. We speculate that this conflict may also have manifested as an increase in self-harm by frustrated young females trapped between the conservative past and the promise of a liberated future. The psychological distress produced by family conflicts associated with these pressures merits serious consideration as a precipitator to suicide among young Indian females.

The youth suicide pattern experienced in a number of Indian states, especially in the South, may well be the pattern followed by other regions in coming decades. Paradoxically, increased levels of human development for the great majority of the population bring with them increased risk of death by suicide for a small but significant number of individuals of both genders.

Finally, we may note that the overall age patterns of suicide in India do not conform to those we would expect for a society at a relatively low level of economic development. The convex age-pattern, with the peak incidence of suicides in the economically productive middle-years of life, which characterises most Indian states, is that which we would ordinarily expect to find in more highly industrialised societies.

Notes

1 We are especially grateful to Sri Sharda Prasad, then director of National Crime Records Bureau, for providing us with a special run of the 1997 India suicide data broken down by state and age.
2 A. Venkatoba Rao indicates that elderly male suicides were three times more frequent than those of females in a suicide autopsy study undertaken in Madurai between 1979 and 1982 (Venkoba Rao 1991).
3 Source: Data quoted here are 1993–1995 suicide rates per 100,000, taken from the WHO *World Health Statistics Annual, 1996*.
4 Source: Study data and Diekstra 1989: Tables 4a and 4b.
5 This section summarises findings presented in (Steen and Mayer 2003).
6 Data for 1997 provided by the National Crime Records Bureau.
7 It should be noted that the four age categories used in this period (0 to 17, 18 to 29, 30 to 49, 50+ years) are not the same as those which have been used elsewhere in the chapter.
8 A limitation in this method when used in a society like India which is undergoing rapid social change is that the 'index of change' methodology does not necessarily convey whether the base suicide rate was high or low compared to the index year. The very large increase in the suicide rates for young females in Maharashtra from a relatively lower base provides a clear example of this. In contrast, base rates for similar aged females in Karnataka and Kerala were already high at around 22 per 100,000. Their increases of 71 per cent and 14 per cent respectively are not as drastic as the increase in Maharashtra. Nevertheless their high rates continue to be cause for serious concern.
9 Data obtained from Centers for Disease Control (http://www.cdc.gov/ncipc/wisqars).
10 The Registrar General's Department indicated to us in private communication that comparable figures for urban causes of death are not compiled.

9   Urbanisation and suicide

Urbanisation in India

India has the second largest population in the world, with an estimated total population of 1.18 billion in 2010; approximately 28 per cent of this population lives in an urban setting (Census of India 2002). It has been suggested that if urban India were a separate country in itself, it would rank as the fourth most populous country in the world (Visaria 1997). Although the pace of urbanisation has slowed in recent times (Krishan 1993), in absolute terms an extra 68.15 million people entered the urban population between 1991 and 2001. Thus, enormous pressure is placed on the existing urban infrastructure; the provision of housing, sanitation, basic public utilities as well as such things as schools, hospitals and transport. It is estimated that 14.6 per cent of urban India (approximately 31 million people) were living in slums in 1988–1989 (Visaria 1997). In some of India's major cities this figure is much higher, with up to 30.6 per cent of Mumbai's population living in slums (Visaria 1997).

Such rapid and impoverished urban growth has produced many social problems, not least of which are public health issues concerning pollution and disease (Mutatkar 1995). In Delhi, the fourth most polluted city in the world where an estimated 7491 pollution-related deaths occur annually, 64 per cent of its air pollution is attributed to vehicular emissions – an estimated 1300 tonnes of vehicular pollution are released into the air per day (Agarwal, Sharma *et al.* 1996). India's overcrowded cities contribute other environmental pollutants; it is estimated that the coliform (faecal bacteria) count in the Yamuna, Delhi's main river, increases 3000-fold in its passage through this city (McMichael 2000). Disease in these cities is also rife. For example, deaths caused by pneumonia in 1989 in urban areas of Maharashtra state were nine times those in rural areas. Deaths by tuberculosis were over two times, and deaths caused by heart disease were more than four times, those in rural areas (Mutatkar 1995: 978). Bearing in mind that Maharashtra is considered to be one of India's most progressive states, the comparative lack of quality of life that urban dwellers face is significant regardless of the supposed benefits that proximity to public services should bring.

The crowding and adverse conditions under which so many poor city-dwellers live has led many theorists to argue that these conditions encourage suicide (for a discussion of the linkage between urbanisation and suicide in the nineteenth century, see, Kushner 1984: 14). Morselli made reference to the suicidogenic social disruption caused by industrialisation and urbanisation, via the 'progressive' nature of urban residents and the 'friction of city life', and provided data from across Europe that supported his position (1881: 169).

As we have noted in earlier chapters, Durkheim also argued that modernisation and urbanisation disrupt social integration through migration and loss of traditional beliefs and support mechanisms, and lead to higher levels of either anomic or egotistic suicide (Durkheim 1951, e.g. 377–378). Rural society, on the other hand, was considered to uphold traditional belief systems and lifestyles – that is rural society was considered to be 'integrated' – and as such, to protect against suicide. Halbwachs further developed Durkheim's hypothesis, attempting to demonstrate empirically that French suicide rates were higher in urban areas than in rural areas (Halbwachs 1978). Although he struck problems of reliability which (favourably) biased his work, Halbwachs concluded, as had Morselli before him, that the fundamental social differences between the urban way of life and the rural way of life contribute to a distinct divergence in suicide rates (Douglas 1967). Ever since, research into suicide differentials between urban and rural suicides have been couched in terms of these hypotheses and few dissenting voices have been heard (see Beskow 1979; Capstick 1960; Labovitz and Brinkerhoff 1977; Micciolo, Willams *et al.* 1991).

Urban and rural suicide in India

Few studies of suicide in India examine national data, most preferring instead to limit their investigations to individual states, cities or even districts and specific villages. Given the large discrepancies both between and within states (for example Banerjee, Nandi *et al.* 1990), this was probably a wise approach. In addition, many of these studies examine the data in the context of the psychological/aetiological antecedents of the event rather than looking at the broader sociological forces involved. Nonetheless, these highly specific studies make definite contributions to more general discussions of suicide.

Ganapathi and Venkoba Rao (1966) in their study of suicides in Madurai suggest that there are very high rates of suicide in this large urban centre, more than ten times the national figure, and that this figure may well be an underestimate of the true rate. Social isolation and the breakdown of the traditional family structure are blamed for the noted increase in suicides in the aged, but it also reported that the actual peak in suicides occurs in the 21 to 30 age group.

Research into the suicide rate in Panji, the capital of Goa, found that this urban centre had an average annual suicide rate of 16 per 100,000 for the period 1966–1975 (Phal 1978). Suicide rates increased after 1970 and unusually for India, many more men than women committed suicide over the entire study period. These increases are thought to reflect the rapid urbanisation and industrialisation of the city after the liberation of Goa in 1961, in agreement with Durkheim's theories regarding social integration and the urban environment (Phal 1978).

A study of urban suicide rates in Jhansi, Uttar Pradesh, reported an annual suicide rate of 29 per 100,000. Of these, 55 per cent were female suicides (Shukla *et al.*

1990, cited in Desjarlais, Eisenberg *et al.* 1995), which supports other reports of approximately equal male–female suicide rates in Indian urban areas (Ponnudurai and Jeyakar 1980). In particular, the Jhansi study demonstrates, as we note in Chapter 3, that perhaps because different standards of proof are used, field research often reveals much higher rates of suicide than those reported by official sources.

Urban and rural comparisons

Early research into suicide in the Saurashtra region of Gujarat (between 1952 and 1955) suggested that urban areas in this region had higher rates of suicide than rural areas. While the urban population represented 34 per cent of the total population of Saurashtra, 38 per cent of the suicides in these years occurred in urban areas (Shah 1960). Other early studies have also reported finding higher rates of suicide in urban areas as opposed to rural areas (Singh *et al.* 1971, cited in Hallen 1989; Varma 1972).

Recent research into accidental and suicidal poisoning in the Telengana region of Andhra Pradesh directly compared the incidence of these cases in the urban setting, the semi-urban and the rural settings (Gautami, Sudershan *et al.* 2001). These authors found that the number of deaths due to chemical poisoning (including suicides and accidental poisonings) is higher in rural areas than urban and semi-urban areas. Semi-urban areas also had higher numbers of poisoning/suicide deaths than urban areas (Gautami, Sudershan *et al.* 2001). As in similar studies overseas (for example, Maniam 1988), the authors noted that the number of attempted suicides (unsuccessful) was strikingly small, an indication of the high toxicity of the substances consumed. Interestingly, this study reported that actual cases of suicide/poisoning dealt with in the three study districts of Andhra Pradesh were far greater in number than those officially reported for the entire state.

All-India research suggests that for data collected in 1994, urban suicide rates, as indicated by data from the 23 major Indian cities, appear to be marginally higher than rural suicide rates (Lester, Agarwal *et al.* 1999). Investigation of social correlates of regional suicide rates using the Indian data and data from the continental US found that while in India suicide rates were higher in the *more densely populated states*, in the US rates were higher in the *less densely populated states*. Other social variables (such as per capita income) were insignificant (Lester, Agarwal *et al.* 1999).

A study of particular interest is that by Chauhan (1984), which attempted to measure directly the sociological variables of integration and their impact upon Indian suicide rates. Variables collected from various government statistical sources were used to operationalise the concepts of urbanisation, industrialisation and social integration and these were measured against the suicide statistics for the year 1972. Variables pertaining to industrialisation revealed positive but insignificant correlations with suicide whereas one of the variables representing urbanisation (non-agricultural population) was positively and significantly correlated with the suicide rate. Unexpectedly, the percentage of Scheduled Castes in a state was (significantly) negatively correlated with the suicide rate, running counter to the hypothesis that low proportions of Dalits in a given population should contribute to social integration and as such be protective against suicide. No other variables representing the concepts of social and political integration were in any way significantly correlated with suicide, and interestingly neither was the other measure of urbanisation – urban population. Measures of literacy were highly positively correlated with suicide, leading Chauhan to state that 'education is the single most important predictor of the suicide rate in India' (Chauhan 1984: 27).

Chauhan concluded that his data supported the traditional Durkheimian Social Integration hypothesis, a surprising finding given the conspicuous lack of significant correlations between suicide rate and the many sociological variables tested. Because of our sceptical assessment of Chauhan's conclusions, we decided to conduct our own analysis of Indian suicide, using more recent data. As Chauhan suggested that 'it is quite possible that with the further industrialization of the country this . . . [weakly positive industrialisation-suicide correlation] . . . relationship may correspondingly become significant' (Chauhan 1984: 27), we therefore hoped to be able to demonstrate any significant relationship that may exist.

Suicides in rural and urban India

We examined data for the years 1993–1999 (prior to 1993 data were not reported in sufficient detail to be comparable between years). These report suicide rates for major cities in different states. 'Rural' suicide rates were calculated by subtracting the reported city suicides from the state totals. We are aware that many smaller urban areas are thus included in what we now present as 'rural' data, but this could not be avoided. However, as the 23 cities for which we do have data are the largest cities in the nation, we assume that any urban trends would be exaggerated in this sample (cf. Lester, Agarwal *et al.* 1999). Aggregate average rates for these seven years were then calculated from the individual annual data.

Using data obtained from a variety of sources (Agrawal and Om Varma 1997; Census of India 2002; National Crime Records Bureau 2001a, 2001b; Tata Services 1999), sociological concepts were operationalised following Chauhan (1984), where state-wise data were available.

Few variables were significantly correlated with either urban or rural suicide rates 1993–1999 (see Table 9.3 below). Interestingly, and puzzlingly, only the percentage of suicides by self-employed farmers or agriculturists returned a significant, though weak, positive correlation with urban suicides ($r = 0.59$, sig. < 0.04). No other variables tested, including measures of industrialisation and urbanisation, appeared to be correlated with urban suicides. Equally puzzling was the finding that the variables that were found to be significantly correlated with rural suicide rates include measures of urbanisation (change in urban population) ($r = 0.64$, sig < 0.001) and human development (total literacy ($r = 0.61$, sig < 0.003) and female literacy $(r = 0.58$, sig < 0.006)). These correlations are positive and indicate that increases in these measures will concomitantly see increases in the rural suicide rate. However, our social integration variable (crimes

Table 9.1 Sociological variables used

Concept	Variable
Urbanisation	• Percentage urban population, 1991 • Percentage urban population, 2001 • Percentage change in urban population • Percentage increase in urban population, 1981–1991
Industrialisation	• Per capita income, 1996–1997 • Per capita State Domestic Product, 1997 • Average daily number of workers employed in factories, 1997 • Percentage villages electrified, 1996
Social integration	• Percentage Scheduled Castes, 1991 • Riots 1999 (rate/100,000 population) • Property crime (theft & burglary) 1999 (rate/100,000 population) • 'Crimes against person' (murder & rape) 1999 (rate/100,000 population) • Total IPC crimes, 1999 (rate/100,000 population)
Human development	• Percentage female literacy, 1991 • Percentage (all) literacy, 1991 • Average household size
'Rural stagnation'	• Percentage suicides by 'self-employed (farming/agriculture)', 1999

against person) ($r = -0.46$, sig < 0.02) returned a significant negative correlation with rural suicide rates, contrary to what we would expect given the Durkheimian model. An additional significant negative correlation between rural suicide rate and average household size ($r = -0.48$, sig < 0.05) supports previous findings that suicides are less frequent in states where larger (joint) families are prevalent (Lal and Sethi (1975) cited in Hallen 1989).

These results are largely in agreement with those presented by Chauhan (1984), but we choose to interpret the results differently. Instead of concluding that the presence of some significant correlations provides enough evidence to support Durkheimian theory, our analysis shows that very few variables are correlated with urban suicide rates while most of the significant correlations are between our sociological measures and rural suicide, which runs counter to the predictions made by social integration theory. We also find it extraordinary that the only variable to produce a significant relationship with the urban suicide rate is an essentially rural one (percentage suicides by 'self employed (farming/agriculture)'). Hence, we concluded that there is no support for the traditional view regarding development and suicide and therefore felt that there was enough evidence to warrant further investigation.

Factor analysis conducted upon the urban and rural suicide rates, and what we consider to be the most sociologically relevant variables, extracted three distinct factors. Rural suicides, percentage change in urban population, average household size and female literacy are heavily loaded in factor one. We interpreted this factor to represent a development factor. Factor two we took to be an industrialisation factor, since it loaded heavily in on per capita State domestic product and average daily number of workers employed in factories. Factor three represents the same unexpected relationship between urban suicides and suicides by self-employed farmers/agriculturists, as was revealed in our correlation matrix above. We have termed this the urban suicide factor.

Variables representing the concepts of urbanisation, industrialisation, and human development were then regressed against our rural suicide rate. Six regression models were generated. The model which included female literacy only (Model 6 in Table 9.3 below) gave an adjusted R^2 of 0.72, which agrees with Chauhan's assertion that education plays a singularly important role in suicidal behaviour. (We will examine in detail the role of education in Chapter 10.)

However, we have concluded that the model that best explains the Indian rural suicide rate is Model 3, which includes measures of female literacy, percentage suicides by 'self employed (farming/agriculture)', the average daily number of workers employed in factories, and the percentage increase in urban population. This model gives an adjusted R^2 of 0.79 and minimises the standard error.

By splitting our suicide rate data into two subsets – urban and rural – we have assumed that the factors considered to be the most important contributors to suicide: urbanisation, industrialisation and (lack of) social integration would become even more apparent through significant correlations with urban suicide in

Table 9.2 Factor analysis rotated component matrix

Component	Development factor	Industrialisation factor	Urban suicide factor
Urban suicide rate, 1993–1999	0.14	0.005	0.75
Rural suicide rate, 1993–1999	0.90	0.15	0.005
Percentage change in urban population, 1981–1991	0.78	−0.004	0.34
Percentage female literacy, 1991	0.95	0.18	−0.008
Per capita State domestic product (net) at 1993–1994 prices	0.32	0.86	0.12
Percentage suicides by 'self employed (farming/agriculture)', 1999	−0.01	−0.004	0.94
'Crimes against person' (murder & rape), 1999 rate/lakh	−0.71	−0.27	0.47
Average daily number of workers employed in factories, 1997	−0.0052	0.97	−0.13
Average household size	−0.64	−0.63	−0.002
Percentage of the variance explained	37.5%	24.6%	20.1%

Note: Extraction method: principal component analysis. Rotation method: Varimax with Kaiser normalization. Rotation converged in 5 iterations.

Table 9.3 Regression models summary

Model	1	2	3	4	5	6
	Beta (S.E.)	Beta (S.E.)	Beta (S.E.)	Beta (S.E.)	Beta (S.E.)	Beta (S.E.)
(Constant)	15.66 (20.05)	16.06 (18.49)	−0.39 (5.19)	−4.16 (4.49)	−7.55 (4.15)	−3.41 (3.02)
Per capita state domestic product (net)	0.00 (0.01)					
Percent increase in urban population, 1981–1991	−0.31 (0.18)	−0.31 (0.16)	−0.33 (0.16)	−0.21 (0.14)		
Percent suicides by 'self employed (farming/agriculture)' in 1999	0.51 (0.24)	0.51* (0.22)	0.54* (0.22)	0.42 (0.20)	0.25 (0.18)	
Average daily number of workers employed in factories	0.00 (0.00)	0.00 (0.00)	0.00 (0.00)			
Average household size	−2.23 (2.76)	−2.33 (2.51)				
Percent female literacy	0.44** (0.11)	0.44** (0.10)	0.50** (0.08)	0.45** (0.07)	0.39** (0.07)	0.38** (0.07)
R²	**0.87**	**0.87**	**0.86**	**0.83**	**0.78**	**0.74**
Adjusted R²	**0.75**	**0.78**	**0.79**	**0.77**	**0.74**	**0.72**
Std. Error of the Estimate	**3.87**	**3.59**	**3.56**	**3.70**	**3.94**	**4.11**
F	**6.89**	**9.59**	**11.98**	**14.27**	**17.86**	**31.09**

particular. If the protective factor of traditional rural life holds sway, we would expect that few significant results, or negatively correlated relationships, would be produced in relation to the rural suicide rate. This has not happened. Contrary to Durkheimian theory, increasing measures of urbanisation, industrialisation and human development appear to contribute to increasing levels of *rural* suicide. Geographical analysis supports these findings (see Figure 9.1 below). Indian states with the highest average rural suicide rates per 100,000 coincide with the industrialised, urbanised south and west while the less industrialised, rural northern states have comparatively low rural suicide rates. Interestingly, Figure 9.1 also illustrates the comparatively high urban suicide rates in the North, a subject to which we will return to later in this section.[1]

A brief review of the literature finds many reports from other countries returning similar findings. As we noted in the introduction, earlier works have generally found that urban suicide rates were higher than rural rates (Capstick 1960; Durkheim 1951; Halbwachs 1978; Labovitz and Brinkerhoff 1977; Morselli 1881), the noticeable exception being studies from the US in the 1950s (for

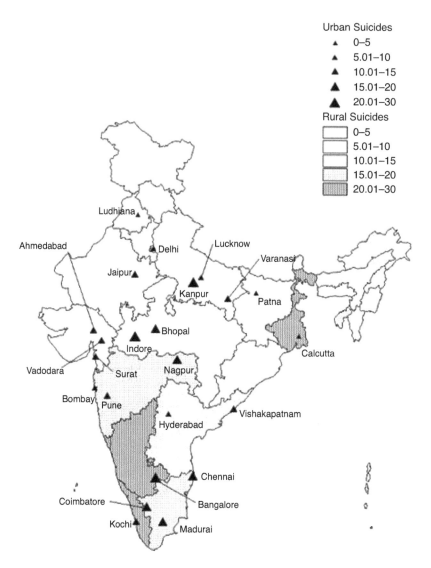

Figure 9.1 Urban and rural suicides in India 1993–1999 (average rate per 100,000 population).

example Schroeder and Beegle 1953). Now an increasing number of international studies are reporting a preponderance of rural suicides.

Contemporary studies of suicide in Sweden (Otto and Spate 1975, Coombs *et al.* 1977 and Lönnqvist 1977 cited in Beskow 1979; Ferrada-Noli 1997) report a shift in high suicide rates from highly urbanised areas to suburban and rural areas. This finding is confirmed by similar results from the UK (Hawton, Harriss *et al.* 2001; Malmberg, Simpkin *et al.* 1999).

A study by Rancans *et al.* (2001) of suicide in Latvia before, during and after its incorporation by the Soviet Union found that suicide rates in rural areas were consistently higher (up to 2.2 times higher at times) than those in urban areas throughout the study period.

Research in Greece – a nation that has one of the lowest national suicide rates in Europe – found that rural suicides were more frequent than urban suicide for both sexes (Zacharakis, Madianos *et al.* 1998; see also Beratis 1986).

Research from the US has also found that suicide rates rise with increasing 'rurality' (Singh and Siahpush 2002), supporting the findings of earlier studies (Schroeder and Beegle 1953; Wilkinson 1984; Wilkinson and Israel 1984). Reviewing data from all US counties 1970–1997, Singh and Siahpush (2002) found that suicide rates for rural men were twice those of their urban counterparts.

In a study of suicide rates of the elderly in Japan, Watanabe *et al.* found that in 1988 the suicide rate for elders in urban Kawasaki was 38.3 per 100,000, while in rural Higashikubiki the 1988 rate was an astounding 240.4 per 100,000 (1995; see also Kurosu 1991: 603).

Of particular relevance to the situation in India is the data emerging from China. The Chinese data show that suicide rates are not only higher in rural areas than in urban areas but, as we saw in Chapter 7, female suicides are far more frequent than male suicides. Phillips, Liu *et al.* (1999) report rates in rural areas more than three times the magnitude of those in urban areas, while suicide rates for women are 40 per cent higher than those for men (see also Ji, Kleinman *et al.* 2001; Phillips, Li *et al.* 2002). Work by Yip, Callanan *et al.* (2000) supports these findings, reporting that the suicide rate for the rural areas of Beijing is higher for both genders than for urban residents.

These findings support the proposition of Stack (1982) that urban suicide rates may be viewed as being curvilinear over time, being higher in the earlier stages of modernisation but decreasing over time as the urban 'way of life' becomes the norm. Stack also posits that urban rates may ultimately become lower than rural rates 'once the mass media and other institutions diffuse urban culture into rural areas' (Stack 1982: 52). It stands to reason that if the suicidogenic factor of modernisation/urbanisation is the disruption of the traditional (rural) way of life, once urbanisation becomes the norm this should cease to be a disrupting influence. Furthermore, if the urban way of life becomes a disrupting influence in rural society (changing cultural expectations, social relationships or economic behaviour), an increase in suicide rates similar to those noted in early-stage urbanisation should be expected. That is, the social isolation principle traditionally invoked to explain increased urban suicides, which may have had valid application in the past (for example see Capstick 1960), may now be more relevant in rural areas, as has been demonstrated in Scotland (Crombie 1991) and Poland (Jarosz 1985). Schroeder and Beegle suggest that 'the decision of such individuals to commit suicide may have its origin in an incomplete reconciliation of rural and urban values' (Schroeder and Beegle 1953: 50), and while this statement could be equally made regarding higher urban suicide rates, these emergent trends emphasise the need to re-evaluate our common assumptions regarding the directional nature of sociological variables contributing to suicide in urbanised/urbanising nations.

Murphy Haliburton noted acutely that suicide rates in Kochi (Cochin), Kerala, were about half those of the state as a whole (Halliburton 1998: 2342). When we compare urban to rural rates across the nation, a more complex pattern is apparent. The findings of our Indian analysis indicates that higher, though statistically insignificant ($t = 1.27$, $p = 0.23$), ratios of urban–rural suicides occur in the north, where development scores as derived from our factor analysis are also low. The relationship is, however, a complex and, as Stack suggests, a curvilinear one. If we transform the urban–rural rate by taking its fourth root and compare it with the log of the rate for the whole state, we find a strong and striking linear relationship ($r = 0.86$). As can be seen in Figure 9.2, in those, primarily northern, states where suicide rates as a whole are low, they are very much higher in urban than in rural areas. In the south and in West Bengal, where overall suicide rates are high, rural suicide rates exceed those in the cities.

The explanation for this pattern is indicated by the geographical distributions that can be seen in Figure 9.3. As we have seen, factor analysis of the Indian suicide data and a number of sociological variables generated three orthogonal factors: a development factor, an industrialisation factor and an urban suicide factor. Of these, only the development factor scores were significantly correlated ($r = -0.634$, $p = 0.036$) with the ratio of urban to rural suicide rates (used to

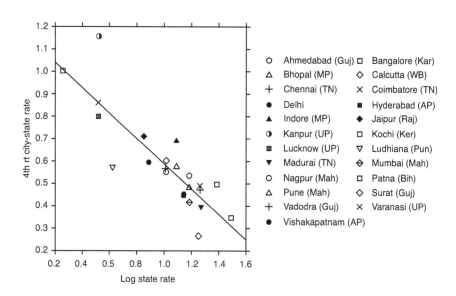

4th rt city-state rate = 1.153 – 0.563 * Log state rate; R^2 = 0.742

Figure 9.2 Urban–rural suicide rates vs state suicide rates.

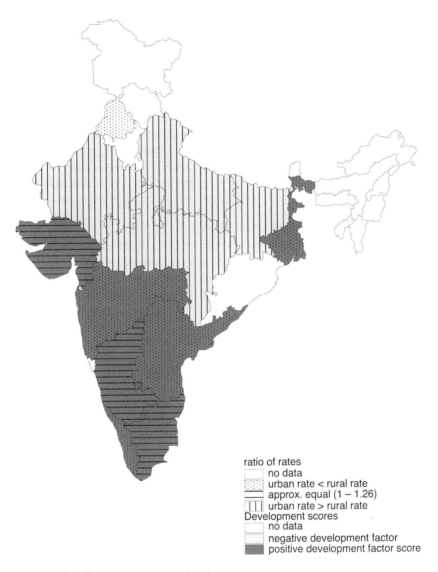

Figure 9.3 Indian suicide rates and development scores.

eliminate effects of magnitude). Development scores have a negative value in the northern states (Figure 9.3 light shading), for those states where there is data available. In every one of these states urban suicide rates are higher than the rural suicide rate (vertical shading). In the south however, development scores all have positive values (dark shading) and urban suicide rates are all less than or equal to the states' rural suicide rates (horizontal or stippled shading). Thus, if increasing development scores are taken to be analogous to the idea of development over time we see a similar effect – decreasing relative rates of urban suicide – to that posited by Stack (1982).

Partial confirmation that economic stagnation may in part explain the relatively higher urban to rural ratios we find in the north is provided by Figure 9.4. Here the transformed urban–rural ratio is regressed on the natural log of the ratio of the numbers of urban dwellers employed in the construction industry in 1991 to that employed in services. A relatively large service sector is taken to be a proxy for a relatively weak manufacturing sector and a city with a small construction sector is understood to be one in which overall economic growth is sluggish. A larger negative number is taken as an indicator of a stagnating urban economy while a smaller number indicates one in which manufacturing is a significant sector and which is experiencing greater economic growth. What we find is that apparently stagnating urban economies such as Kanpur, Patna, Varanasi and Lucknow also have relatively high urban–rural suicide ratios. Rural suicide rates are higher than urban ones in apparently more dynamic urban economies, including Kochi, Pune, Bangalore, Nagpur, Ludhiana and Hyderabad.

Taken together, instead of finding social disruption in the urban centres with increasing modernisation it appears from our findings that it is the rural sector that is now bearing the brunt of these disruptive forces (for example Bhalla, Sharma *et al.* 1998). We have termed this 'rural stagnation'. As studies have found in other nations, lifestyle changes associated with urbanisation have permeated rural areas leaving disjointed family structures, raised expectations without the means to fulfil them and a rapid erosion of traditional values (for example Ji, Kleinman *et al.* 2001; Ratnayeke 1998). As Kurosu comments in relation to Japan 'higher suicide rates are observed in areas with a sparse population, a stagnant economy, and a population over-represented by elderly people' (Kurosu 1991: 603) – in short, the rural areas

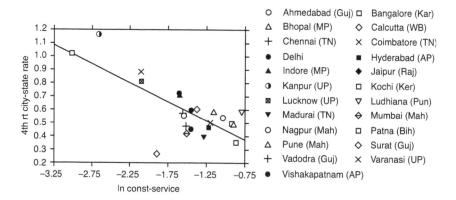

4th rt city-state rate = 1.15 − 0.287 * ln const-service; R^2 = 0.565

Figure 9.4 Urban–rural suicide ratio vs urban economic stagnation index.

of a developed nation. As India shows, even with dense populations, economic stagnation can produce the same phenomenon in a developing economy.

Numerous authors have suggested that modernisation may have disadvantageous socio-economic ramifications in India (see Bardhan and Bardhan 1973; Jena 1960). Patterns of urban–rural and rural–rural migration have been found, unsurprisingly, to alter the social composition and heighten the gap between rich and poor in Indian villages (Connell, Dasgupta *et al.* 1976). So while we cannot say conclusively that this necessarily increases the suicide rate, our statistical findings do indicate that rural life is adversely affected by modernisation and that the traditional assumptions of the Social Integration theory are not wholly valid in India. As our geographical analysis attests, the less developed regions of India conform, at least to some degree to the Social Integration theory, but not the more developed, southern regions. Like Stack (Stack 1982) we feel that there is evidence to suggest that modernisation may have a curvilinear effect on suicide differentials in India.

Conclusion

Many past studies have reported evidence that the processes of urbanisation and industrialisation increase the suicide rate in urban areas while the traditional value system in rural areas is protective against suicide (Capstick 1960; Chauhan 1984; Durkheim 1951; Halbwachs 1978). However, many recent studies suggest that these same processes are increasingly contributing to a sense of social isolation and radical changes in social values in rural areas, and as such are aggravating suicidal behaviour in these areas (Bhalla, Sharma *et al.* 1998; Crombie 1991; Ji, Kleinman *et al.* 2001). As Kurosu (1991) reports regarding suicide in rural Japan, there is an element of socio-economic stagnation in rural areas with increasing levels of urbanisation and this is characterised by higher suicide rates. Similar causes appear to operate in India. Statistical analysis indicates that processes of urbanisation, industrialisation and human development are correlated with, and contribute to, rural suicide rates in India, which is not the case for urban suicide data. Following Stack (1982) we believe that after a certain level of modernisation has been reached in a developing country, elevated urban suicide rates, arising from social isolation, recede while the disruptive elements of modernisation continue – at an increasing rate – to create suicidogenic conditions in rural communities. Thus, the traditional view of city life being a life of isolation and suicidogenic conditions may need to be inverted and the city in the urbanised nation be considered as rural communities have been in the past: cohesive communities with dense social networks that mitigate the occurrence of suicide.

Note

1 We had hoped check the validity of our approach by comparing our data with district-wise urban and rural data on suicide deaths contained in the *Statistical Abstract of Maharashtra State, 1995–96 & 1996–97* (Directorate of Economics and Statistics 2003: 185). However, as the *Statistical Abstract* reports only 22 per cent of the suicides recorded by the NCRB; consequently we felt a detailed analysis of urban and rural suicides based on the Maharashtra data was meaningless.

10 Education and suicide

The earliest researchers on the relationship between education and suicide in Europe felt certain that increases in the one went hand in hand with the other. Morselli reported that 'mental aberration' and suicide seemed to be related. He offered it as a general rule that:

> *it is those countries which possess a higher standard of general culture which furnish the largest contingent of voluntary deaths.* Although sometimes great differences may be observed in the degree of instruction, but equal intensity in the suicides, yet the geographical distribution of these violent deaths goes in a general way *pari passu* with instruction. [Emphasis in original]
>
> (Morselli 1881: 131)

More recent studies, as we noted in Chapter 7, have found that the literature on the relationship between education and suicide is more equivocal.

On the one hand, in a study of 43 nations Lester found a positive association between education and suicide (Lester 1996). On the other hand, in a study restricted to the 50 States in the US Saucer found no significant correlation between education levels and suicide rates (Saucer 1993).

In Chapter 7 we noted that increasing gender equality in educational attainment in India is strongly and significantly correlated with higher total and male suicide rates. If we summarise that finding by looking at the relationship between literacy, the most basic marker of education, and suicide we find that there is a very strong, positive and highly statistically significant relationship. In Figure 10.1 we have used the percentage of male literates for the 14 major Indian states from the 1991 census and regressed the suicide rates for 1997 on to it (the results are virtually identical for female literacy rates). In states such as Bihar and Uttar Pradesh where literacy is lowest, suicide rates are also quite low. There is a nearly linear relationship between increasing rates of literacy and suicide rates, the extreme case being Kerala, which has both the greatest literacy and the highest suicide rates of the major states. The regression equation indicates that a 10 per cent increase in literacy is associated with a 5 per cent increase in the suicide rate.

The strong relationship between literacy and suicide in India raises the question of whether it is simply literacy by itself that is responsible for this linkage. Or are increasing levels of education associated with higher levels of suicide?

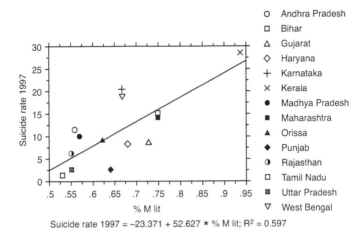

Suicide rate 1997 = −23.371 + 52.627 * % M lit; R² = 0.597

Figure 10.1 Male literacy, 1991 vs suicide rate, 1997.

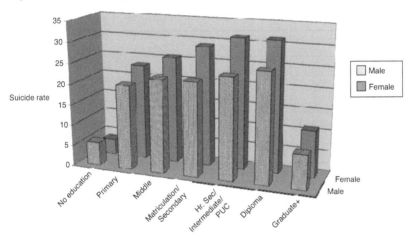

Figure 10.2 Suicide rates by education level – all India, 1997.

All-India pattern

The pattern of suicide rates for each educational level is given in Figure 10.2. There are a number of striking features of the figure. We may note, first of all, that the lowest rate for males occurs amongst those with no education. Second, suicide rates rise with each increase in the level of study – with the remarkable exception of those who have undertaken tertiary or postgraduate study: suicide rates for the university educated are the lowest of all educational categories. It is not clear why tertiary-level training should so markedly reduce the risk of suicide. The third remarkable feature of the figure is that except for those with no education, female suicide rates are higher, and increase more rapidly at each educational level, than do suicide rates for males.

As can be seen in Table 10.1, the female–male suicide ratio rises with increasing levels of education, the exception being diploma-level study where, because female rates remain static, there is a minor decrease in the ratio.

No education

When we look at the state-wise patterns of suicide for those who have had no education (some of whom, nevertheless, are literate) we see a wide range of vulnerabilities to suicide (Figure 10.3). On the whole, as we would anticipate from the national figures, suicide rates for those who have never been to school are very low. Suicide rates for those without educational experience are very low indeed in several large north Indian states: Bihar (0.8), Uttar Pradesh (1.6), Punjab (2.5) and Rajasthan (3.3). In four states and one territory male rates are well above the national average: Pondicherry (53.7), Goa (17.4), Karnataka (17.2), Kerala (15.6) and Tamil Nadu (13.8). The rates for females in Pondicherry (19.2) are also well above the national average.

Table 10.1 Female to male suicide ratio by education level

Education level	Female–male ratio
No education	0.686
Primary	1.146
Middle	1.150
Matriculation/Secondary	1.284
Hr. Sec/Intermediate/PUC	1.294
Diploma	1.201
Graduate+	1.336

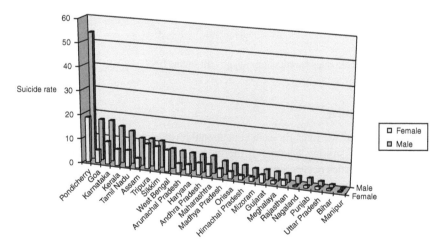

Figure 10.3 Suicide rates for males and females with no education.

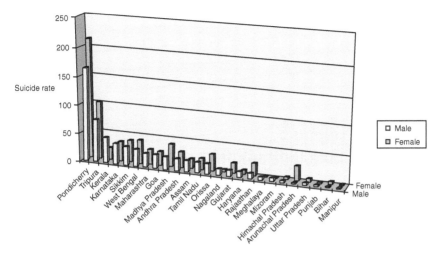

Figure 10.4 Suicide rates for males and females with primary education.

Primary education

The basic pattern and relationships of suicide rates for those with primary education is very similar to that for those with no formal education (Figure 10.4). The most significant difference is that both the average rates are considerably higher and the extreme values are very much higher. For over half the states the male suicide rates are over 20 per 100,000. The state with the highest male suicide rates is Pondicherry at 167.4.

We begin to see here, too, the pattern of female suicide rates exceeding those for males. In some cases, most notably, Pondicherry, female rates are very high (210.9). In the northeastern state of Arunachal, female suicide rates for the primary educated are five times higher than those for males. The female–male rates are also reasonably strong in several Hindi-speaking states: Bihar (1.8:1), Rajasthan (1.8:1) and Madhya Pradesh (1.6:1).

Middle education

A very similar pattern exists for those who have reached middle standard in education (Figure 10.5). The highest rates are observed in Pondicherry and the southern states (plus Tripura). The suicide rates for most states are slightly higher than for the primary educated. The excess of female over male suicide rates in the Hindi belt is higher for those with middle education and the list now includes Uttar Pradesh as well.

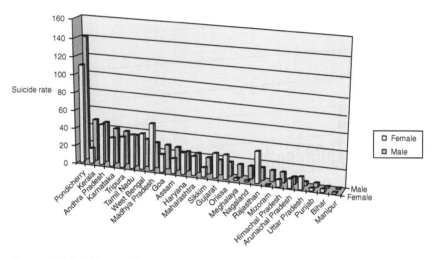

Figure 10.5 Suicide rates for males and females with middle education.

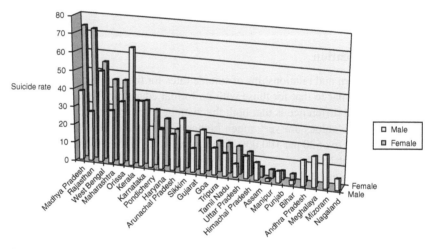

Figure 10.6 Suicide rates for males and females with matriculation/intermediate/
          pre-university education.

Matriculation

The pattern of suicides in the states for those with matriculation (or equivalents
such as Intermediate or Pre-University Course) is quite different from those seen
so far (Figure 10.6). Here the preponderance of the highest suicide rates in each
state is clearly among females. And the southern states that exhibited the highest
rates for the previous educational categories have slipped, relatively speaking,
down the rankings. At the most extreme end are an oddly assorted group of
northern states: Madhya Pradesh, Rajasthan, West Bengal, Maharashtra and

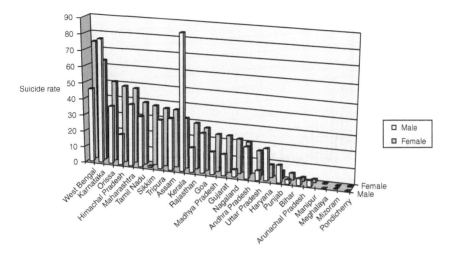

Figure 10.7 Suicide rates for males and females with higher secondary education.

Orissa. In about half the states, both female and male suicide rates are at or above 20 per 100,000.

Higher secondary

The pattern of suicide deaths amongst those who have studied to higher secondary level is complex. Unlike previous levels, where there was a rough correspondence between male and female magnitudes, here two somewhat different rankings are apparent. As can be seen in Figure 10.7, which is arranged in terms of female rates, West Bengal, Karnataka, Orissa, Himachal Pradesh, Maharashtra, Tamil Nadu, Sikkim, Tripura, Assam and Kerala all have female rates over 30. When sorted by male suicide rates Kerala, Karnataka, West Bengal, Maharashtra, Orissa, Assam, Tamil Nadu and Tripura have rates over 30. Most notable of all, Pondicherry, which so frequently has India's highest suicide rates, had *no* suicides with higher secondary education.

Diploma

The pattern of suicide deaths for those holding some form of technical diploma or certificate not equal to a graduate degree is the most singular of all (Figure 10.8). While it may not be immediately apparent, given the different scale of the figure, some male suicide rates in this category are quite high: West Bengal, Assam, Nagaland, Rajasthan, Andhra Pradesh, Madhya Pradesh and Meghalaya all have male suicide rates higher than 30 per 100,000. What is completely arresting, of course, are the extraordinarily high suicide rates for women with technical qualifications: West Bengal (495.1) Rajasthan (258.3) Assam (215.3) Pondicherry

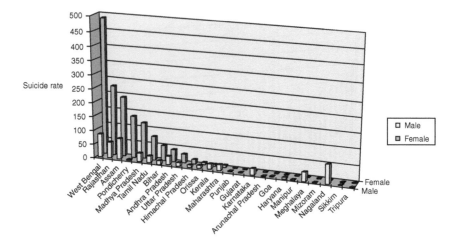

Figure 10.8 Suicide rates for males and females with technical diploma or certificate.

(152.7) Madhya Pradesh (131.0) Tamil Nadu (84.5) Bihar (54.5) Andhra Pradesh (47.1) and Uttar Pradesh (36.5) all have rates over 30. One can only speculate that the acquisition of non-traditional qualifications by women may place them at increased risk of suicide.

University graduate and higher

The contrast of those with university or postgraduate degrees with diploma holders is a sharp one (Figure 10.9). In only four states do women graduates have suicide rates over 20: Sikkim, West Bengal, Tamil Nadu and Rajasthan. And only in Kerala is the rate for males over 20. In the majority of states (including Pondicherry) graduate suicide rates are under 10. Once again we can only conjecture why the holders of a university degree should be, relatively speaking, at lower risk.

Conclusion

It is striking that those who have had no experience of formal education and those who have attained the highest educational levels have the lowest risk of suicide in India. For all others, as we have seen, each increase in educational attainment is accompanied by an increased risk of suicidal death. For women the risks rise more rapidly than for men. At higher levels of education, the risk for women appears to be relatively higher in areas of northern India where female suicide rates are generally low.

Since overall educational levels for women are lowest in the North it suggests that it may be that those women who first obtain more advanced qualifications –

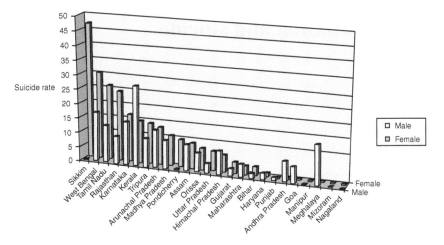

Figure 10.9 Suicide rates for male and female university graduates or postgraduates.

whom we may term the 'fuglemen [leaders] of modernisation' – are at greatest risk of suicide. Partial confirmation of this view may be the very high risk of the relatively limited number of women who obtain technical qualifications. When the log of the suicide rate of female holders of technical qualification is regressed onto a measure of how many hold the qualifications, there is a fairly strong negative correlation $(r = -0.63; p = 0.01)$, indicating that the risk of suicide is lower where relatively more women in a state hold technical qualifications.[1] As general levels of education increase, the gender-specific risk appears to decrease.

As noted earlier, it is not clear why this general pattern does not apply to those who graduate from university. It may be that it is a consequence of the greater prestige of the occupations open to graduates. As we note in the next chapter, Stack has argued that those with more prestigious occupations are at reduced risk of suicide.

Note

1 The measure is the ratio of holders of technical degrees to those with no education. Goa and Haryana were excluded from the analysis as neither reported any suicides by holders of technical qualifications in 1997.

11 Occupation and suicide

Among the very earliest observations made by observers in Europe about the social characteristics of suicide was that different occupational groups were at very different levels of risk. At one pole were agriculturalists (who were also, of course, largely residents of rural districts) and at another were the most highly educated and trained members of society, such as lawyers, doctors and civil servants. Morselli found that in Italy between 1866 and 1876 those employed in the 'letters and science' professions had exceptionally high suicide rates of 61.83 per 100,000 (Morselli 1881: 244). Italian civil servants (all male) had a suicide rate of 32.43. Those 'classes addicted to agriculture, pastoral life [and] forestry' had very low suicide rates (2.5) (Morselli 1881: 243).

In a recent review of research on occupations and suicide, Stack notes that studies are 'often marked by inconsistent findings' (2001: 384) with different studies reporting high, medium or low risk of suicide for the same occupational groups. Stack also notes that i) 'the link between occupation and suicide is not well understood', ii) 'suicide rates are not available for most occupations' and, iii) 'many of the studies do not address female suicide risk' (Stack 2001: 385). Much may depend upon the historical period being studied or the nature of the economy of the country under investigation. Thus, while many early studies such as Morselli's reported low suicide rates amongst European farmers, many more recent studies report relatively high suicide rates for farmers (for example, Schroeder and Beegle 1953; Capstick 1960; Booth and Lloyd 1999; Malmberg, Simpkin *et al.* 1999).

In a case control study of suicides in the UK, Charlton found elevated relative risk of suicide in some occupations for men such as veterinarian, pharmacist, dentist, farmer and doctor, and for women, such as veterinarian and doctor (Charlton 1995: S51–52).

In a study of suicide in Australia, Hassan reported elevated suicide rates among men in agriculture, sales, those in trades and in transport and communication (Hassan 1995: 102). He observes:

> The general pattern, as far as men are concerned, appears to be that those in blue-collar occupations which are also characterized by less job autonomy, greater external supervision, less on-the-job training, poorer promotion

possibilities, lower wage levels and greater sensitivity to market forces, tend to have higher suicide rates . . .

(Hassan 1995: 103)

In a logistic regression study which controlled for the major demographic covariates of occupation, Stack found that dentists, doctors, mathematicians, scientists and artists were at elevated risk of suicide, as were machinists, auto mechanics, electricians, plumbers, carpenters, welders and labourers. Occupations in which there was a low risk of suicide were primary school teachers and postal workers (Stack 2001: 391).

Despite his finding of high suicide risk amongst dentists and doctors, Stack offers a summary 'rule of thumb' from the existing literature concerning occupational risk of suicide:

Generally speaking, there is an inverse relationship between occupational prestige and the risk of suicide.

(Stack 2001, n.1: 386)

Unemployment – the absence of occupation – has also been the subject of intensive investigation. Charlton, in a case control study in the UK, found the paradoxical result that unemployed men over 45 who lived in areas with *low* unemployment were at increased relative risk of suicide (Charlton 1995: S52). This finding is, however, consistent with Platt's detailed study of parasuicide (attempted suicide) and unemployment in Edinburgh. Platt found that although 'in recent years as much as half of the overall parasuicide rate in Edinburgh may be "attributable" to unemployment', nevertheless 'there is a marked tendency for relative risk to fall as the unemployment rate rises' (Platt 1986: 401). Platt's explanation for the apparent paradox is that:

as economic recession worsens, the stigma associated with unemployment would be expected to be less marked, [and thus] unemployed people would be more integrated in the social order, and their parasuicide potential would decrease . . . when mass unemployment becomes endemic, the change might indeed become negative [i.e. parasucide rates might fall].

(Platt 1986: 403)

In a review of 156 published studies of the relationship between employment and suicide and attempted suicide, Platt found that 'significantly more (para)suicides [i.e. both attempted and completed suicides] are unemployed than would be expected among general population samples. Likewise, (para)suicide rates among the unemployed are always considerably higher than among the employed' (Platt 1984: 107–108). Nevertheless, Platt argues that psychiatric illness must be considered as a causal factor influencing *both* unemployment and suicidal behaviour:

Rather than unemployment leading to psychiatric illness and thereafter to suicide, there is more evidence in favour of the alternative model . . . that unemployment in suicide victims is to a large extent a consequence or reflection of an underlying psychiatric disorder: rather than unemployment being a cause of psychiatric illness and suicide, it is more likely that the risks of both unemployment and suicide are elevated by the presence of major psychiatric illness (in particular, depression).

(Platt 1984: 109)

Occupation and suicide in India

It is difficult to speak with complete certainty about occupation and suicide in India. Except for Satyavathi's studies of students and the unemployed, discussed below, there do not appear to have been any systematic studies of occupation and suicide in India. Data on occupation have only been reported since 1995 and the categories under which they are consolidated at the national level correspond only imperfectly with the National Industrial Classification (NIC) scheme used by the Census of India and the Central Statistical Organisation. Consequently, rates for only a few occupational groups reported by the National Crime Records Bureau can be calculated. The results from these calculations are, however, very striking and add a significant dimension to our understanding of the social origins of suicide in India.

Unemployment

As we have seen, one of the most consistent findings of studies of the relationship between occupation and suicide in developed economies is that those who are unemployed have elevated suicide rates. This finding also holds true in a very serious way for India. In a unique study of suicide in Bangalore, Satyavathi found that 65 per cent of 171 unemployed suicides studied were 'either due to the sole reason of unemployment or for other reasons in addition to the reason of their unemployment' (Sathyavathi 1977: 387). As can be seen in Figure 11.1, suicide rates for unemployed people are extremely high, especially in a number of Indian states. Unemployed women in Pondicherry have suicide rates of over 650 per 100,000 while the rates for males in the Union Territory are 1600. Male suicide rates are also extremely high in Mizoram (1277), with very high rates for females as well (186), though these reflect only 20 male and three female suicides in 1997. Other states in which male unemployed suicide rates are over 200 per 100,000 are Karnataka, Meghalaya, Himachal Pradesh, Gujarat, Andhra Pradesh, Punjab, and Haryana. While high suicide rates in Pondicherry are not surprising, those in some of the northwestern and northeastern states that have very low overall suicide rates, are. They are particularly notable in the Punjab and Meghalaya both of which have overall suicide rates of less than 4 per 100,000.

Another notable aspect of the data on unemployed suicides is the relatively low rates observed in Kerala and West Bengal which both have high overall suicide rates.

Finally we may note that female unemployed suicide rates exceed those for males in Tamil Nadu and Sikkim. Male and female rates are virtually identical in Manipur.

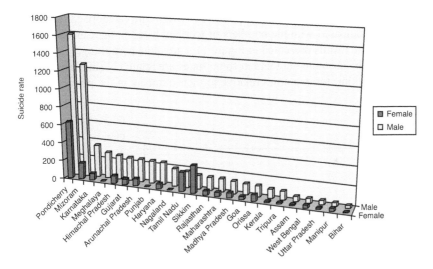

Figure 11.1 Suicide rates for unemployed males and females.

The pattern of very elevated suicide rates for the unemployed, especially for unemployed males, may underscore the psychological toll exacted by the slow growth of employment in the Indian economy.

A possible explanation for the especially elevated suicide patterns that we observe in some otherwise relatively low suicide states may be due to the curvilinear relationship suggested by Platt (Platt 1986). That is, we might expect suicide rates to increase sharply at relatively low rates of unemployment and to fall where unemployment is widespread. Partial confirmation of this hypothesis is given by Figure 11.2, which shows the relationship between unemployment rates in 1996 and suicide rates for unemployed males in 1997. This indicates that there is a rapid increase in unemployed male suicide rates as unemployment rates increase in states such as Rajasthan and Madhya Pradesh. Rates tend to peak at middle levels of unemployment in states such as Haryana and Punjab. At the far end of the distribution, where unemployment is high in Kerala, unemployed suicide rates are relatively lower. There are, of course, some very significant outliers in the distribution, especially Karnataka and West Bengal.

The figure, while suggestive, must be treated with caution. First, the data for unemployment on which it rests, while the best available, may report only those formally registered as unemployed. In addition, the correlation is a moderate one ($r = 0.42$) and is not statistically significant.

Government employees

Although it is a general finding in industrialised economies that educated workers are at elevated risk of suicide, it is no longer common to have the deaths by suicide of government employees listed separately from other professional, administrative or clerical workers. In India such deaths are categorised separately and may be compared with the numbers of workers listed in the Census as state employees. The results presented in Figure 11.3 are quite perturbing.

Although the absolute numbers in some states are relatively small (only three females in Sikkim, for example) relative to their numbers in the population, the

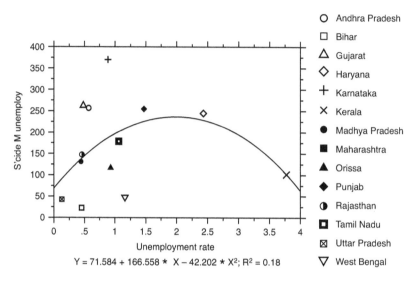

$$Y = 71.584 + 166.558 * X - 42.202 * X^2; R^2 = 0.18$$

Figure 11.2 Unemployment rate, 1996 vs unemployed male suicide rate, 1997.

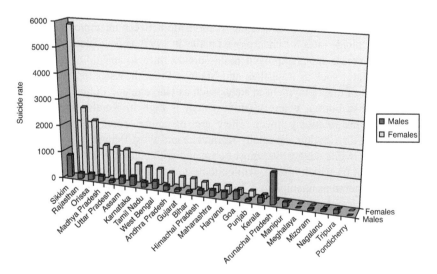

Figure 11.3 Suicide rates for government employees, males and females.

suicide rates for government employees appear to be extraordinarily high, especially for female public servants. Suicide rates for government employees in Sikkim are unbelievably high: the rate for women is nearly 6000 per 100,000 while for males it is nearly 870. In four other states the suicide rates for female public servants is over 1000: Rajasthan, Orissa, Madhya Pradesh, Uttar Pradesh, and Assam. The corresponding rates for males in these states, while far lower, are still far above those for the population taken as a whole, ranging from a low of 76 in Uttar Pradesh to 280 in Assam.

As in the apparently opposite case of the unemployed, securely employed civil servants take their lives at very elevated rates in states in which the overall rates are relatively low, but at very much lower rates in states such as Kerala and Andhra Pradesh where overall rates are relatively high. Most unexpected of all, perhaps, there were no suicides, male or female, by public servants in Pondicherry in 1997.

These figures for government employees pose a dual puzzle. The first is why they are so extremely high. The second is why the levels for female employees are so astronomically high. It is noticeable that a number of the states in which overall rates are low but those for female civil servants are high are also states in which female literacy is lowest, family size is largest and the preference for male children is greatest. This syndrome suggests that female government employees face especial risks in these states where the expectations are strongest that women will adhere to traditional gender roles.

A multiple correlation model in which suicide rates for female civil servants in the 14 major Indian states were regressed on the percentage of female literates (a strong proxy for female emancipation) and perceptions of levels of corruption in the Indian states (a proxy for the esteem in which civil servants may be held) yields a very high correlation coefficient ($r = 0.80$). The correlation with female literacy is negative, indicating that where (as in Rajasthan, Uttar Pradesh, Madhya Pradesh and Orissa), female empowerment is low, suicide rates among female civil servants are high. Where, as in Kerala, female empowerment is most advanced, suicide rates for female government employees are relatively lowest.[1]

A comparable multiple regression for male civil servants regressed their suicide rates on the corruption perception index and a proxy for economic development in a state (the percentage of poor people in the population). The model had a moderately high correlation coefficient ($r = 0.65$). Although the model explains more than 40 per cent of the variance in observed suicide rates, it contradicts hypothesised causes and does not lend itself to simple interpretation. The sign of the correlation between suicide rates and corruption perceptions is negative ($r = -0.44$), contrary to the predicted positive relationship. Similarly, there is only a weak direct relationship between male civil servant suicide rates and the percentage of the population living in poverty.

Retired individuals

Another category for which it is possible to compute suicide rates is the rather undifferentiated body of those who are retired. This category appears to be

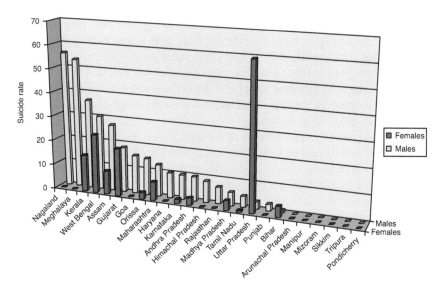

Figure 11.4 Suicide rates for retired males and females.

restricted to those who were once in formal sector employment, since there were estimated to be only some 6.1 million retirees in all of India in 1997. Inspection of Figure 11.4 shows that in some states the suicide rates for this group is quite high.

Retired males appear to be at greater overall risk of suicide, though there are some striking exceptions to this observation. The suicide rate for retired females in Uttar Pradesh is very high (61 per 100,000) and is quite high in West Bengal (25) and Kerala (15). For males the states with the highest rates among retirees are Nagaland, Meghalaya, Kerala, West Bengal and Assam.

We need to have additional information to understand more clearly why retirees kill themselves at relatively elevated levels. It may be simply a concomitant of old age. Or, as has been suggested by articles discussing the growth of abuse of parents by their children in contemporary India, it may be a despairing response to the failure of expectations of support (see for example Mitra 1998).

Farmers

As we have noted in the Introduction, a great deal of attention has been devoted in recent years, especially in 1998, to suicides among what is one of India's largest occupational groups – farmers (Time International 1998; Our Principal Correspondent 1998; Assadi 1998, 2000; Bhalla, Sharma *et al.* 1998; Sharma 1998; Siddiq 2000; Sundar 1999; Venugopal and Jagadisha 2000; Shiva 2000; Harlankar 2003; Ramesh 1998; Rao 1998; Waldman 2004). Since the implication in much of this writing is that very large numbers of farmers commit suicide, frequently as a result of economic distress, it is important that we attempt to understand the risk of suicide faced by farmers in India.

Farmer suicides are also often reported in the popular media. As we noted in the introduction, recent spates of suicides in farming communities have received much attention. Between December 1997 and June 1998 nearly 400 Indian farmers committed suicide, mostly in the southern states of Andhra Pradesh and Karnataka (Time International 1998). The failure of cotton crops due to pest infestation, compounded by the widespread supply of adulterated pesticides, is suggested as the leading cause of this suicide epidemic (Karp 1998; Venugopal and Jagadisha 2000). Drought, cuts to subsidies and indebtedness are frequently mentioned as precipitating causes, affecting farmers growing groundnut (peanut) crops as well as cotton (Siddiq 2000; Karp 1998).

G. S. Bhalla *et al.*: *Suicides in Rural Punjab*

One of the most detailed social science studies of suicide for any part of India is *Suicides in Rural Punjab,* written by G. S. Bhalla, S. L. Sharma, N. N. Wig, Swaranjit Mehta and Pramod Kumar (1998) and published by the Institute for Development and Communication of Chandigarh (IDC). The IDC study was prompted by alarming claims made in a letter to the Indian President K. R. Naryanan by the Movement Against State Repression (MASR) that 93 farmer suicides in the Punjab 1998 were the result of poverty resulting from indebtedness, economic injustice and low official prices for agricultural products (Swami 1998). A limited investigation conducted by the newsmagazine *Frontline* found that a number of claimed suicides did not appear in village registers of births and deaths while almost all deaths in certain age groups had been claimed as suicides (Swami 1998). The *Frontline* investigation also found that much indebtedness that existed in the countryside was incurred for unproductive purposes such as the payment of dowry. It found 'no evidence of widespread poverty in the countryside' (Swami 1998).

Their analysis of seasonal patterns to suicide showed no tendency to peak at times when crop failures might have occurred. Their broader analysis of economic trends in the Punjab shows that small farmers are coming under increasing financial stress. The size of operational holdings is falling, and, with them, incomes are declining for small holders. Total indebtedness is rising to worrisome levels and debt levels are higher in the districts with high suicide rates. The IDC investigators found that alcohol use was high and drug addiction was increasing in their study area. They also document a pattern of increasing unemployment among increasingly well-educated rural young men (Bhalla, Sharma *et al.* 1998: 33–44). Consistent with this pattern, the IDC study found that 45 per cent of suicide victims were landless, followed by marginal and small farmers; as the size of holdings rose, the percentage of suicides declined (Bhalla, Sharma *et al.* 1998: 45–46).[2]

Despite this disturbing pattern of economic and social trends in the Punjab, the social background of suicide victims reveals an unexpected pattern. Nearly 60 per cent, for example, were illiterate and nearly 90 per cent were young (Bhalla, Sharma *et al.* 1998: 49). Furthermore just over 80 per cent were married

(Bhalla, Sharma *et al.* 1998: 51). Three quarters of suicide completers had troubled personal relationships with family members and nearly 90 per cent were described by family members as 'loners' who did not share their feelings with others (Bhalla, Sharma *et al.* 1998: 52). Nearly 70 per cent of completers were reported to be heavy drinkers and just over 25 per cent were drug abusers (Bhalla, Sharma *et al.* 1998: 54–55).

The IDC study also concluded that the accounts that had appeared in the press were exaggerated.[3] The most important single cause of the deaths they studied was family discord, the reported cause of 36 per cent of cases. Drug addiction was the principal factor in 18 per cent of cases and indebtedness was responsible for an additional 18 per cent (Bhalla, Sharma *et al.* 1998: 64). While 41 per cent of completers had some level of debt, 71 per cent of the general household survey reported indebtedness (Bhalla, Sharma *et al.* 1998: 68). The authors of this study concluded that the rise in Punjabi suicides 'cannot be termed merely an agricultural crisis. It is a crisis of overall stagnation of the economy, decline in peasant movements, retrogressive social practices and conspicuous consumption, rising unemployment and inequalities' (Bhalla, Sharma *et al.* 1998: 84).

Finally, we may note that the Punjab study throws light on an obscure corner. There have been no systematic studies of the impact of religion on suicide in India, despite the prominence of religion in Durkheim's seminal study. The reason is simple: because of fears of the political misuse of the information, data on religion have not been collected or made available in official data reported since Independence. The Punjab study indicates that these political fears are probably groundless: Bhalla and his colleagues found little discernible difference between religious communities in their tendency to commit suicide. As can be seen in Table 2.4, Sikhs formed the overwhelming majority of suicide cases (72 per cent) that were investigated; this proportion is virtually identical with the percentage of Sikhs in the general population survey. Hindus were slightly over-represented and Muslims somewhat under-represented in the cases that were studied (Bhalla, Sharma *et al.* 1998: 53).

The IDC study of *Suicides in Rural Punjab* also asked those in its general sample whether they approved or disapproved of suicide 'as an escape route'. The overwhelming majority (86 per cent) of respondents disapproved of suicide; only 4 per cent approved and a further 10 per cent offered no opinion (Bhalla, Sharma *et al.* 1998: 78). The authors report that the vast majority of those surveyed regard suicide:

Table 11.1 Punjab suicide victims and general sample population by religion

	Suicide victims	*General population*
Hindu	26.4	19.91
Sikh	71.7	72.75
Muslim	1.9	7.15
Others	–	0.19

Source: Bhalla, Sharma *et al.* 1998, Table 4.9: 53.

. . . as an act of cowardice. In fact, they showed scant regard for the victims of suicide. Struggle is the name of [the] game called life, according to several respondents. Anybody who runs away from it deserves no sympathy said many of them.

(Bhalla, Sharma *et al.* 1998: 77–78)

K. Gopal Iyer and Mehar Singh Manick: *Indebtedness, Impoverishment and Suicides in Rural Punjab*

Many other studies have explored in detail or lesser detail the causes of farmer suicides in central India in the closing years of the twentieth century and the early years of the new millennium (Vidyasagar and Suman Chandra 2003; Vaidyanathan 2006; Mishra 2008, 2006a, 2006b, 2006c; Nagaraj 2008; Gruère, Mehta-Bhatt *et al.* 2008; Choudhary 2009). Iyer and Manick, for example, investigated farmer suicides in Punjab's Sangrur District, their focus being the years 1991–1997. They found that landless labourers, marginal farmers and smallholders comprised the largest portion of their sample of 80 cases, though these were not adjusted for the distribution of holdings in the general population (Iyer and Manick 2000: 13). Two-thirds of those who took their own lives were illiterates (Iyer and Manick 2000: 14). An equal proportion were Jat Sikhs (Iyer and Manick 2000: 16). While focusing on the significance of debt, they note, significantly:

It is necessary to mention here that while indebtedness was the necessary condition . . . the intervening social factor was the sufficient condition for causing suicide. The constant pressure by lending agencies to repay the loan emerged as an important precipitant social factor for committing suicide by the deceased.

(Iyer and Manick 2000: 43)

Their study is also to be noted for its attention to the circumstances of the dependents of suicide victims (Chapter 6). Just over 50 per cent of suicide completers had between four and six dependents, two-thirds of whom were females, mainly children, older adults or adult females (Iyer and Manick 2000: 82). They also point to the role played by social change as a factor in the rising levels of suicides in the district:

The breaking up of the joint families and the emergence of nuclear families has adverse implications on the landholdings. The landholdings of the family are being partitioned among different brothers and consequently the[re] is accentuated fragmentation of holdings. There is also a simultaneous change in the underlying value system of the rural society. This also strengthens the economic process of pauperisation and proletarianisation.

(Iyer and Manick 2000: 100)

The role of the traditional institutions like the *Biradari*, the village *Panchayat*, religious and other humanitarian institutions which were providing mutual help and social security are now under great stress. The economic development, commercialisation and monetisation of the economy, dominance of the capitalist value system, emergence of consumerist culture and the role of mass media have contributed jointly to the degeneration of [the] traditional value system and [society] is overtaken by the value of individualism (Iyer and Manick 2000: 101).

Dandekar, Narawade *et al.*: *Causes of Farmer Suicides in Maharashtra: An Enquiry*

Ajay Dandekar and colleagues at the Tata Institute of Social Sciences (TISS) presented a report to the Mumbai High Court in 2005 (for media reports of the TISS study, see Katakam 2005; Thakkar 2005). The report investigated 36 of 644 Maharashtra farmer suicides that occurred between January 2001 and December 2004 in some depth, concentrating on the Vidharba region. The authors also considered two broad alternative explanations for the agrarian crisis in central India:

> One strand attributes the suicides to the agro-economic problems, namely crop failure, indebtedness and the macro-policy issues arising out of the WTO-led economic regime . . .

The second strand attributes the suicides to the failure of the state and its politico-economic policy . . . (Dandekar, Narawade *et al.* 2005: 4, 5)

Dandekar *et al.* report that all of those investigated were household heads (Dandekar, Narawade *et al.* 2005: 10). They found that 81 per cent of suicides they investigated were of small and medium-sized farmers who came from a range of caste backgrounds (Dandekar, Narawade *et al.* 2005: 17–18). Virtually all who killed themselves were male (97 per cent), married (89 per cent) and literate (81 per cent) (Dandekar, Narawade *et al.* 2005: 10–19).

The study also found that significant changes in the economic and climatic conditions of agriculture seemed to have been responsible for placing many farmers into debt. Their research showed that farmers were caught in a cost-price squeeze, receiving prices that fail to meet the rising costs of cultivation. The retreat from lending to agriculture by the formal banking sector access had forced about half of the sample to take loans from relatives and moneylenders (Dandekar, Narawade *et al.* 2005: 32). They also found that state government subsidies to agriculture did not benefit small farmers who are overwhelmingly dependent on rain-fed agriculture (Dandekar, Narawade *et al.* 2005: 35). The crisis in rain-fed agriculture was most acute in the cotton-belt of Vidharba.

Vidyasagar and Suman Chandra: *Farmers' Suicides in Andhra Pradesh and Karnataka*

Another study that examined farmer suicides is that of Vidyasagar and Suman Chandra of the National Institute of Rural Development, Hyderabad, which covered the period 1998–2003. Like the Tata Institute study, the Andhra and

Karataka study found most who took their own lives were male (95 per cent), with caste, class and education playing little observable part (Vidyasagar and Suman Chandra 2003). The institutional factors identified in the NIRD study were also very similar to those found in Maharashtra: institutional failures, especially the growing dependence of farmers on private sources of credit. They note that tenant farmers who lease in land are ineligible for either formal credit or crop insurance. They conclude:

> Suicide of farmers in such phenomenal scale cannot be just dismissed as personal and psychological problems or mass hysteria. This would amount to psychological reductionism. The central issue of farmers' suicides is the debt trap.
>
> (Vidyasagar and Suman Chandra 2003)

Male and female farmer suicide rates

With the exception of the work of Srijit Mishra, most studies of farmer suicides examine only raw numbers and do not express the results in terms of rates, as we do here. The most forcible conclusion that emerges from an inspection of Figure 11.5 (based on Census of India 1991 figures for self-employed in agriculture) is that, especially in comparison with the occupational groups we have considered so far, with a few exceptions, suicide rates are relatively low. Even in states such as Andhra Pradesh, where farmer suicides have featured regularly in press coverage, suicide rates (14.4), while not low, are certainly not at the very elevated levels of some other occupations. The two states where farmer deaths by suicide *are* very high are Pondicherry and Kerala. The very high suicide rates of female

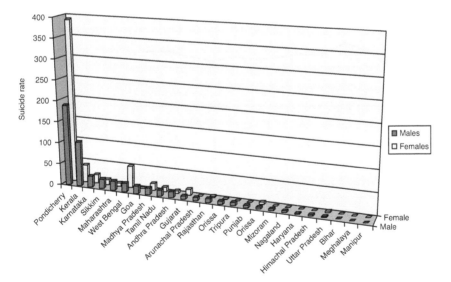

Figure 11.5 Suicide rates for male and female farmers.

and male cultivators in Pondicherry would be of greater concern were the actual numbers (one and four individuals respectively) not so small. The numbers for both males and females are relatively far larger in Kerala, and the suicide rates for male cultivators (107.8) are very high; those for female cultivators are also elevated (42.9). It should be noted that the detailed studies of farmer suicides do not examine female farmer suicides. The other state with very high female farmer suicide rates is West Bengal where the rate is 52.0 per 100,000 (see also Mishra 2008).

Although the absolute numbers of farmers taking their own lives is, as we might expect given the number of cultivators in India, quite large (11,150 males and 2,376 females in 1997), male farmer suicide numbers are little over half those of housewives.

Trend of farmer suicides

The aggregate numbers of farmer suicides have been a continuing cause for concern in the media (for example, Sainath 2007). Although the numbers are alarming, it must be borne in mind that agriculture employs 57 per cent of what the Census terms 'main workers' (Census of India 2007). The trend of cultivator suicide rates between 1997 and 2008 can be seen in Figure 11.6 (see the Appendix to this chapter for a comparison of estimated rates). Rates rose from around 10 per 100,000 in 1997 to 12 in 1998 and the following six years. Since 2004 they have declined to near their level in 1997.

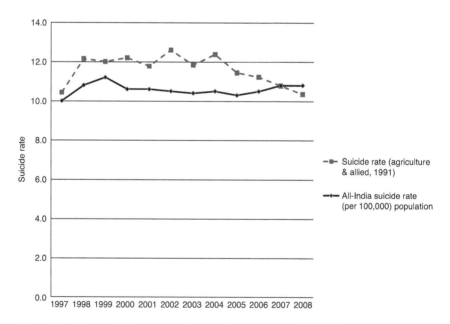

Figure 11.6 Trend of all-India suicide rates for cultivators, 1997–2008.

Housewives

Although some 3,012,047 men were listed by the Census of India, 1991, as having 'household duties' as their occupation, not a single male is included under the occupational category 'housewife' in the suicide statistics compiled by the National Crime Records Bureau.

It can be seen in Figure 11.7 that suicide rates for housewives are relatively low, compared to other occupations. On the whole they are comparable to those for farmers, though in general they are higher than those for female farmers. The highest rates are those found in Pondicherry (54.1), Maharashtra (31.1), Karnataka (27.0), Andhra Pradesh (24.5), Kerala (22.01) and Goa (21.0). It is clear that these are all southern and western states. One would predict that one or another variable associated with modernisation and female empowerment would be associated with this pattern. The best predictor was found to be average household size, a measure of the strength of the traditional family. The regression of suicide rates for housewives in the fourteen major Indian states on average family size is given in Figure 11.8. Where family size is relatively large, housewife suicide rates are low and vice-versa.

Students

There have been only a few serious studies of student suicides. Venkoba Rao and Chinnian reported on 35 attempted and seven completed student suicides, which were registered with the Department of Psychiatry, Erskine Hospital, Madurai in the first 10 months of 1971 (1972). To their surprise there were no instances of depressive illness, nor did any cases arise from the frequently cited 'failure in

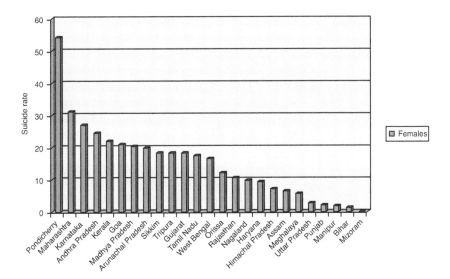

Figure 11.7 Suicide rates for housewives.

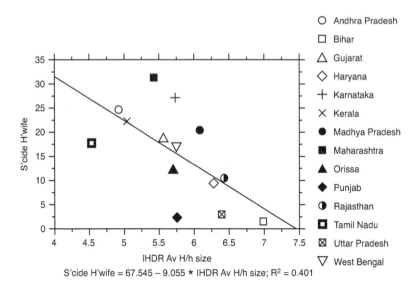

Figure 11.8 Housewife suicide rate vs average household size.

examinations'. On the other hand about one quarter of all cases were schizophrenics (Venkoba Rao and Chinnian 1972: 394).

Every year around the time that examination results come out, the media carry stories of students taking their lives because they did not secure the results which they, or their families, expected, or because a mistake has been made in reporting examination results (see for example *Indian Express* 1998; Washington Report on Middle East Affairs 2002; Nair 2004; Our Staff Reporter 2002). Lurid headlines suggest 'Andhra Students on Suicide Spree' or that there is a 'wave of suicide mania sweeping over the adolescent scene in the post-SSLC scenario' each year in Kerala (Menon 2002). The facts suggest that a more sober conclusion is warranted.

It is evident from examination of Figure 11.9 that despite their prominent media coverage, student suicides occur at relatively low rates. The highest rates for both females and males occur in West Bengal and Tripura. In most states the student suicide rate is much lower than the comparable rates for young men and women aged up to 14 or between 15 and 29 which were examined in Chapter 8. As with the intense media coverage given at certain periods to farmer suicides, media reporting of student suicides tends to magnify these tragic deaths well beyond their true severity as a threat to public health and may even, inadvertently, promote 'copycat' behaviour.

Conclusion

Different occupations expose individuals to varied degrees of risk of suicide. Because of the inexact match between the categories used by Indian police to record the occupations of suicide deaths and the categories used in the Census of India, we can

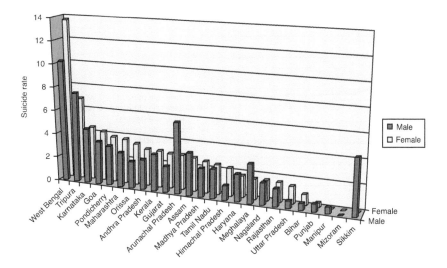

Figure 11.9 Male and female student suicides.

determine suicide rates for only a few occupations. Many others which are of importance, such as agricultural labourers, or which feature in media coverage, such as weavers, are not recorded as separate categories. We know nothing about the suicide numbers of businessmen or occupational groups such as doctors and dentists who have been shown to be at elevated risk in developed economies. Without such records we cannot determine whether the risks of suicide for such groups are high, or low.

Nevertheless, what we have discovered about the risk of suicide of a number of occupational categories helps us understand the differing social forces that seem to create increased suicide risk in India. As in many other societies, those without employment in India are at very much higher risk of taking their own lives. So too are government employees, whose potential vulnerability may be a pointer to the broader risk of suicide of other professions which require higher levels of education and professionalism.[4] On the other hand, neither farmers nor students, often the subject of alarmist coverage in the media, have an especially high risk of suicide. This may make a more sobering story than those that seek to dramatise genuine economic distress by giving prominence to the suicide deaths of a number of distressed individuals, but it is also a more scientifically accurate one. It is probably fruitless to hope that the media might devote its attention in rough proportion to the actual risk, but on that basis, the suicides of housewives should receive many more times the press coverage than they do now.

Appendix

The Census of India enumerates cultivators, not farmers. From one Census to another, the definitions of who is a cultivator have changed, making the precise

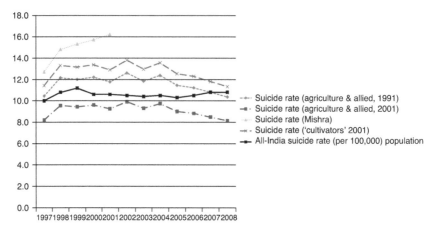

Figure 11.10 Comparison of cultivator suicide rate estimates, 1997–2008.

use of Census a subject best left to experts (for a discussion of the problems with the 1961 and 1971 Censuses, see Rudolph and Rudolph 1987). In addition, the police do not utilise the precise Census categories in recording suicides. In this chapter we utilised the numbers from the 1991 Census, indexed up by the estimated mid-year population figures provided by the National Crime Records Bureau. The number of cultivators enumerated in the 2001 Census was very much higher than our estimated figures. In Figure 11.10 we compare the 1991-based suicide rates with those based on the 2001 figures (labelled Agriculture & allied), a second 2001 estimate based only on main and marginal cultivators, as well as Mishra's figures for 1997–2000 (Mishra 2006a) which, because they are based on smaller age-adjusted population figures, have a higher estimated rate.

Notes

1 The relationship with corruption perceptions is not clear-cut, with low suicide rates at either extreme, and a range from low to high suicide rates at middle corruption perception rates.
2 Bhalla and his colleagues neglect to point out that distribution of suicides is almost exactly the same as the distribution of holdings themselves (c.f. Bhalla, Sharma *et al.* 1998: 34). It seems likely that the rates are quite similar for all categories.
3 Swami concludes from comparing the IDC findings with the original claims that 'presumably only 11 cases in [the MASR] list [of 93 suicides] were real ones' (Swami 1998).
4 Hundreds of workers in the Information Technology (IT) and business process outsourcing industries were reported to have contacted an on-line suicide counselling service after it was opened in late 2005. 'About 20 per cent of the mailers talk about how "life is worthless" and why they want to end it. "They are angry, frustrated and depressed. They don't even get time to talk it out with their family or friends because of the night shifts and work pressure," says [Sneha's Director] Mr Sankaranarayanan' (Soman 2005).

12 Marriage, the family and suicide

If there is a single finding in suicide research that approaches the status of a sociological law, it is that marriage everywhere reduces the risk of suicide. Emile Durkheim found that for those over the age of 20, marriage cut the risk of suicide in half (Durkheim 1951: 179). Many subsequent findings have come to the same conclusion. Several studies of suicide in the US (Henry and Short 1954; Breault 1986) reported that marriage protects while divorce increases risk. Hassan (1983: 54–60) found a similar pattern in Singapore. The 'sociological law' of marriage is aptly summarised by Ruzicka and Choi:

> In all societies for which there are statistics available, suicide mortality has been considerably higher among those who are not married than among those who are married.
>
> (Ruzicka and Choi 1993: 108)

There has been little study of the relationship between suicide and marital status in developing countries such as India (Latha, Bhat *et al.* 1996).

The all-India picture

In a previously published paper that used data from 1995, the first to classify suicides by marriage status, we sought to test whether marriage was protective in India (Mayer and Ziaian 2002).[1] We also explored whether widows who have traditionally faced severe discrimination in Indian society, and separated or divorced individuals who experience social disapproval would both have higher rates of suicide.

Our results were surprising in several areas (Table 12.1). First, we found that marriage does not convey protection: two-thirds of all completed suicides were married. This was principally the case for Indian men. Men in India are at lower risk of suicide before rather than after marriage. Except for the category of 'never married', the suicide rates for males exceed those of women in every marital category. Married women in India do enjoy the protection found elsewhere in the world.

When marriage ends in separation or divorce, the risks of suicide rise sharply. The rate for men is an extremely high 347 per 100,000; for women a very high 126 per 100,000.

Table 12.1 Number of suicide victims, ratio of suicide victims and suicide rates classified by marital status and gender per 100,000, India, 1995

	Male		Female		Persons		% Suicide victims	% Male to total	% Female to total	M/f ratio
	Number	Rate	Number	Rate	Number	Rate				
Never married	12,244	14.9	7,889	21.9	20,133	17.0	23.00	60.8	39.18	.7
Married	35,241	17.3	24,691	11.9	59,932	14.6	67.0	58.8	41.2	1.5
Widow/-er	2,314	25.2	2,297	8.1	4,611	12.2	5.0	50.2	49.8	3.1
Divorced/ separated	2,558	346.8	19,44	126.4	4,502	197.9	5.0	56.8	43.2	2.7
Total suicides	52,357	17.7	36,821	13.4	89,178	15.7	100.0	58.7	41.3	1.3

Source: Mayer and Ziaian 2002: 300.

Table 12.2 Index of preservation, by marital status, India, 1995

	Index of Preservation	
	Male	*Female*
Never married	0.86	1.84
Married	1	1
Widow/-er	1.46	0.68
Divorced/Separated	20.05	10.62

The relative relationships between marital categories are often captured by the 'coefficient of preservation', presented in Table 12.2. The coefficient was named and first utilised by Durkheim in 1897 (1951: 177); it is computed by the following ratios: $\frac{\text{Never married}}{\text{Married}}$, $\frac{\text{Widowed}}{\text{Married}}$, $\frac{\text{Divorced/Separated}}{\text{Married}}$. These ratios may be considered as indicators of the relative immunity conferred by marriage in comparison with not being married, being divorced or widowed. If any of these ratios is larger than 1, the incidence of suicide for the relevant group is higher than for those who are married. For men, the lowest relative risk is for the never married. Suicide risk increases at marriage and at the death of a spouse. Divorced men are twenty times more at risk than married men. For women, marriage reduces the rate of suicide by almost half. Some studies have suggested that issues relating to marriage and sexuality such as familial disputes and proposed marriage and problems relating to pre-marital relationships help to explain why suicide rates are higher in females before their marriage (Deoki, 1987, Haynes, 1984, Karim and Price, 1975, cited in Booth 1999b). Loss of a partner reduces it further still – something we will discuss in greater depth below. As with men, divorce greatly increases the risk of suicide, divorcees being at ten times the risk of married women.

The impact of social forces

In our published paper we also explored the impact of literacy, industrialization and life expectancy on different gender and marital categories. We found a significant correlation between industrialization and divorced male suicide rates ($r = 0.59, p < 0.05$). Life expectancy was associated with suicide rates for married ($r = 0.67, p < 0.01$) and widowed ($r = 0.69, p < 0.01$) men (Mayer and Ziaian 2002: 300). The variable with the strongest correlation was literacy. The correlation coefficients were: single men ($r = 0.61, p < 0.05$), married men ($r = 0.76, p < 0.001$), widowed men ($r = 0.71, p < 0.01$). For married women the correlation was ($r = 0.64, p < 0.01$) (Mayer and Ziaian 2002: 301).

Marital status and suicide at the state-level

Let us now turn our attention to the relationship between marital status and suicide as it appears at the level of the Indian states. On the basis of what we have learned about the all-India picture, it is logical to expect that we will find a repetition of the national pattern that married men do not experience the same immunity from suicide as women. We may also expect to find that widowed women have the highest immunity against suicide, and that both sexes are highly vulnerable in a divorce situation. On the basis of all-India findings, we would also predict that suicide rates for males and females in the Indian states would be noticeably larger for single females than they are for single males and these ratios would be larger for divorced or widowed males.

In our analysis of the impact of marital status on suicide at state-level we utilised official suicide data for 1997 that were made available to the authors by the National Crime Records Bureau. As anticipated, at the state level, also, we do not find the common European and North American rank ordering of marital suicide rates: married < single < widowed and divorced. The relationship between the various categories varies according to sex and to the different states of India can be seen in Table 12.3.

In the Indian states as a whole, as indicated in Table 12.3, the average female suicide rates in 1997 for those who were married, never married, widowed, and divorced were, 12.1, 23.3, 9.1 and 136.7 respectively. The suicide rate for widowed women was the lowest (9.1). However, there were noticeable variations among the different states. For example, suicide rates for widowed women in Haryana, West Bengal, Tamil Nadu, Tripura and Karnataka were much higher than in other states. Nonetheless, widowed women's rates were still lower than those for widowed men in these states. Further, the suicide rates for married women were also lower than for never married, and divorced/separated women. This suggests that for women, widowhood and marriage provide the best protection against suicide in the Indian states, whereas divorced and single women appear to be elevating the suicide rate within these categories of marital status.

The state-level pattern for men is different from that for women. In the Indian states as a whole, as indicated in Table 12.3, the average male suicide rates in 1997 for those who were married, never married, widowed, and divorced were 17.7, 16.0, 27.6 and 367.8 respectively. Never-married men were better protected against suicide than married men. The divorced/separated suicide rate was highest for men, namely, 367.8 per 100,000. However, there were significant variations among the different states. For example, suicide for this group in Punjab, Kerala, Assam, Karnataka and Tamil Nadu occurs at astonishingly high rates, whereas in some very small states such as Arunachal Pradesh, Goa, Manipur, Meghalaya and Sikkim with small numbers of divorced/separated persons, men were apparently completely immune from suicide. In most states where the divorced male suicide rate was high, the divorced female suicide rate was also high. The exceptions were small eastern Indian hill states: Sikkim (male rate: 0, female rate: 106.7), Mizoram (male rate: 44.6, female rate: 0) and Nagaland (male rate: 81.2, female rate: 0). In the Indian states as a whole, men who had never married had lower suicide rates than the married and the widowed.

One notable if incidental finding of our study is that the divorce rate for females is much higher than for males in all states with the exception of Himachal Pradesh,

Table 12.3 Indian states and suicide rates classified by sex, marital status, 1997

States	Males				Females				Total suicide rates for marital categories for each state
	Never married	Married	Widowed	Divorced or separated	Never married	Married	Widowed	Divorced or separated	
Andhra Pradesh	16.3	20.6	51.1	146.2	23.8	15.2	8.9	58.5	18.2
Arunachal Pradesh	13.3	12.2	0.0	0.0	18.4	7.9	0.0	0.0	10.8
Assam	28.0	21.8	25.7	1027.6	27.3	8.7	6.7	116.0	20.1
Bihar	2.0	2.0	5.0	393.7	5.5	1.7	2.2	147.4	2.4
Goa	25.3	23.9	82.5	0.0	16.2	17.8	10.0	0.0	21.0
Gujarat	10.4	12.9	27.1	87.8	18.3	13.1	8.7	71.2	13.3
Haryana	12.0	16.2	82.7	192.1	9.1	9.0	19.4	113.7	13.8
Himachal Pradesh	8.7	10.3	6.0	124.2	8.3	5.3	1.9	84.8	8.0
Karnataka	30.2	40.7	75.2	836.9	43.3	21.4	13.5	178.9	32.0
Kerala	33.3	67.0	108.3	1267.8	22.5	24.7	10.2	142.2	40.7
Madhya Pradesh	17.6	17.2	21.2	111.3	34.9	13.0	8.6	70.1	16.5
Maharashtra	16.8	26.6	39.0	518.0	31.4	18.2	8.3	110.1	22.3
Manipur	1.3	0.7	0.0	0.0	0.4	1.2	0.0	0.0	0.9
Meghalaya	12.8	6.7	15.7	0.0	2.9	2.5	2.3	0.0	5.8
Mizoram	9.0	8.9	0.0	44.6	2.9	1.3	0.0	0.0	5.7
Nagaland	7.8	10.3	0.0	81.2	2.0	2.3	0.0	0.0	6.0
Orissa	16.9	14.6	14.4	196.7	21.5	11.4	8.6	89.1	14.5
Punjab	3.5	3.8	4.6	2864.0	1.5	2.5	0.2	443.3	4.1
Rajasthan	14.0	9.6	20.4	399.0	27.5	6.9	8.6	433.2	10.6
Sikkim	19.3	22.4	0.0	0.0	40.7	13.7	0.0	106.7	20.5
Tamil Nadu	15.3	26.1	49.8	840.0	19.4	16.9	15.0	240.0	22.1
Tripura	32.4	28.7	69.8	595.3	56.5	25.4	15.4	269.3	32.7
Uttar Pradesh	5.1	4.4	5.3	79.3	7.8	3.9	2.8	180.6	4.6
West Bengal	27.3	27.3	81.5	622.8	44.3	26.0	16.3	210.3	29.4
Total States	16.0	17.7	27.6	367.8	23.3	12.1	9.1	136.7	16.3

Source: National Crime Records Bureau 1999, Government of India (special data runs).

Table 12.4 Comparison of coefficients of preservation for divorced suicides in Southern and Northern kinship systems

State	Coefficient of Preservation
South India	
Andhra Pradesh	3.9
Karnataka	8.3
Kerala	5.8
Tamil Nadu	14.2
Average	*8.05*
North India	
Bihar	89.1
Haryana	12.7
Himachal Pradesh	15.9
Madhya Pradesh	5.4
Punjab	174.2
Rajasthan	62.8
Uttar Pradesh	46.7
Average	*58.1*

Note: $F = 0.006$; $p = 0.0007$.

Rajasthan and Uttar Pradesh (for all states, the male divorce rate is 251.7; the female divorce rate is 562.3 per 100,000).[2] By contrast, the divorced suicide rate is much higher for males than females in all Indian states except for Rajasthan, Sikkim and Uttar Pradesh (for all states, the divorced male suicide rate is 367.8; the divorced female suicide rate is 136.7 per 100,000). While it is a general finding of studies worldwide for divorced suicide rates to be higher than for other marital categories, the very high suicide rates among those who have divorced in India are unusual and may reflect the relatively stigmatised status of those who are divorced in a society where it is still exceptional and rare.

We sought to explore the significance of these high divorced suicide rates using Pearson product–moment correlations. We utilised the divorce rate as a proxy measure of the social acceptability of divorce in Indian society. We hypothesised that where divorces are uncommon they are relatively unacceptable and that suicide rates among divorced individuals would be higher. We found, as predicted, that the relationship between the male divorce rate and the female divorced suicide rate was negative yet statistically significant ($r = -0.41$; $p < 0.05$), indicating that in a state where the male divorce rate was low – and hence relatively less socially acceptable – the divorced female suicide rate was high. It was of interest to note that a weak negative but not significant relationship existed between the male divorce rate and male suicide divorce rate ($r = -0.34$), and between the female divorce rate and the female suicide divorce rate ($r = -0.39$), indicating the possibility that in states where divorce is more common for males and females, divorced men and divorced women are less prone to suicide.

Widows and suicide

Perhaps the most unexpected finding to emerge from our investigation of the relationship between marital status and suicide rates concerns those who are widows and widowers. We predicted, on the basis of studies elsewhere in the world, that those who had lost a partner would be at higher risk of suicide. We expected that this would be especially the case for widowed women in India, since they have traditionally been stigmatized. Many studies have found widows to experience discrimination in the provision of basic social supports. It is commonly suggested that many widows suffer from psychological hardships as a consequence. Chen states that widows and their children constitute a financial burden to their extended family and kinship groups (1997). Traditionally, unlike widowers, widows were not permitted to remarry. Because they had no right to inherit their husbands' property, they were usually financially dependent, received little support from their families or communities, and had severe restrictions on job opportunities (Chen 1997; Drèze and Sen 1998). Mackinnon (2000) reported that in most parts of India widows are still considered harbingers of bad luck. In the light of the very low status of widows in traditional Indian society, we expected that widows would have very high suicide rates.

Our hypothesis was only partially confirmed. The conventional relationship does appear to apply to widowed men who are at over three times greater risk of completing suicide than widowed women. However, *the suicide rates for women were utterly unexpected.* We were astonished to find that they have the *lowest* suicide rate for any marital category, male or female.

Not only is the finding striking because of its unexpected nature, it also poses a significant challenge to our conventional understanding of the role of women in Indian society. Overall, widowed women are one-third as likely to commit suicide as widowed men (9.1, and 27.6 per 100,000 respectively). This finding confirms in detail our all-India survey and reinforces the finding that low social status, poor health, financial problems and loneliness of widowed women in India, which were identified by many studies (for example, Chen and Drèze 1995; Chen 1997; Drèze and Sen 1998; Mackinnon 2000), do not increase the risk of suicide for this group of women.[3] Our findings appear to completely contradict previous studies (Freed and Freed 1989; Mehta, 1990, cited in Booth 1999a; Diekstra 1992), which have claimed that Indian women have a high female suicide rate because of their low status and powerlessness. The difference in suicide rates of widowed men and women may suggest that social environment may not be more important than economic environment in suicide, as was suggested by Yip (1996: 499).

In only three states (Haryana, Bihar and Rajasthan) were ratios of widowed-to-married greater than one for widowed women. For widowed men, ratios were greater than 1 in 17 states, indicating that married men had significantly lower suicide rates than widowed men in the majority of the Indian states. This may reflect age patterns in Indian suicides (Chapter 8). The low suicide rates of widows may well be related to this pattern as Drèze and Sen (1995: 173) noted that 63 per cent of Indian women over the age of 60 are widowed.

Conclusion

The existing suicide literature based on experience in Western nations suggests that in almost all cases the suicide rates of those who are married are lower than those of the unmarried, widowed, or divorced. It also indicates that men in every marital category are at greater risk of suicide than women. The suicide data for Indian men and women reveal different patterns.

Taking the Indian states as a whole, single males had lower suicide rates than single females (16.0 and 23.3 per 100,000 respectively). This is an unexpected finding; in Europe and North America unmarried women generally have lower suicide rates than men. One may speculate that the difference between single men and women may be that single men in Indian culture are more likely to have closer interpersonal ties with their mothers, and that such ties may be very important in maintaining a sense of support and well-being.

We found that overall, married women are slightly more immune to suicide than married men (12.1 and 17.7 per 100,000 respectively). Here again the Indian experience is at variance to the findings reported in a number of more industrialised societies. For example, Hassan reported that in Australia in 1981, the male suicide rate (18 per 100,000) was three times higher than that for females (1995: 113). These results may be the other side of the coin of the relative preservation of unmarried men – the intense bond between Indian mothers and sons.

The distinctly lower suicide rates of unmarried compared with those of married men show another striking difference between Indian and Western experience. A possible explanation for the Indian pattern emerges from Kathinka Sinha-Kerkhoff's study of young men in Ranchi, Jharkhand (2003). She argues that these young, unmarried men:

> did not despair, nor were they depressed, and certainly not passive. They were active in day-to-day life, trying to cope with hierarchies, ignore them or even reverse them. What is more, sometimes and in certain places, life is but a dream for young men in Ranchi. They often expressed relief at the fact that they did not have to shoulder 'adult responsibilities' yet. Not only age but also the fact that they were still studying and unmarried often defined them as 'mere boys' with corresponding masculinities that encompassed privileges that neither adult men nor male children enjoyed. In other words, they often perceived 'being a boy' as an asset, but feared 'becoming adults'.
>
> (Sinha-Kerkhoff 2003: 434–435)

The future hung as a sword of Damocles above their heads. Whereas, 'girls do not have to think of anything. Their husband will think for them'. Boys on the other hand 'have to carry all the burdens. We have to think about the family's physical, mental and economic needs. We also have to look after our sisters' well being'. (Sinha-Kerkhoff 2003: 438).[4]

Although marriage may offer some degree of protection to women, we must not lose sight of the fact that a clear majority of those who commit suicide in India are, in fact, married. The high percentage of the married in the total of suicides may itself be a reflection of the prevalence of arranged marriages in Indian society. The strains that emerge from arranged marriages in circumstances of social change are a theme that emerges with especial clarity in studies of the Indian diaspora.[5] Booth noted in the context of Fiji, for example, 'Previous studies indicate that marriage (which is usually arranged) is not protective against suicide because of disharmony with husband and/or in-laws' (Booth 1999a: 444; see also Haynes 1984: 436).

The evidence suggests that in contemporary India the changes that are taking place in family relations are not, or at least not at present, leading to the reduced suicide rates. As we will see in the final chapter, movement towards the nuclear family in India is associated with higher rather than lower suicide rates. The relatively frequent association of 'quarrel with kin' as an immediately precedent cause of suicide which we noted in Chapter 4, and which we will see is the most frequent aetiology of suicide in Pondicherry in Chapter 15, may be evidence that some young Indians in states where literacy levels and exposure to the media are high, find themselves in intense familial conflict. The darker side of the conflict may be revealed in newspaper accounts which suggest that pressures exerted by in-laws over levels of dowry may be responsible for high levels of suicide deaths in some regions. Prabhjot Singh, for example, reported in 2000 that 'harassment by in-laws for various reasons, including insufficient dowry, accounts for 80 per cent of suicides by women in Punjab, where the incidence of ending one's own life has been alarmingly on the rise in the recent past' (Singh 2000).

Our findings concerning the impact of divorce on suicide are one area where behaviour in India is parallel to that reported elsewhere. We saw in Tables 12.1 and 12.3 that the suicide rates for divorced men and women are far higher than for other marital categories. Durkheim drew similar conclusions from his late nineteenth century European data (1951: 262). Hassan's figures for Australia, in an era when divorce had become relatively common, show that suicide rates for those who are divorced are about three times higher than those who are married (1995: 113).

The high divorced suicide rate among Indian men may indeed be due to society's excessive influence over men as was claimed by Durkheim (1951). However, we feel unable to accept Durkheim's explanation of the lower suicide rates of women because of their lack of involvement in society (1951: 385). In one of his more outrageously patriarchal passages he stated that the mental life of women was 'less developed' and that

> ... being a more instinctive creature than man, woman has only to follow her instincts to find calmness and peace. She thus does not require so strict a social regulation as marriage, and particularly monogamic marriage ... So divorce protects her and she has frequent recourse to it.
>
> (Durkheim 1951: 272)

The sharp lines of gender discrimination in India seem to us to offer more plausible grounds of explanation. For example, as Chen pointed out (1995) the consequence of separation from one's spouse is very different for men and women. Men have more freedom to remarry, more extensive property rights, wider opportunities for employment, and a more authoritative claim on economic support from their children. Secondly, the social meaning of divorce and the level of social support and independence for men and women in Indian society may be a major factor in producing this pattern. Divorced men may be placed under greater stress by the increased probability of role-conflict or role-tension, financial debts or legal action for maintenance, in particular for men with children. Divorced women, despite the strong social disapproval they experience, may retain stronger ties with their parental communities. While this may be especially true in southern kinship systems where close ties with their parental homes are the rule, Patricia Jeffrey's evidence from Uttar Pradesh indicates that women there must rely on their parents in the event of marital breakdown (Jeffrey 2003). Partial confirmation of this hypothesis emerges from a comparison of the coefficients of preservation in the southern states (in which marriage with affiliated families such as the 'cross-cousin' marriage pattern in Tamil Nadu was traditional) with northern states (where village exogamy was traditional) (Table 12.4). Although there is some overlap in levels, on the whole the relative levels of divorced suicides are significantly lower where brides do not traditionally sever ties with their parental homes.

Notes

1 The material in this section has been summarised from Mayer and Ziaian 2002.
2 This result may be no more than an artefact of a greater propensity of divorced men to remarry.
3 This is of special interest because, according to Chen (1997: 311), 'the proportion of widows in female population rises sharply with age, reaching over 60 per cent among women aged sixty and above'. Mari Bhat (1994, cited in Drèze and Sen 1998), for example, reports that mortality rates are, on average, 86 per cent higher among elderly widows than among married women of the same age. This may indicate that although there is a low suicide rate for widows, the death rate for this group is high due to other causes. However, social conditions of widows vary greatly between different age groups, regions, communities and classes.
4 We are indebted to Niharika Gupta for drawing Sinha-Kerhoff's work to our attention.
5 We discuss the suicide experience of Indian migrants in Chapter 14.

13 Alcohol and suicide

As part of his development of the justification for the sociological analysis of suicide, Durkheim considered, and rejected, any association with the consumption of alcohol, noting that if one compared maps of regions of suicide and alcohol 'almost no connection is seen between them' (Durkheim 1951: 77). Consistent with the Durkheimian tradition, early suicide literature tended to ignore alcohol consumption as a possible risk factor for suicide. More recently, however, Lester (1995) has shown that there is considerable documentation to support the idea that there is a positive association between alcohol consumption and suicide. Most research has investigated this issue in industrialised nations and there has been little that has focused on less developed countries, such as India.

Durkheim and alcohol

Alcohol consumption was not discussed in early suicide research literature because Durkheim (1951: 81) contended that as alcoholism was a psychiatric disorder, and therefore an individual social problem, it could not be used to explain variations in a population-level social problem, such as suicide (Skog 1991). However, explanations of the role that alcohol may play in suicidal behaviour do appear to be consistent with Durkheim's (1951) ideas, even though he did not specifically consider an association. Skog et al. (1991; Skog, Teixeira et al. 1995), for example, have indicated that alcohol abuse generally leads to the social isolation and disintegration that Durkheim said was a prerequisite for suicidal behaviour. This is also consistent with more recent explanations about how alcohol might encourage suicidal behaviour (Stack 2000). For example, chronic alcohol abuse typically leads to reduced self-esteem and thus to the disintegration of marriages, family, work and social networks (Lester 1992). With increased alcohol abuse, the alcoholic tends to lose social ties, becomes increasingly socially isolated with fewer social supports and therefore more vulnerable to suicide (Stack 2000).

There are other explanations that relate more specifically to how alcohol affects psychological well being. For example, alcohol consumption often promotes depression, which has been indicated as a key risk factor for suicidal behaviour (Lester 1992). At the same time, it may also be a form of self-medication for depression. In industrialised countries, it has long been recognised that depression is associated with suicide completion (Klerman 1987, 1988). For example, in Australia, about 70 per cent of all suicides committed each year are by depressed individuals (Burrows 1994). According to Wasserman (1989), when the general level of alcohol consumption in an area changes, for example, during times of prohibition or war, levels of depression are concurrently altered, significantly affecting suicide rates.

Besides its association with depression, alcohol consumption may also encourage emotional disinhibition (Stack 2000). This can subsequently lead to reckless or impulsive behaviours that might result in suicidal death (Skog 1991). In many cases, it may be unclear which comes first. Another explanation focuses on the pharmacological consequences of mixing otherwise safe sedative medication with alcohol, resulting in a possible lethal cocktail (Stack 2000).

Alcohol and suicide

Research findings to date appear to support a positive relationship between alcohol consumption and suicide. For example, Hawton, Fagg *et al.* (1989) reported that suicides tended to be high alcohol consumers and abusers while Wilhelmsen, Elmfeldt *et al.* (1983) also reported that alcoholics commit suicide at a higher rate than do non-alcoholics. In Mexico, Escobedo and Ortiz (2002) found that there was a significant, positive correlation between the number of liquor outlets and suicide rates in 11 Mexican counties. A major review of clinical studies by the Centers for Disease Control (1990) reported that 28 per cent of suicides in the US in 1987 were related to alcohol. In other research, Britton and McPherson (2001) reported that during 1996 in England and Wales, suicide was the main cause of alcohol-related deaths in both males and females aged 25 to 34 years. It was also the second and third cause of such deaths in those aged 16 to 24 years and 35 to 44 years respectively, as well as the third cause of death in males 45 to 54 years.

There have also been some notable results from time-series research investigating the population-level association between alcohol and suicide. For example, Lester (1995) examined data from 13 nations for the years 1950–1972, and found ten countries, including Canada, Finland, Norway, Sweden and the US, reported a positive association between alcohol consumption and suicide rates. Similarly, Norström (1988) reported that in Norway and Sweden, during the years 1930–1980, there were significant, positive associations between per capita alcohol consumption and suicide. It was shown that when consumption of alcohol increased by one litre per capita, there was a significant accompanying increase in the total suicide rate of 16 per cent for Norway and 15 per cent for Sweden.

In another study, Skog (1993) found that there was a significant and positive relationship between alcohol consumption and suicide in Hungary in the post-World War II period, 1950–1990. Skog (1993) also analysed alcohol consumption and suicide data from Denmark for the years 1911–1924. In this 'natural experiment', alcohol taxes, and therefore the price of alcohol, increased dramatically during the years 1916–1917, resulting in a considerable fall in alcohol consumption. It was found that as the alcohol consumption decreased, there was a direct proportional decrease in suicide among alcohol abusers while there was no such result for the suicide rate among non-abusers. Skog (1993) reported that when consumption of alcohol decreased by one litre per capita in Denmark, there was a significant reduction in the suicide rate by 2.5 per cent. Skog (1993) noted, however, that the effect in Denmark was not as marked as Norström (1988) had found for Sweden and Norway.

In more extensive research, Ramstedt (2001) studied the relationship between alcohol consumption and suicide in 14 European countries. This study tested the hypothesis that such a relationship would be more likely to be positive in 'dry' rather than 'wet' drinking cultures. A dry drinking culture is generally typified by 'low per capita consumption, explosive drinking on weekends and a restrictive alcohol control policy' (p. 60). Alternatively, a wet drinking culture usually refers to an area with a generally high level of drinking all the time and fewer restrictions on alcohol availability. Ramstedt (2001) found that the suicide rate for males in dry cultures was more related to alcohol consumption than for males in wet cultures, while for women, the effect was more obvious in medium and low consumption areas. It was concluded that the relationship between alcohol and suicide is influenced by culture, particularly so in non-drinking or low-consumption cultures.

Rossow cites an earlier review, which reported that a range between 10 and 54 per cent of suicides were associated with alcohol abuse (Roy and Linnoila, 1986 cited in Rossow 2000: 415). Rossow cites another review that found that 30–40 per cent of male suicide attempters and 15–20 per cent of female attempters were alcohol abusers (Rygnestad *et al.*, 1992 cited in Rossow 2000).

Caces and Harford (1998) reported time-series analysis of suicide and alcohol consumption for the US for the years 1934–1987. Although significant associations between suicide rates and alcohol consumption could not be demonstrated, it was found that when unemployment was introduced into a multivariate model, alcohol consumption was significantly associated to overall suicide deaths, particularly among those aged up to 59 years. When alcohol consumption increased by one litre per capita, the suicide rate increased by 3 per cent overall, and 5 per cent for those aged under 60 years. Other research found that suicide might be related more to alcohol 'type', rather than actual alcohol consumption. For example, Gruenewald, Ponicki *et al.* (1995) reported time-series analysis of suicide and alcohol consumption for the US from 1970–1989. This investigation concluded that suicide rates were more related to the sales of spirit-type alcoholic beverages than to sales of wine or beer. However, it was also reported that the relationship between alcohol and suicide was more complicated as suicidal behaviour was influenced by other factors, such as employment levels, religion, the general age composition of relevant populations and per capita land area.

Alcohol and the Indian experience

Although alcohol has been consumed in India for centuries, it is only in recent decades that amounts and patterns of consumption have changed to the extent that alcohol-related social problems have been noticed (Saxena 1999). Chopra and

Chopra (1965) have commented on ancient Indian literature that mentions different types of intoxicating beverages popular in Indian culture. For example, the elite classes appear to have consumed *soma*, a beverage that played a key role in the ritual ceremonies of the Vedic peoples. Soma is thought to have been derived from plant roots or stems or 'magic mushroom' (*amanita muscaria*) type plants and was purported to have an intoxicant, hallucinogenic effect. However, there is still debate about its origins and the use of *soma* continues to be shrouded in mystery (Hajicek-Dobberstein 1995; Staal 2001).

Another, less mysterious, alcoholic beverage mentioned in the ancient texts is *sura*, made from fermented sugarcane and rice, supposed to increase the courage of warriors (cited in Saxena 1999). While later historical writings make little further mention of *soma*, they indicate that the consumption of *sura*-type beverages has continued into the present day. Examples include *toddy*, a wine fermented from palm sap and similar to that consumed in South India in ancient times (Dikshitar 1951). Another is *arrack* or 'common spirit', distilled from various plants, for example, fermented sap from palms, cane-molasses or rice, depending on the region (Yule and Burnell 1886). Traditional medical preparations also included alcohol among their ingredients and this practice continues today.

It is apparent from the old medical texts that ancient Indian cultures were aware of the dangers of excessive consumption of fermented beverages (Saxena 1999). For example, Hindu culture prohibited drinking among Brahmins, although in contemporary culture, prohibitions are weaker for Hindus than other religious groups such as Muslims, whose religious beliefs forbid alcohol consumption. Nowadays, the Sikhs have a less prohibitive stance toward alcohol than some groups and the Punjab, their traditional homeland, has one of the highest levels of alcohol consumption in India (Saxena 1999). Traditionally, there is some suggestion that areas of a more tribal nature have been culturally predisposed to alcohol consumption and that such areas continue to condone it (Saldanha 1995). However, until more recently in most other areas, alcohol consumption was not routinely encouraged and abstinence was considered a virtue by most of the populace. Furthermore, during the years of India's struggle for independence, there was a strong voice from Congress Party leadership for the prohibition of alcohol and this was integral to the fight for independence (Saxena 1999). After Independence, prohibition was introduced in some states and territories.

Over time, alcohol consumption has become more accepted in Indian culture, initially encouraged by the British attitude favouring alcohol over the more popular traditional intoxicants of Indian society, such as opium and cannabis. Licensing laws therefore changed over the years, contributing to increased alcohol production. This also encouraged more refined methods of alcohol distillation producing 'foreign-made alcohol' beverages of much higher alcohol content than the traditional fermented beverages. All these factors ensured that by the time India became independent, alcohol had become synonymous with Western mores as well as a recognised element of Indian society (Saxena 1999).

Today, the alcohol industry is 'big business in India' (Mahal 2000: 1) and there has been a significant rise in the rate of alcohol consumption, compared to a general downward trend in most other countries of the world. Alcohol has become an important source of tax revenue, especially in some of the southern states (Abraham 1995). As mentioned, alcohol use has also been a significant political issue in India and there continues to be a strong voice for prohibition, originating mainly from more traditional sections of society (Saxena 1999). Such condemnations range from its implication in road accidents to its deleterious effects on consumers' health and finances as well as their 'moral fibre' (Mahal 2000).

India is characterized by striking disparities across its states in terms of attitudes toward alcohol. As mentioned, levels of alcohol consumption can be influenced by the dominant religious and tribal nature of states but also by literacy levels and the social prominence of females (Mahal 2000). There is some suggestion that increased literacy should lead to lower consumption of alcohol because with education, people become more aware of the health implications of excessive alcohol consumption. Furthermore, there has always been a strong anti-alcohol voice among women in India and it has therefore been suggested that alcohol consumption might be lower in areas with a prevalence of female-headed households (Mahal 2000). Alcohol policy is the province of state, not federal, jurisdictions and therefore legal drinking age and tax laws vary between the states. In addition, in some states certain types of alcohol have been banned and in others, prohibition or partial prohibition has operated at different times. For example, 'country spirit' or 'arrack' was banned in Andhra Pradesh (Abraham 1995) during the 1990s, although that has since been repealed (Mahal 2000). Tamil Nadu was 'dry' until the early 1990s and alcohol could only be acquired with a permit, however it now ranks as the state with the highest level of alcohol consumption per capita in India (Niven, Honan *et al.* 1999). Neighbouring Pondicherry, on the other hand, has always had a more moderate attitude towards alcohol, probably partly because of the French influence. Alcohol is also much cheaper there than in states such as Tamil Nadu. As with Andhra Pradesh, prohibition was introduced in Haryana during the 1990s but has since been repealed. Gujarat, on the other hand, has banned alcohol since 1949 and is reported to have had few apparent social problems (Mahal 2000).

These discrepancies raise the question of whether prohibition works in terms of reducing social health problems such as suicide. As mentioned, Skog (1993) demonstrated a significant relationship between a time of prohibition, falling alcohol consumption and suicide rates for Denmark during 1911–1924. There have been arguments against prohibition in countries such as the US (Thornton 1991), but the situation is less clear in India (Mahal 2000). Does this relate to a lack of available data that may inform about consumption and effects on health? It is expected that the debate will increase in intensity given that alcohol consumption is increasing. For example, in the Punjab, it is estimated that about 13 per cent of males aged 15 to 24 years now 'often' consume alcohol (Mahal 2000).

There has been some research into the association between alcohol and suicide in some parts of India. For example, according to Kumar (1995), alcoholism is an important contributor to suicide in Kerala. In a study conducted at the Trivandrum Medical College, many males who attempted suicide reported that their alcoholism and associated problems were the most important causes of suicidal attempt. These included problems related to medical conditions, occupation-related and socially related issues. However, families of alcoholics appeared to suffer more than the alcoholics themselves in terms of attempting suicide, especially spouses. They found that 18 per cent of females who attempted suicide reported that the cause of their attempt was heavy drinking by their husbands. Kumar (1995) noted that families of alcoholics were particularly subject to embarrassment and social isolation, as well as financial and social upheaval.

Consistent with this, Antony (cited in John 1995) observed that psychiatric illness was evident in about 80 per cent of suicide attempters admitted to the medical college in Kozhikode, Kerala. Of these about half were diagnosed with depression, while in 25 per cent of cases the primary diagnosis was chronic alcoholism. John (1995) also notes that in Kerala, increased alcoholism has far outpaced the increase in population. Males with a long history of alcohol abuse and previous suicide attempts are considered to be at greater risk of completing suicide. Such drinkers are likely to become steadily more socially isolated with greater physical, financial, family and social complications. In addition, prolonged alcohol abuse affects brain functioning, possibly leading to deficits in control of aggressive, impulsive behaviour that may precede suicide attempts (John 1995).

Latha *et al.* (1996) report that of 73 suicide attempters assessed in a psychiatric unit of the General Hospital in Manipal, Karnataka, 27 per cent had used alcohol. That is, alcohol was implicated in suicide attempts because of habitual excessive consumption, intoxication or elements of withdrawal. Eleven per cent were actually diagnosed as alcohol abusers, while 19 per cent 'had consumed alcohol during or prior to their suicidal attempt' (Latha, Bhat *et al.* 1996: 27). Latha (1996) notes that India continues to be a male-dominated society and that males have all the responsibilities associated with that position. When there is a familial or financial crisis of some type, many males are more likely to seek solace in the 'bottle' rather than actually ask for assistance from others, an action not generally condoned in Indian society, especially among males.

In a study of 2,651 suicides that occurred in Bangalore between 1996 and 1999, Gururaj and Isaacs report that 14 per cent of completed suicides were regular and chronic users of alcohol (Gururaj and Isaac 2001: 20). In addition, 56 per cent of completers were under the influence of alcohol at the time of their deaths (Gururaj and Isaac 2001: 20). In a further psychological autopsy of 30 randomly chosen cases from amongst their larger sample, Gururaj and Isaac found that alcohol use by the individual themselves or their parents was a factor in 14 (46 per cent) cases (Gururaj and Isaac 2001: 47). This is almost the same level as those with a history of depression (43 per cent) (Gururaj and Isaac 2001: 48). In their psychological autopsy of 100 suicides in Chennai (Madras), Vijaykumar and Rajkumar found alcoholism involved in 34 per cent of cases (Vijayakumar and Rajkumar 1999: 409).

As we have seen earlier, the upsurge in suicides by farmers, particularly in Kerala, Karnataka, Andhra Pradesh and the Punjab in the late 1990s – often due to increased rural debt – has received increased media attention. Bhalla and his colleagues (1998) reported on a study conducted among 14 Punjabi villages of 53 cases of confirmed suicide, aged mainly from 15 to 29 years. They found that 68 per cent of the victims had been heavy drinkers, with a majority considered to be chronic alcoholics. Furthermore, 90 per cent of the victims were described as 'loners' with little social support. Concerning their pre-suicidal behaviour, nearly 55 per cent were described by family members as 'depressed'. However, of the victims, only about 30 per cent had been receiving some type of medical help and only 11 per cent were being treated for a psychiatric disorder.

There has been some research into the relationship between alcohol consumption and suicide among Indian communities in other countries. For example, Morris (2001) reported that alcohol abuse was not significantly involved in suicides among Malay Indians, although excessive drinking was a common social problem in the Indian community in Malaysia. Malay Indians believe that alcohol provides 'strength for manual labour' (Morris and Maniam 2001: 61). This is not consistent with findings reported from Western societies (Lester 1995).

There is limited all-India data that address suicide as it relates to alcohol abuse. However, if increased consumption is related to increased suicide, we expect that suicide rates will be higher in those states with higher levels of consumption. We also therefore expect, in accord with previous research, that suicide rates will be positively related to percentage of tribal consumers per state. If alcohol consumption is negatively related to the Muslim religion, and female-headed households, we would expect there to be a negative relationship between suicide rates and these variables. That is, these consumers are likely to consume less alcohol and so there is a reduced risk of suicide. With respect to literacy, Mahal (2000) suggests that alcohol consumption rates fall with increased literacy, however we know from the results presented in Chapter 10 and previous research by Mayer (Mayer 2003) that in India, literacy itself is strongly associated with suicide. Therefore, if both literacy and consumption are positively related to suicide, we would expect that literates who consume alcohol should also be at an elevated risk of suicide. Finally, we also expect that states with higher excise revenue from alcohol will show higher suicide rates.

Data for the percentage of consumers of alcohol per state, proportion of Muslim, tribal and literate consumers as well as the proportion of consumers from female-headed households are shown for 15 of the Indian states in Table 13.1. This data related to persons aged 15 years and over in all categories and was obtained from a report by Mahal (2000) from survey data collected by the National Council of Applied Economic Research (NCAER), covering 1750 villages in 15 major Indian states in 1994. Table 13.2 provides excise revenue data also provided by the report from the NCAER by Mahal (2000). This data was in the form of fiscal year data and we show suicide rates calculated for the same fiscal years to provide consistency with the revenue rates.

We found a significant, but negative, correlation between percentage of consumers for each state and the suicide rates for 1994 with $r = -0.53$. Even though the sample size was small, reference to Cohen (1992) showed that this was a large effect size.[1] For each of the time periods in succession, the correlations

Table 13.1 Suicide rates and state alcohol consumption by socio-economic and demographic characteristics (percentages) for 1994

State	Suicide rate (1994)	Consumers	Muslim consumers	Tribal consumers	Literate consumers	Female h/head consumers
Andhra Pradesh	10.3	11.8	13.2	11.5	9.4	8.8
Bihar	1.6	17.4	6.1	44.8	15.6	19.7
Gujarat	8.7	3.9	1.0	9.9	2.6	3.5
Haryana	5.2	8.3	6.4	4.8	10.1	3.6
Himachal Pradesh	4.6	16.7	8.2	16.8	17.5	4.1
Karnataka	19.1	3.3	3.3	6.2	3.0	2.6
Kerala	28.3	7.5	1.8	3.2	6.9	5.1
Madhya Pradesh	10.1	12.1	6.7	22.9	12.1	8.3
Maharashtra	12.9	5.8	1.8	13.8	5.3	1.9
Orissa	9.0	10.2	7.6	31.2	5.1	9.6
Punjab	2.5	17.4	17.4	39.7	19.4	10.0
Rajasthan	5.7	8.6	1.6	20.2	9.4	.6
Tamil Nadu	16.0	8.1	5.2	11.8	7.7	2.3
Uttar Pradesh	4.7	4.0	3.1	3.7	4.9	2.9
West Bengal	17.4	4.5	1.0	20.2	3.9	12.2

Source: Alcohol consumption data from Mahal 2000.

were $r = -0.52, -0.57, -0.54$ and -0.53 respectively. This indicates that high consumption is significantly correlated with *lower* suicide rates, which is contrary to previous research findings and our predictions. We also expected negative correlations between the suicide rates and percentage of Muslim consumers and though the correlations were negative, they were not statistically significant. However, the correlations of $-0.42, -0.45, -0.43$ and -0.38 respectively, are all medium to large effect sizes, demonstrating that there is substantial effect. We expected that those states with high levels of tribal consumers would have high suicide rates due to increased alcohol consumption, but we found significant and negative correlations of $-0.47, -0.54, -0.51$ and -0.53 respectively. Contrary to predictions, too, the percentage of literate consumers was significantly correlated in an inverse direction, for all time periods. The correlations were $-0.56, -0.58, -0.56$ and -0.54, respectively.

There were no significant correlations between suicide rates and the percentage of consumers who lived in female-headed households. However, the correlations were all in the expected, negative direction but these were of low effect size, so more research into this is needed before firmer conclusions can be drawn.

Another hypothesis was that revenue for each time period should be positively correlated to percentage of consumers, as these are both indicators of consumption. Although the correlations were not significant, perhaps due to the small sample size, they were in the right direction and the effect sizes (ES) were medium to large, being $0.42, 0.36, 0.39$ and 0.45 respectively for each time period.

Table 13.2 State excise revenue as share of state tax revenue versus suicide rates for four time periods

State	1992–1993		1994–1995		1996–1997		1998–1999	
	Revenue	Suicide rate	Revenue	Suicide rate	Revenue	Suicide rate	Revenue	Suicide rate
Andhra Pradesh	27.2	10.45	10.5	9.84	1.3	10.97	12.3	13.3
Bihar	3.4	1.60	3.5	1.28	3.5	1.17	3.7	1.8
Gujarat	0.4	8.16	0.4	8.85	0.4	8.87	0.4	10.0
Haryana	27.2	5.67	28.0	7.84	3.0	7.33	21.6	10.0
Himachal Pradesh	34.1	2.86	31.7	4.63	32.3	4.39	29.4	4.4
Karnataka	16.6	17.48	16.6	21.29	14.6	19.22	13.7	22.8
Kerala	11.8	27.17	12.6	26.95	10.7	27.15	10.8	29.9
Madhya Pradesh	19.0	9.82	19.3	9.70	18.1	9.57	17.1	12.2
Maharashtra	10.5	11.84	10.0	13.30	9.1	13.56	10.8	15.2
Orissa	8.2	9.90	6.4	8.95	6.8	8.85	7.7	10.1
Punjab	33.7	2.41	34.0	2.72	36.6	2.68	36.8	3.9
Rajasthan	23.9	5.43	24.2	6.19	25.1	5.79	24.7	6.7
Tamil Nadu	13.6	13.95	10.5	15.52	13.3	15.28	15.0	18.3
Uttar Pradesh	22.8	3.22	22.7	3.69	21.0	2.82	18.1	3.1
West Bengal	7.8	17.21	6.2	17.35	7.7	18.70	6.9	18.1

Source: Alcohol revenue data from Mahal 2000.

We predicted that if alcohol consumption, as indicated by the percentage of state revenue derived from excise, were related to suicide rates, there would be significant, positive correlations for each time period, but this was not found. The correlations were –0.38, –0.33, –0.32 and –0.35 respectively. The correlations were thus in an inverse direction and effect sizes were medium, indicating a substantial, underlying effect, despite a lack of significance. This suggests that increased consumption is not related to increased suicide rates, but rather to low suicide rates.

It can be seen in Table 13.2 that those states with the highest state excise revenue, for example, Himachal Pradesh and the Punjab, do not have high suicide rates. Figure 13.1 shows data for the latter and it can be seen that, despite consistently high revenue from the sale of alcohol, suicide rates are not correspondingly high as a consequence. Conversely, those states with low excise revenue do not have corresponding low suicide rates. For example, West Bengal derives a low percentage of state revenue from excise and yet its suicide rates are generally high.

If prohibition protects against suicide, then it would be expected that states where prohibition was in force would have lower suicide rates than those without such restrictions. A case in point is Gujarat where prohibition has been, and still is, the norm, but as can be seen in Table 13.2, suicide rates are moderate, and not especially low. In addition, Gujarat does not demonstrate lower suicide rates than the Punjab for example, where prohibition has not been enforced.

The state that particularly demonstrates the lack of relationship between alcohol consumption and suicide is Haryana, where partial prohibition was in force during the 1996–1997 revenue period. As can be seen from Figure 13.2, there is no striking change in the suicide rates despite a significant drop in state excise revenue from alcohol during that period. A similar conclusion can be drawn from the experience of Andhra Pradesh, which introduced prohibition in the 1996–1997 fiscal year. As can be seen from Figure 13.3, this did not cause a

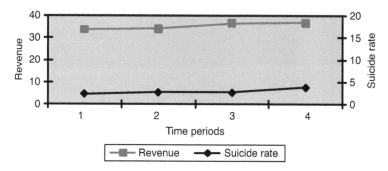

Figure 13.1 Punjab – Alcohol revenues versus suicide rates over four time periods.

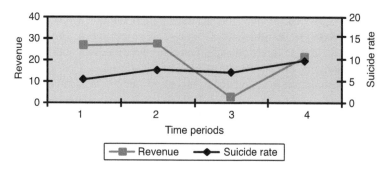

Figure 13.2 Haryana – Alcohol revenues versus suicide rates over four time periods.

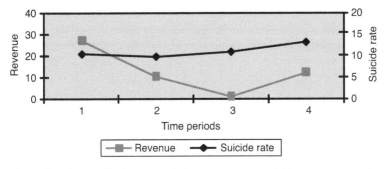

Figure 13.3 Andhra Pradesh – Alcohol revenues versus suicide rates over four time periods.

slump in suicide rates, which could have been expected, but rather suicide rates increased marginally.

Conclusion

It is clear from these results that the relationship between alcohol consumption and suicide in India is difficult to compare to that of other places, especially Western countries. Not only is the sociological debate about this issue in its infancy, but there is limited available data from India that allows us to draw firm conclusions. There is only weak social acceptance of alcohol in India, unlike most Western countries where alcohol consumption is generally socially accepted. In India, by contrast, alcohol consumption is more gender-specific and society accepts drinking among males while discouraging drinking among females, who generally do not condone alcohol consumption. Although alcohol production and consumption have become more widespread over the last few decades, there are still areas and certain classes of the populace for whom alcohol consumption is anathema.

Although the data are limited and our statistical analyses rudimentary, our effect sizes were substantial, and we could find no evidence, to date, that higher levels of alcohol consumption are related to increased suicide rates across India. For example, we found that percentage of consumers was inversely related to suicide rates, which is not consistent with previous research by Norström (1988) and others such as Hawton, Fagg *et al.* (1989).

We expected that suicide would be negatively related to percentage of Muslim consumers and this was found, although the correlations were not significant. However, the effect sizes show that there was a substantial, underlying effect. This is best exemplified in the Punjab, which had the highest percentage of Muslim consumers yet one of the lowest suicide rates for 1994. Although we expected that states with higher percentages of tribal consumers would have similar high suicide rates, we found the reverse. If tribal populations consume the large amounts of alcohol that Mahal (2000) has indicated, then this has not apparently translated to an increased risk of suicide (see also Skog 1993 for a discussion of the alcohol/suicide link in Hungary). Does tribal affiliation in some way counter the effects of alcohol consumption in terms of suicide risk? More research about this is warranted.

We predicted that the interaction between literacy and alcohol consumption would lead to increased suicide risk. Our finding of a strong negative correlation is puzzling. Inspection of the geographical patterns of relatively high alcohol consumption by literates, however, indicates that they are clustered in north India where suicide levels as a whole are relatively low. Thus, it appears that geographical and cultural factors are stronger than the impact of increased consumption.

Although we did not find significant correlations between the number of consumers living in female-headed households and suicide, the relationship was inverse as expected, suggesting that a larger sample size may have provided stronger evidence that where females are in charge of the household there is less consumption and therefore a reduced risk of alcohol-related suicide.

Excise revenue from alcohol and percentage of alcohol consumers were positively associated, which is to be expected if they are both indicators of alcohol consumption. However, the correlation was not significant which may have been due, again, to the small sample size. The weak correlation may also be due to variations in the level at which alcohol consumption is taxed in different states. It is interesting to note that both revenue and the percentage of alcohol consumers were inversely related to suicide rates, although only the latter had a significant relationship. This suggests that although both indicators were related inversely to suicide, the latter measure may be a more precise measure of consumption.

Some state examples were particularly notable for demonstrating a negative relationship between consumption and suicide rates, with respect to revenue. For example, the Punjab records high revenue from alcohol but this is not associated with high suicide rates. Furthermore, we could show no relationship between changes in alcohol consumption, as evidenced by times of prohibition, and suicide rates. Unlike Skog (1993), our 'natural experiment' failed to find a relationship between suicide and alcohol consumption in states where prohibition was in effect, i.e. Gujarat, or where prohibition has been implemented for short periods, i.e. Haryana and Andhra Pradesh.

Clearly it is still 'early days' in terms of collecting data to determine how increasing alcohol consumption will affect suicidal behaviour among the Indian populace. In addition, levels of alcohol consumption are still relatively low in India, compared with more developed countries. Furthermore, the availability of alcohol and its consumption are not as socially condoned or acceptable in India as in other countries. However, given the experience with other more developed nations, Indian health authorities may need to keep a close eye on this situation in the future, especially given that alcohol consumption is increasing rapidly among some specific groups, such as young males. This group has been referred to elsewhere as a group that is increasingly vulnerable to risky behaviours that may precede suicidal behaviour. Alcohol consumption is unlikely to be an exception.

The findings presented in this chapter sit uneasily with the individual-level results of clinicians who, as we have seen, consistently find that alcohol abuse is involved in a very significant percentage of suicides in India. Our findings are also inconsistent with aggregate-level studies overseas, which frequently find that higher levels of alcohol consumption are associated with increased incidence of suicide. The resolution of the apparent inconsistency may lie in what are still relatively low levels of alcohol use in India compared with Europe. Significant alcohol abuse may be concentrated in a relatively small number of at-risk individuals. For argument's sake, if alcohol abuse were involved in 30 per cent of suicides, it would mean approximately 30,000 individuals in a population of 1 billion (0.0003), which may simply be too small a number to register at the aggregate level of analysis.

Note

1 Effect sizes are explained in the appendix to Chapter 3.

14 Suicide in the Indian diaspora

It is estimated that in the late 1980s there were 8.7 million persons of south Asian ethnicity living overseas (Clarke, Peach *et al.* 1990: 2). By 2001 a Report by the High Level Committee on the Indian Diaspora to the Indian Government estimated that the total population in the diaspora was nearly 17 million (High Level Committee 2001). Since the High Level Committee appears to have omitted figures for several countries, most notably Martinique, this total appears slightly understated. The south Asian diaspora was created in three principal phases: from the 1830s, Indian indentured labour was drawn to plantations across the British Empire; from the 1840s there was a second stream of voluntary migration from Gujarat to east Africa; finally since 1947 there has been a major stream of migration from the sub-continent to the UK, the US and Canada (Brennan 1998: 1). The emergence in European colonies of commercial plantations growing – above all – sugar, but also tea and coffee, rice, tobacco, cotton, rubber and a host of other tropical commodities produced a strong international demand for labour in the eighteenth and nineteenth centuries and to a certain extent, the twentieth. The banning of the landing of slaves in British colonies in 1808 was a significant step in the eventual abolition of slavery in 1834 (Tinker 1974: 1–2). The prohibition of the trade in slaves created a strong demand for alternative sources of labour which during the nineteenth century came to be filled by indentured labourers, many of whom were recruited in India (for an account which focuses on the experiences of the indentured themselves, see Lal 1998). Bihar and eastern Uttar Pradesh in the north and present-day Tamil Nadu and Andhra Pradesh in the south furnished many of those recruited for plantation labour overseas (Brennan 1998: 3). Tinker estimates that between 1830 and 1870 one to two million Indians embarked for periods of virtual capitalist slavery in Sri Lanka (Ceylon), the West Indies, South and East Africa, Burma, Malaya, Mauritius and Fiji (Tinker 1974: 115). The abusive system of indentures was eventually ended in 1917, to be replaced by a scheme of 'assisted passage' – the need for imported labour, after all, did not end until the Great Depression. Of those who boarded ship and survived their period of indenture, perhaps only one-quarter returned to India (Tinker 1974: 232). Those who remained behind became traders or smallholder agriculturalists and pursued a host of other professions and trades. By 1921 there were significant Indian communities in a number of colonies and former colonies. As can be seen in Table 14.1, the largest communities were in Burma, Ceylon and Malaya (which included Singapore).

The third wave of migration has brought hundreds of thousands of south Asians – many but by no means all from what is independent India – to first world countries, most notably the UK (for a study of the culture of the post-war migrants, see Shukla 2003). The estimated numbers of persons of south Asian origin are given in Table 14.2.

Clarke, Peach *et al.*, drawing on Speckmann's (1965) periodisation of the experience of Indian migrants in Suriname, identify five critical episodes in the experiences of migrant communities:

(1) immigration (causing social disarray and anomie); (2) acculturation (a reorientation of traditional institutions and the adoption of new ones); (3) establishment (growth in numbers, residential footing and economic security; (4) incorporation (increased urban social patterns and the rise of a middle class); and (5) accelerated development (including greater occupational mobility, educational attainment, and political representation).

(Clarke, Peach *et al.* 1990: 3)

Plainly, these experiences not only set the experiences of migrant communities apart from the societies from which they had their origins, but also have placed migrants under stresses that might be expected to lead to elevated rates of suicide.

It has been frequently noted that among the aspects of culture that migrants bring with them to a new country are their attitudes to the taking of one's own life (see for example Prosser 1996). Kushner, for example, commented that in the US in the nineteenth century 'the distribution of suicide among immigrants reflects, in an inflated fashion, the suicide rates in their homelands . . . What is most surprising is that even today the incidence of suicide among European ethnic groups in America continues to reflect the patterns first noticed in the mid-nineteenth century' (Kushner 1984: 11, 14). As we shall see, Indians abroad and their descendants share similar rates of suicide to Indians in the subcontinent. Figures on suicide rates are available for only a handful of the nations to which those of Indian origin have migrated.

Table 14.1 Indian communities in the British commonwealth, 1921

Burma	887,077	Jamaica	18,610
Ceylon	635,671	Zanzibar	13,500
Malaya	479,180	Tanganyika	10,000
Mauritius	265,524	Uganda	3,518
South Africa	161,329	Hong Kong	2,000
British Guiana	124,938	Southern Rhodesia	1,184
Trinidad	122,117	Canada	1,016
Fiji	60,634	Australia	300
Kenya	22,822	United Kingdom	5,000

Source: Tinker 1976: 36.

Table 14.2 Overseas South Asians by major area, by country, 2001

UK	1,200,000		United Arab Emirates	950,000	
Netherlands	217,000		Oman	312,000	
France	65,000		Kuwait	295,000	
Germany (FRG)	35,000		Iraq	110	
Spain	29,000		Saudi Arabia	1,500,000	
Portugal	70,000		Qatar	131,000	
Sweden	11,000		Bahrain	130,000	
Austria	11,945		Yemen	100,900	
Norway	5,630		Lebanon	11,025	
Switzerland	13,500		Iran	800	
Denmark	2,152		Jordan	930	
Other	103,055		Other	47,700	
Total Europe		1,770,082	Total Middle East		3,483,665
Mauritius	715,756		Trinidad & Tobago	500,600	
South Africa	1,000,000		Guyana	395,350	
Kenya	102,000		Surinam	150,456	
Reunion	220,000		Jamaica	61,500	
Tanzania	90,000		Guadeloupe	40,000	
Libya	12,400		*Martinique	10,000	
Malagasy	29,000		St Vincent & the Grenadines	160	
Zambia	13,000		*Grenada	4,000	
Mozambique	20,870		St Lucia	200	
Zimbabwe	16,700		Panama	2,164	
Nigeria	25,000		Other	22,168	
Seychelles	5,000		Total Caribbean and Latin America		1,178,598
*Malawi	5,000				
*Liberia	3,066				
Algeria	45		USA	1,678,765	
Ethiopia	734		Canada	851,000	
*Congo	2,711		Total North America		2,529,765
Other	42,980				
Total Africa		1,353,229			
			Fiji	336,829	
Malaysia	1,665,000		Australia	190,000	
Burma	2,902,000		New Zealand	55,000	
Singapore	307,100		Other	1,070	
Bhutan	1,500		Total Pacific		582,899
Afghanistan	500				
Indonesia	55,000		Grand Total:		16,968,357
Hong Kong	50,500				
Philippines	38,000				
Thailand	85,000				
Brunei	7,600				
Japan	10,000				
Other	17,208				
Total Asia		6,070,119			

Source: High Level Committee 2001. Items indicated by asterisk from (Clarke *et al.* 1990, Table 1: 2).

Singapore

Recruitment of Indian labour for work in Malaya and Singapore occurred only early in the twentieth century. Before the bicycle and automobile driven 'rubber boom',

> ... there was a larger Indian population in British Guiana than in Malaya. But with the rubber boom, the demands of Malaya seemed insatiable. Madras supplied virtually all the labourers for the Malayan rubber estates.
>
> (Tinker 1974: 57)

Kua and Tsoi (1985: 227) reported that the contemporary Singapore community is comprised of 76 per cent Chinese, 15 per cent Malays, 7 per cent Indians and 2 per cent other ethnicities. The Singapore citizens of Indian origin are primarily Tamil speakers. Hassan (1983, Table 3.1: 38) reported that between 1968 and 1971, the average annual suicide rate was 11.2 per 100,000 for the Chinese, 10.8 for Indians and 1.4 for the indigenous Malay. People of 'other ethnicities' had an average annual rate of 7.2 in the same period (Hassan 1983, Table 3.1: 38). Interestingly, Hassan reported that Singapore-born Indians and Chinese commit suicide less frequently than their peers born elsewhere do. For the period 1968–1971, 73 per cent of suicides from the Indian ethnic group were of those born somewhere other than Singapore (54 per cent being Indian-born)(Hassan 1983: 40). This finding supports the theory that migrants generally have higher suicide rates than those born in the new home country (Hassan 1995: 123).

The suicide rate for the Singapore population as a whole in 1970 was reported as 9.6 per 100,000 (Hassan 1983, Table 3.1: 38) and ten years later the reported rate was no different, at 9.5 per 100,000 (Kua and Tsoi 1985: 228). In 1989 the suicide rate reached a peak at 14.7; it fell to a relative low of 7.9 in 1996, rising again to be at 10.4 in 1998 (Parker and Yap 2001, Table 1: 12). What has changed over this period, however, is the rank order of the different ethnic groups in the population; the suicide rate for the Indian ethnic group is much higher at 13.7 per 100,000 and the rate for ethnic Chinese is similarly high, but marginally lower than the Indian rate, at 13.5 (Kua and Tsoi 1985: 229). The suicide rate for indigenous Malays remains extremely low, dropping to 1.0 per 100,000. The reasons suggested for this disparity are that the indigenous Malays have strong Islamic beliefs that prohibit suicide, while the immigrant Indians and Chinese tend to be more competitive and business-orientated and tend to believe that career failures bring shame upon themselves and their community (Kua and Tsoi 1985: 229).

More recent figures regarding suicide rates in Singapore reflect a minor increase in actual rate, but no further change since 1980 in the rank order for ethnic group. Lester (1998 cited in Lester 2000) reports that in 1984 the suicide rate of Indians was 17.8 per 100,000, 14.6 for Chinese and 2.7 for indigenous Malay.

Wai and his colleagues reported that there were 1.4 female suicides for every male suicide in those under 21 years, irrespective of community (Wai, Hong *et al.*

1999: 129–130). Young Singaporeans of Indian origin have higher suicide rates than those of other ethnicities: 'Although Indians comprise only 6.5 per cent of the population of Singapore, they comprise 21 per cent [i.e. 3.2 times higher than their population percentage] of the recorded cases.' (Wai, Hong *et al.* 1999: 130). Wai and his colleagues also found aetiologies quite similar to those reported in India:

> The most common problems reported by the cases were conflicts with members of the family (24.5 per cent), followed by interpersonal difficulties with friends (23.6 per cent). These included arguments with siblings or significant others, disagreements with parents over their choice of partners or friends, the imposition of lifestyle restrictions, the break up of a love relationship, and bullying by school peers.
>
> (Wai, Hong *et al.* 1999: 130)

Somewhat unexpectedly, elderly Singaporeans of Chinese background have the highest suicide rates. Kua and Ko reported that among those over 65 in 1985–1989 the rate for those of Chinese ethnicity was 61.2 per 100,000, for Indians 30.5 and for Malays 3.2 (Kua and Ko 1992: 558).

These differences in suicide propensity are also reflected in rates of attempted suicide. Wai and Kua studied admissions to a Singapore teaching hospital between 1991 and 1995 (1998; for an earlier study of attempted suicide in Singapore, see Tsoi 1974). Predictably, Wai and Kua found that Singaporeans of Indian origin were 260 per cent more likely to attempt suicide than would be expected from their proportion of the population (6.5 per cent). Chinese attempters were at 95 per cent of their proportion in the population (75 per cent) and attempters of Malayan background were only 48.6 per cent of their population percentage (15 per cent) (figures computed from Table 1, Wai and Kua 1998).

Malaysia

As we have seen, Malaysians of Indian origin came primarily from Tamil Nadu during the early twentieth century to work in the rubber plantations. They remained predominantly a poorer, working class stratum of the Malaysian population (Kaur 1998).

The suicide rates reported in this section are for West (Peninsula) Malaysia and do not include the rather unreliable data from East Malaysia (Sabah and Sarawak). Suicide rates in Malaysia have dropped consistently since 1966. The average crude suicide rate for West Malaysia as a whole (1966–1969) was reported by Maniam (1995: 182) as being 7.1 per 100,000, dropping to 3.7 between 1970–1979 and down to 1.5 for the period 1980–1985; by 1990 it had fallen to 0.4 per 100,000. Of the different ethnic groups in Malaysia, those of Indian descent had the highest suicide rate in the population, at 42.4 per 100,000 in 1969 (by contrast, the rate for Chinese was 15.6, and for Malays, 4.3). Suicide rates for all ethnic groups declined in a similar fashion to the average population rates above, with the main explanatory factor for this trend being a change in reporting meth-odology after 1975 (Maniam 1995: 182–184). The large apparent drop in the suicide rate after 1975 is mirrored by a large increase in the number of 'undeter-mined violent deaths' at this time, with the Indian ethnic group again being over-represented in this rate. Maniam argues that there is no evident reason why Indians should have such high rates of undetermined violent deaths and suggests that high proportions of these are misclassified suicides. As such, a Corrected Suicide Rate for the 1980s suggests that the true suicide rate for the West Malaysian population was in the realm of 8–13 per 100,000 rather than the official figure of 1.5. The corrected 1990 figures for the three ethnic groups in the population are given as 35 per 100,000 for Indians, 12 for Chinese and 6 for indigenous Malays, (Maniam 1995, Figure 9: 184).

Suicide rates within West Malaysia vary considerably with region. Maniam (1988) reports that for the hill resort district of the Cameron Highlands, suicide rates are much higher than those for West Malaysia as a whole. Moreover, although they constitute only 25 per cent of the population, Indians have particularly high suicide rates in this region. In a study of 95 cases of suicide between 1973 and 1984, 81 per cent of these involved ethnic Indians, giving an average suicide rate of 157 per 100,000 of the population aged over ten years (Maniam 1988: 222–223). Reasons suggested for these extreme values include the 'popular' use of highly lethal agricultural poisons in suicidal behaviour in this farming community, which may see many intended parasuicides become actual suicides (Maniam 1988: 224).

In a follow-up study in the Cameron Highlands between 1984 and 1993, Maniam (cited in Morris and Maniam 2001: 57) reported persistently high suicide rates for the Indian ethnic sub-population, at 135 per 100,000 population aged over ten years. During this time there was also an appreciable increase in the rate of suicide in the Malay population and an increase in the use of paraquat as a method of self-poisoning.

A study of attempted suicides in Kuala Lumpur in 1989 by Habil and his col-leagues showed a broadly similar patterns (Habil, Ganesvaran *et al.* 1992/1993; for earlier studies of attempted suicide in Malaysia, see Yeoh 1981; Murugesan and Yeoh 1978). Those of Indian origin were 320 per cent more frequent among attempt-ers (48 per cent) than their proportion of the population (15 per cent). Attempters of Chinese background were 88 per cent relative to their population (46 per cent) and those of Malay background were at 26 per cent of their representation in the popula-tion (38.5 per cent) (calculated from Table 1, Habil, Ganesvaran *et al.*: 5). Maniam has reported that in the Cameron Highlands, the attempted: completed ratio is not the usual 14:1 but closer to 1.4:1 because of the common use of highly deadly pest-icides and the absence of adequate medical facilities (Maniam 2001).

Fiji

Like Malaya, Indian emigration to Fiji occurred primarily in the twentieth century, following the accession of Fiji to the British Crown in 1875 (for a pioneering study of the origins of the migrants to Fiji, see Lal 1983). The driving force for the importation of Indian labour was the Colonial Sugar Refining Company (CSR) of Australia, which produced over 90 per cent of the sugar in Fiji. Most Indian migrants were recruited either from south Bihar and the eastern districts of the North Western Provinces (modern day Uttar Pradesh) in the North or from the Madras Presidency, primarily from amongst Tamil-speaking Untouchables (Brennan, McDonald *et al.* 1998: 44 ff.; see also Tinker 1974: 57–59). Siegel states that between 1879 and 1916 'more than 60,000 people were transported from India to Fiji ... About 60 percent of them stayed on after their indenture' (Siegel 1998: 181). Tinker notes that 'although the scale of the operation was relatively limited, it was sufficient to increase the Fiji Indian population to the point where it equalled the indigenous Fijians' (Tinker 1974: 57). Today the balance between the two communities is still roughly equal with Fijian Indian slightly outnumbering indigenous Fijians (Lal 1990: 115; Siegel 1998: 181).

Amongst the emerging aspects of the indentured labour system in Fiji to attract concern and criticism was their high rate of suicide. In 1871 the rate amongst indentured Indian labourers was reported to be 78 per 100,000, rising to 83.1 in 1910 (Tinker 1974: 201). Gandhi's associate, the Reverend C. F. Andrews, an outspoken critic of the abuses of the system of indentured labour, 'went on to analyse [James] McNeill's statistics [contained in his 1914 *Report on the Condition of Indian Immigrants in the Four British Colonies: Trinidad, British Guiana or Demerara, Jamaica and Fiji, and in the Dutch Colony of Surinam of Dutch Guiana*] [calculating that] "In 1911 and 1912 ... one in every nine hundred indentured coolies in Fiji committed suicide – one in every nine hundred!" ...' (Tinker 1974: 337). This was a rate of 111.1 per 100,000.

Suicide rates in the Pacific Island region are amongst the highest in the world. In particular, the Indian population of Fiji has extremely high suicide rates, reported as being 34 per 100,000 for the years 1982–1983 (Booth 1999a, Table 2: 437). By comparison, native Fijians had a suicide rate of 3 per 100,000 for the same period. However, previous research reports much lower suicide rates for the Fijian population: 15.1 per 100,000 for Indians and 1.3 for native Fijians for the period 1971–1972 (Price and Karim 1975 cited in Lester 2000, Table 1: 245). Rates of suicide for female youth in the Fijian Indian population are extremely high (60 per 100,000, for 1982–1983). Booth suggests that the pressures exerted by a culture in which arranged marriages feature prominently and women are considered to have an inferior status in general, gives rise to this phenomenon (Booth 1999a: 444–445).

Other studies of suicide in Fiji have concentrated on data from the Macuata province (Haynes 1984; and Rees, 1971, in Lester 2000). Rees (1971) reported that Fijian Indians have an average suicide rate of 33.4 per 100,000 in the Macuata province, compared to a rate of 5.7 for the native Fijian population (cited in Lester 2000). Haynes (1984, Table 1a: 434) reports similarly high figures for the period 1979–1982. During this time, Indians had annual suicide rates of 61.0 per 100,000 for males and 71.9 for females, while the native Fijian population had rates of 11.6 (males) and 0.0 (females). By way of contrast, the suicide rates for the general Fijian population were; 45.2 per 100,000 (Indian males), 33.1 (Indian females), 9.2 (Fijian males) and 9.3 (Fijian females) during the period 1981–1982 (Haynes 1984, Table 1a: 434). Again, socio-cultural factors are invoked to explain the high rate of suicide amongst Indians in Macuata, and also the low rate amongst native Fijians. The traditional Fijian way of life is highly communal and extremely supportive (Haynes 1984: 436). Why Macuata has such high rates relative to the rest of Fiji is undetermined, except that it has a particularly high proportion of Indians descended from the large number of indentured workers brought to the province to farm sugar cane between 1879 and 1920 (Haynes 1984: 433).

South Africa

Indian migration to Natal was first approved in 1860 (Tinker 1974: 96–97). By 1880 there were 20,536 Indians, the number rising to 33,494 a decade later (Tinker 1974: 270; see also Brennan, McDonald *et al.* 1998: 43 ff.). In the years following the Boer War, comparatively large numbers of labourers went to Natal, attracted by the high wages in the coal-mines (Tinker 1974: 57, 293). White settlers, concerned at the emergence of competition from Indian merchants and artisans, and concerned that they might be reduced to a 'minority' in the province, began to lobby for restrictions on Indian settlers.[1] The ill treatment of Indian labourers in Natal became an increasing source of concern. Sir Arthur Gordon, Governor of Mauritius, for example, reported to Lord Kimberly, Secretary for the Colonies, his concern at the high rate of suicides among labourers. The rate in Natal, for example, was 64 per 100,000 while in Madras, from which many labourers were drawn, the suicide rate was 4.6 per 100,000 (Tinker 1974: 201). It was, of course, concern over the growing restrictions on Indians in Natal that led to the invitation by members of the Indian community to Gandhi to come to South Africa in 1894.

Suicide rates reported for South African Asians in 1984–1986 give values of 21.11 per 100,000 for men and 6.65 for women (Flisher and Parry 1994, Table 1: 349). In comparison, the same authors cite suicide rates for Whites as 39.93 for men and 10.1 for women. The higher suicide rates in the White population are explained in terms of their higher standard of living than that of other groups in South Africa, as it has been demonstrated that suicide rates positively correlate with quality of life (Flisher and Parry 1994: 351). Cultural factors such as the influence of Islam are suggested as an explanation for the lower suicide rates in the Asian and coloured populations.

Looking at South African Indian women in particular, Wassenaar *et al.* (1998: 83) report an average annual suicide rate of 3.4 per 100,000 for this group. This is lower than the rate of 5 per 100,000 for South African White women. South African Indian women have a peak suicide rate of 11.4 in the 15 to 24 age group, which is thought to be due to the combined stress of adolescence and socio-cultural factors (see also Flisher and Parry 1994: 351).

United Kingdom

Many migrants from the Indian subcontinent have settled in the UK. However, many of the studies of suicidal behaviour in this population report only Standard-ised Mortality Ratios (for example, Soni Raleigh 1996) and are not useful to include for comparison here. This notwithstanding, Soni Raleigh (personal communication, in Lester 2000: 251) does report that the suicide rate for Indian migrants in the UK was 16.4 per 100,000 for the period 1988–1992. In the absence of standardised rates, Soni Raleigh *et al.* used proportional mortality ratios (PMR) for 1970–1978. They found that while ratios for Indian men in the UK were consistently low, there was a higher and statistically significant excess of suicide mortality for Indian women, especially those aged between 15 and 24 (Soni Raleigh, Bulusu *et al.* 1990: 47).

Indian women also chose burning 'much more frequently' than did the general population of the UK (Soni Raleigh, Bulusu *et al.* 1990: 47). In a study of first generation migrants, Soni Raleigh and Balarajan found that Asian migrants to the UK from India and East Africa had a nine-fold excess in suicide by burning, compared to other immigrant groups (Soni Raleigh and Balarajan 1992: 366). In a study of 57 suicides by burning in 1991, Prosser reported that 30 per cent of female suicides and 7 per cent of male suicides were of Asian origin (Prosser 1996: 177). The odds ratio of self-immolation as a method for Asia-born women as compared to non-Asian-born was 20.08 (Prosser 1996: 189).

The great majority (83 per cent) of UK Indian women in the 15 to 24 age group who took their own lives were married (Soni Raleigh, Bulusu *et al.* 1990: 48). UK Hindus and Sikhs were much more likely to commit suicide (69 per cent of men and 83 per cent of women) than were Muslims (26 per cent of males and 15 per cent of women) (Soni Raleigh, Bulusu *et al.* 1990: 49).

Several studies have reported on attempted suicides among migrant communities in London. Bhugra and his colleagues studied 434 cases of 'deliberate self-harm' at four London hospitals in Ealing between 1994 and 1995 (Bhugra, Desai *et al.* 1999; Bhugra, Baldwin *et al.* 1999; see also Neeleman and Wessely 1999; Neeleman, Wilson-Jones *et al.* 2001). The attempted suicide rate for UK women of south Asian background was 375 per 100,000, considerably higher (1.5 times) than the rate for UK whites (234 per 100,000). By contrast, the rate for UK men of south Asian back-ground (169/100,000) was considerably lower than that for the white population (246) (rates recalculated from Table 1 in Bhugra, Desai *et al.* 1999: 1128). Attempted suicide rates for UK women of south Asian background in the 16–24 age group were 7.5 times higher than those for south Asian men (Bhugra, Desai *et al.* 1999: 1128). Bhugra and his colleagues argue that 'Asian women may be especially prone to experience cultural conflict, which includes dealing with changes in family expecta-tions regarding social behaviour' (Bhugra, Baldwin *et al.* 1999: 1132).

Australia

Traditionally, migrants to Australia have been of European origin, however this is changing and recent years have seen an increase in the number of migrants settling in Australia from Asian countries (Burvill 1995: 202). Hassan (1995, Table 11.4: 124) reported that Indian migrants in Australia have an average suicide rate of 13.6 per 100,000, as opposed to an overall national rate of 12.6 in 1990. Indian migrants who have been in Australia for less than ten years have an average suicide rate of 15 per 100,000, while Indian migrants who have been in the country for more than ten years have an average suicide rate of 11.1 (Hassan 1995, Table 11.4: 124). This is compared to the current Indian average suicide rate of 10.6 per 100,000. These figures are supported by research cited in Burvill (1995), suggesting that suicide rates in migrants in Australia resemble those in the country of origin no matter how long the migrants have lived in Australia. However, the methods of suicide used by migrants change to become more like those used by the Australian-born with increasing years of residence.

The Indian migrant suicide rate pattern seems typical of most migrant groups in Australia, whereby sociological factors such as lack of social support, lack of integration and relatively high levels of social isolation contribute to an initially high rate of suicide in migrants in their first ten years in Australia. After this time, suicide rates decline as migrants presumably become better integrated into Australian society (Hassan 1995: 123).

United States

Very little data are available regarding suicide rates of Indian migrants to the US, presumably due to the relatively small size of this migrant group. However, based on 1992 Census Data for seven states in the US, Shiang (1998, Table 4: 244) reports that the suicide rate per 100,000 is 11.2 in total for all races, while the suicide rate for Asian Indians is 4.

Conclusion

The world-wide dispersal of people from the Indian sub-continent in the nineteenth and twentieth centuries offers scope for suggestive comparisons with conditions in India itself. While there appears to be clear evidence that migrants brought attitudes to suicide with them along with other aspects of a complex culture, there are so many confounding factors that one can only draw the most tentative of conclusions.

As can be seen in the summary figures in Table 14.3, reported suicide rates for persons of Indian origin in the diaspora vary widely, and are certainly within the range of variation found between the states in contemporary India, especially if we bear in mind the probability of the wider validity of Hassan's observation that migrants to Australia 'tend to have higher rates compared with the rates for their native countries' (Hassan 1995).

Among the many confounding factors that might have an impact on suicide rates in the diaspora, the most important must be the varied impact of the experience of migration itself. Clarke *et al.* note that factors such as i) the type of

Table 14.3 Comparison of suicide rates for persons of Indian origin

Country	Indian-origin suicide rates (per 100,000)
Singapore (1984)	17.8
West Malaysia (1990)	35
Fiji (1982–1983)	43
South Africa (1984–1986)	14.0
UK (1998)	16.4
Australia (1990)	13.6

migration (indentured, free passage, etc.), ii) extent of continuing ties with south Asia (kinship, marriage, property, etc.), iii) form of economic activity in the country of migration, iv) geographic location of settlement (rural, urban) and v) official policies affecting migrants (migrant policies, housing, loans, race relations policies) all affect the specific migrant experience in a country (Clarke, Peach *et al.* 1990: 5).

Another potentially significant factor may be the specific regional culture that Indian migrants brought with them. Clarke and his colleagues include religion, language, region of origin, caste and degree of 'cultural homogenisation' as important factors that affect the culture of the migrant community (Clarke, Peach *et al.* 1990: 6). We would wish to know, for example, whether migrants from south India brought with them a heightened propensity to take their lives. Another factor whose impact cannot be assessed is the impact of education. Indians in the diaspora are in many countries (but not all, of course) generally better educated than the Indian population as a whole. As we saw in Chapter 10, suicide rates in India generally increase with level of education. Is there the same effect in the diaspora? There are also significant class differences between those who migrated as indentured labourers in the nineteenth century and those, for example, who went as 'Green Card' migrants to the IT industry in the US in the late twentieth century.

These and other possibly significant factors make it impossible to simply or directly compare suicide rates in the Indian diaspora with those of contemporary India.[2] Nevertheless, as we have seen in this brief survey, there are suggestive similarities, which indicate a level of continuity. Almost every study of diasporic communities has found relatively high suicide rates among young women. And many of these studies report tensions in family relationships as causal factors, much as we have found in contemporary India. And although the methods employed in suicide tend largely to reflect available means (jumping from apartment blocks in Singapore, for example) the relatively high rates of death by self-immolation seems to reveal a retained component of culture.

Appendix

Table 14.4 Summary

Country	Source	Suicide rates (per 100,000 population)
West Malaysia	Morris & Maniam (2001)	Teoh (1974) Indians: 23.3 Total pop.: 6.3
West Malaysia	Maniam (1995)	Indians: 35 Chinese: 12 Malay: 6 Total pop: 8–13 per 100,000 'corrected'
Cameron Highlands	Maniam (1988)	Indians: 157
Cameron Highlands	Morris & Maniam (2001)	Maniam (1994a, 1994b) Indians: 135
Kuala Lumpur	Lester (2000)	Ong & Leng (1992) Indians: 10.2
Singapore	Lester (2000)	Hassan (1980) Indian males 11.4 Indian females: 10.0 All Indians: 10.8
Singapore	Kua & Tsoi (1985)	Kua & Tsoi (1985) Indians: 13.7 Indigenous pop.: 1.0
Singapore	Lester (2000)	Lester (1998) Indians: 17.8 Chinese: 14.6 Malay: 2.7
Singapore	Lester (2000)	Chia & Tsoi (1972) Indian males: 10.9 Indian females: 8.7
Singapore	Lester (2000)	Chia (1981, 1983) Indian males: 5.4 Indian females: 11.4
Singapore	Hassan (1983)	Indian males Indian females: 10.0 All Indians: 10.8 Chinese males: 13.4 Chinese females: 8.8 All Chinese: 11.2 Malay males: 1.7 Malay females: 1.0 All Malay: 1.4 'Other' males: 8.9 'Other' females: 5.4 All 'others': 7.2 Total males: 11.4 Total females: 7.7 Total all: 9.6
Fiji	Booth (1999a)	Indians: 34 (M = 41, F = 27) Total pop: 19 (M = 22, F = 15)

(Continued Overleaf)

Table 14.4 continued

Country	Source	Suicide rates (per 100,000 population)
Fiji	Lester (2000)	Price & Karim (1975) Indians: 15.1 Native Fijians: 1.3
Fiji	Haynes (1984)	Indian males 45.2 Indian females: 33.1 Native Fijian males: 9.2 Native Fijian females: 9.3
Macuata, Fiji	Lester (2000)	Rees (1971) Indians: 33.4 Native Fijians: 5.7
Macuata, Fiji	Haynes (1984)	Indian males: 61.0 Indian females: 71.9 Native Fijian males: 11.6 Native Fijian females: 0
Australia	Hassan (1995)	0–9 years in Australia Indian males: 19.7 Indian females: 10.5 All: 15.0 10+ years in Australia Indian males: 15.4 Indian females: 7.0 All: 11.1 All years Indian males: 17.7 Indian females: 8.6 All: 13.6
Australia	Burvill (1995)	Migrants over the age of 65 years Indian males: 14.4 (N = 4) Indian females: 5.3 (N = 2)
United States	Shiang (1998)	Indian: 4.0 All races in US: 11.2 (M = 17.8, F = 4.8)
South Africa	Flisher & Parry (1994)	Asian men: 21.11 Asian women: 6.65 White men: 39.93 White women: 10.10
South Africa	Wassenaar *et al.* (1998)	Wassenaar & Naidoo (1995) Indian women: 3.4 SA women total: 5
UK	Lester (2000)	Raleigh (1998, pers. comm) Indian males: 23.11 Indian females: 10.0 All Indians: 16.4

Notes

1 Tinker reports that in 1894 there were 45,000 Whites, 46,000 Indians and 470,000 Africans in Natal (Tinker 1974: 281).
2 Clarke and his colleagues also note the importance of aspects of social structure and political power as well as the significance of community organisations, leadership, quality of ethnic relations and the size of the migrant community vis-à-vis its hosts (Clarke, Peach *et al.* 1990: 6–7).

15 Suicide in Pondicherry

As we have seen in earlier chapters, the Union Territory of Pondicherry, a former French colonial toehold in southeastern India, has the doubtful distinction of regularly returning India's highest suicide rates. Pondicherry's very high rate of suicides is also many times higher than the rates for most OECD countries. For example, WHO suicide rates for 1996 in the UK were around 6 per 100,000; rates for the United States and Australia were around 10 per 100,000, and for France around 16 per 100,000. In the 1990s, Pondicherry's overall suicide rate was over 60 per 100,000, about six times the all-India rate. It rose to this high level from a relatively high base in the late 1970s, increasing at an annual rate of about 2.5 per cent. In the twenty-first century, suicide rates appear to have returned to the level of the 1970s.

Pondicherry is something of a geographical, as well as an historical anomaly. While the majority of the population of the territory live in Pondicherry proper, a sizeable minority live in the enclave of Karaikal on the coast of Thanjavur District, Tamil Nadu. There are two still smaller, more widely separated enclaves: Mahe on the coast of Kerala state and Yanam on the coast of Andhra Pradesh.

There are two reasons for devoting a separate chapter to suicides in this small territory. The first, of course, is simply because of the exceptionally high rates of suicide that occur there. The second is because of the unique data sources we have for Pondicherry. We have utilised two primary sources of data in this chapter. In examining the historical trend of suicide in Pondicherry, we have drawn as elsewhere in this book upon annual issues of *Accidental Deaths and Suicides* published by the National Crime Records Bureau in New Delhi. The rest of the analysis, however, draws upon primary records, termed in India First Information Reports (FIR), of individual suicides that occurred between 1995 and 1999 maintained by the police in Pondicherry. Volunteers working for the suicide counselling service, Maitreyi, in Pondicherry, transcribed these individual records – which are the basic records from which national reports are derived.[1] Although there is a core of consistent information recorded for each suicide, additional data were collected in some years but not in others. Individual records for 2,093 suicides were analysed. As far as we are aware, this chapter is the first to analyse such a comprehensive data set for any Indian state or territory. In addition to the unique insight that these individual-level data throw on our understanding of suicide in India, they also permit us to make a supplementary assessment of the reliability of official suicide statistics in India.

Historical trend of suicide in Pondicherry

Annual data on suicide rates are available to us since 1967, the first year of publication of *Accidental Deaths and Suicides*. The average suicide rate over the 40 years for which we have data was 55 per 100,000. As can be seen in Figure 15.1, there is some volatility in Pondicherry's suicide rate, in part an artefact, no doubt, of the sensitivity of the rate to its relatively small population. There appear to be three periods in the data. Between 1967 and 1976, we observe short-term fluctuations around the mean, with a sudden fall in 1979. In the second phase we observe a pattern of nearly constant increase in the suicide rates, which rose from 29 to 73 in 1993. Since 1993 Pondicherry has entered a third phase in which rates have declined to the level seen in the 1970s.

Gender, age and suicide

There were very nearly two male suicides (65 per cent of the total) for every female suicide (35 per cent of the total) in Pondicherry for the period covered by our data. This is a significantly different pattern to the near gender equality in suicides reported for India as a whole in Chapter 7.

Suicide rates

In calculating age-specific rates of suicide, we have used suicides recorded in 1997, a year in which our records contain 93 per cent of those reported in *Accidental Deaths and Suicides in India*.[2] For this year also we are able to compare our analysis with some additional tables prepared for us by the National Crime Records Bureau. Because Pondicherry's population has the 'Christmas tree'-shaped age distribution

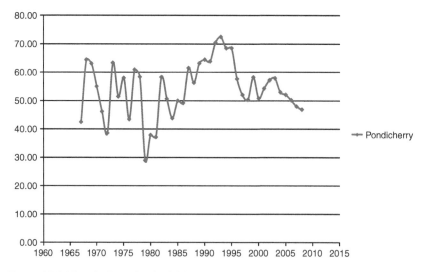

Figure 15.1 Historical trends of suicide in Pondicherry.

typical of a developing country, there is little correspondence between the actual incidence of suicide and standardised rates per 100,000 of the population. It can be seen in Table 15.1 that youth suicide rates are very high for both sexes in Pondicherry; the rate for both is 64 per 100,000. The peak suicide rate is a distressingly high 147 per 100,000 for men in the 45 to 54 age category, more than double that of Finland which has one of the highest OECD suicide rates for that age category.

Incidence of suicide

Pondicherry exhibits a 'classical' age and gender suicide pattern found in many developing nations with a 'downward sloping' pattern for females that peaks in early adulthood and a 'convex' pattern for males, which peaks in middle-age.[3] Nearly 60 per cent of female suicides occur between 15 and 29, the age in which marriages are commonly arranged in south India. As Girard notes, 'men and women in less developed countries are likely to experience identity threats surrounding marriage, child birth, and initiation into adulthood' (Girard 1993: 558).

Plotting the age distribution using five-year categories (Figure 15.2) shows that the incidence of female suicides rises rapidly after 15, peaking around 20 and then falling away rapidly after age 30.

Table 15.1 Suicide rates per 100,000 population in Pondicherry by sex and age, 1997

	< 14	*15–24*	*25–34*	*35–44*	*45–54*	*55–64*	*65+*	*Total*
Male	1.9	63.6	95.6	92.6.3	146.8	92.8	50.6	61.4
Female	1.9	64.0	64.4	44.8	17.2	27.5	17.1	34.3

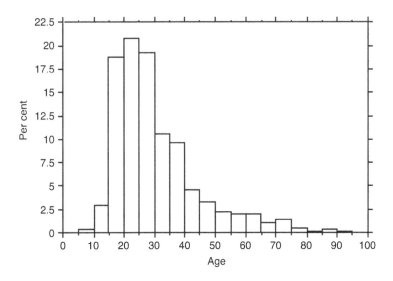

Figure 15.2 Female suicide by age, 1995–1999.

Male suicides in Pondicherry also peak in early adulthood and remain at elevated rates in middle age, roughly 35 per cent of suicides occurring in the 15 to 29 and the 30 to 44 age categories. It is clear from inspection of Figure 15.3 that male suicides reach their peak incidence in the early 20s, a few years later than those of females. The male incidence also declines more slowly with increasing age.

Methods of suicide

The data available for Pondicherry partially contradict the common finding in Western suicidology that women tend to chose less violent methods to commit suicide. As can be seen in Table 15.2, almost 98 per cent of those of either sex who commit suicide use one of three methods. Hanging is most common for both women and men; it is more frequently chosen by men. Nearly equal proportions of both sexes use poisons. Self-immolation, the third most frequent method, is

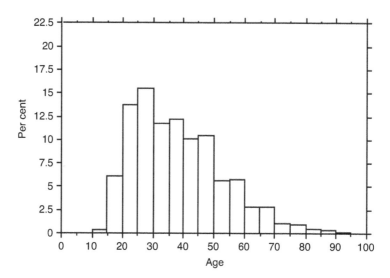

Figure 15.3 Male suicide by age, 1995–1999.

Table 15.2 Percentage of suicides in Pondicherry 1995–1999 by method and sex

	Female	Male	Total
Hanging	43.2	56.8	52.0
Other	2.0	1.0	1.4
Poison	30.0	36.9	34.4
Self-immolation	24.7	5.2	12.1
Total	100	100	100

very much more likely to be used by women than men. Although the differences in distribution are statistically significant ($p < 0.0001$), the differences in choice of method do not seem to have the same character as those found in OECD countries such as Australia where men are very much more likely than women to use firearms. Certainly there is no obvious pattern for women in Pondicherry to use less violent methods of death.

Monthly variations

It can be seen from Figure 15.4 that percentage of total suicides varies slightly throughout the year.[4] Suicides are least frequent in November and December. The greatest number occurs in September, July and August.

Seasonality of suicide

When months are grouped into seasons (Table 15.3), it becomes evident that suicides in Pondicherry are most frequent in the hottest months of the year (April–May) and during the monsoon season (June–October). They are relatively less frequent in winter (November–March). By contrast, Bagadia *et al.* reported in 1974 that more attempted suicides in occurred Bombay [Mumbai] during the

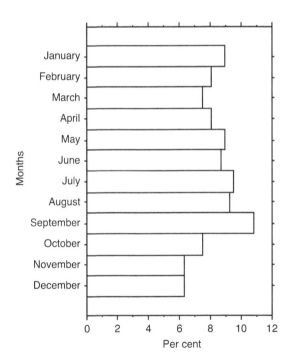

Figure 15.4 Suicides by month, 1996.

Table 15.3 Monthly mean suicides by season

Season	Suicides per month
Summer	44
Monsoon	47.4
Winter	38.4

monsoon (38 per cent) and winter (28 per cent); only 20 per cent occurred in summer (Bagadia, Pradhan *et al.* 1974: 305).

Regional variations

Although the main centre of population of the Union Territory of Pondicherry is in 'Pondicherry itself' (estimated 1997 population 606,000), about 160 km south of Chennai (Madras), the historical accident of French colonial territories in India has resulted in the inclusion of three smaller districts in the territory. These are Karaikal located in the Thanjavur District of Tamilnadu (estimated 1997 population 145,000), Mahe located at the intersection of Kannur and Kozhikode Districts of Kerala (estimated 1997 population 33,400) and Yanam, located in East Godavari District of Andhra Pradesh (estimated 1997 population 20,500). The inclusion of these separate districts within the single administrative territory allows us to explore the significance for suicide rates of different south Indian cultural regions.

Table 15.4 Suicide rates per 100,000 by sex and age for districts of Pondicherry, Karaikal, Mahe and Yanam, 1997

Gender	Age group	Pondicherry	Karaikal	Mahe	Yanam
Male	<15	2.5	0	0	0
	15–24	54.4	115.4	23.7	81.7
	25–34	104.4	88.4	0	44.3
	35–44	103.7	71.9	0	0
	45–54	147.3	142.1	126.0	97.6
	55–64	110.2	91.0	0	0
	64+	55.2	48.4	0	0
	Total	64.3	66.3	15.5	31.1
Female	<15	1.72	3.5	0	0
	15–24	60.4	87.9	0	118.6
	25–34	57.0	120.8	0	0
	35–44	48.6	37.3	35.9	0
	45–54	16.6	25.5	0	0
	55–64	32.9	17.4	0	0
	64+	17.6	0	73.5	0
	Total	33.1	47.1	8.9	24.1

The two districts enclosed within Tamil Nadu state have relatively higher suicide rates than do those which are in Kerala and Andhra Pradesh. Suicide rates for Mahe and Yanam must be treated with caution because of their very small populations.

When we compare the two districts within Tamil Nadu we can see that Karaikal has higher overall rates for both men and women than does Pondicherry proper.[5] The rate for young men in Karaikal is very much higher than the already high rate in Pondicherry. The rates for young women aged 15 to 24 are also higher than their counterparts in Pondicherry. The young adult female (25 to 34) rate is exceptionally high (120.8) and is higher than that for males of the same age in Karaikal.

Aetiology of suicides

Quarrel with kin

Although they have an inevitably stereotypical quality, the brief descriptions of the immediate circumstances of suicides in Pondicherry nevertheless throw light on the lines of stress which affect contemporary Indian society. Contrary to some assertions by critics of globalisation, economic factors were perceived to be the precipitating cause of suicide in only a small proportion of cases. The largest single category is what we have termed 'quarrels with kin'. This subsumes such causes as 'quarrel with husband/wife/mother/father/brother/sister/relative'. It can be seen from Table 15.5 that about 40 per cent of suicides in Pondicherry for the period for which we have data fall into this category.[6] The percentage might be even slightly higher if the more ambiguous 'family problems' were included in this category. Conflict with family members accounts for over 40 per cent of suicides of all those under the age of 55. Quarrels with kin are the leading cause of suicide for young adults in Pondicherry. As can be seen in Figure 15.5, 35 per cent of suicides of females and 31 per cent of suicides of males aged between 15 and 44 were attributed to quarrels with kin.

The frequency of familial strife as a precursor to suicide leads us to hypothesise that changing social roles, exposure to the media and other aspects of development may be producing broad role conflicts between parents and children and between spouses in contemporary India, which on relatively rare occasions become manifest in suicide. Venkoba Rao reported that marital problems were a significant antecedent circumstance in the analysis of 100 female burns cases studied in Madurai (Venkoba Rao, Mahendran *et al.* 1989). Latha *et al.* note similar role conflicts in their study of 73 suicide attempters in Manipal (Latha, Bhat *et al.* 1996). They remark that 'the general picture of these adolescents and young adults appears to be one of vulnerability caused by many life stresses or their struggle to cope with threatening situations. . . . [T]hose individuals who are prone to suicide attempts appear to be in conflict with themselves, significant other members of their family and the world around them' (Latha, Bhat *et al.* 1996: 29).

Table 15.5 Immediate circumstances or factors affecting suicide in Pondicherry, 1995–1999

	Female	Male	Total
Economic causes	2.4	6.7	5.2
Family problems	0.5	0.6	0.6
Quarrel with kin	39.9	41.7	41.0
Illness	6.8	9.2	8.4
Mental disorder	5.1	3.3	4.0
Stomach pain	27.8	20.8	23.3
Not known	2.7	5.5	4.5
Other	4.2	2.7	3.2
Total	100	100	100

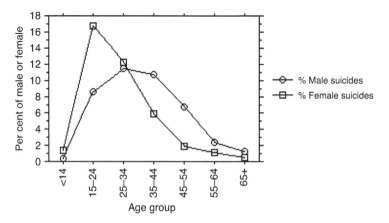

Figure 15.5   Percentage of suicides arising from quarrel with kin, by sex, age group, 1995–1999.

Frustration with life

Another major circumstance of suicide is that most frequently recorded as 'frustration with life', in which we have also included what we perceive as related causes such as 'failure in examinations'. Suicides attributed to this cause are most frequent among those under 14 years of age (19 per cent). They decline monotonically and are the attributed cause of death for only 7 per cent of those over 55.

'Stomach pain'

The most enigmatic category of circumstances of suicide is that repeatedly termed in the reports as 'stomach pain' or much more rarely 'chest pain' or something similar. It is cited as a circumstance in over 23 per cent of all suicides. It is least frequently given as a cause among the very young (6.5 per cent) and most frequently among those aged 55 to 64 (34.5 per cent). As we noted in Chapter 4, it seems likely that in many instances these somatic symptoms are expressions of depressive illness, which for a variety of cultural reasons cannot be expressed in directly psychological terms.

Religion and suicide

The apparent association between religion and rate of suicide is perhaps the most celebrated aspect of Émile Durkheim's *Suicide*. Although contemporary interpretation has largely dismissed the association between Protestantism and high rates of suicide, the question of the association between religion and suicide is of perennial interest. Our Pondicherry data permit us to undertake a unique systematic investigation of the relationship in India using individual level data.[7]

As discussed in the Appendix, 492 cases recorded in 1997 were coded for religion on the basis of the name of the suicide and their listed relative in the records. The calculated suicide rates for Hindus of both sexes (Table 15.6) are strikingly higher (58 per 100,000 for females and 106 for males) than those for either Muslims (12 and 14 per 100,000) or Christians (16 and 18 per 100,000) (Table 15.6). Despite the stark contrast, the differences are not statistically significant, primarily because Hindus constitute such a high proportion (80 per cent) of the population.

If the differences between the propensity to commit suicide between different religious groups which have emerged in this initial investigation are sustained in a broader investigation, it may reignite interest in one of the classical issues in suicide studies.

Conclusions

In a comparative international perspective, suicide is a major social problem in the Union Territory of Pondicherry. In an OECD country such as Australia rates of youth suicide half as high as those we have found for Pondicherry are considered to be at 'crisis' levels and have generated widespread public health interventions in response.

Our study has shown that suicides are particularly concentrated within the majority Hindu community. Two principal causes encompass around 70 per cent of suicides, one social, the other possibly psychological. Conflict within families

Table 15.6 Suicide per 100,000 by sex and religion, 1997

Gender	Religion	Suicide rate
Female	Hindu	37.7
	Muslim	11.6
	Christian	15.8
Male	Hindu	68.4
	Muslim	14.2
	Christian	18.0

Note: $X^2 = 13.7$; not significant.

is identified as the precipitating circumstance in around 40 per cent of all cases we have studied. In another 20–30 per cent of cases it appears that undiagnosed depression may have been the precipitating cause.

In our opinion there is an urgent need for public health authorities to recognise the gravity of what we must term the 'suicide epidemic' in Pondicherry and develop programmes which promote awareness of the risk of suicidal tendencies especially in young adults. Much more effort and far greater resources need to be given to suicide prevention programmes in all districts. Education of medical personnel in the poorly articulated symptoms of depression and the availability of appropriate anti-depressant medications could also assist in reducing the very high incidence of suicide in the territory.

Appendix: Coding of additional data

We have utilised internal evidence to add codes for a number of variables in our data set.

Season

In coding season we have used the dates of death for 1996, the only year for which we have a complete year of records. We have coded the months November to March as winter, April to June as summer and July to October as monsoon.

Religion

No record is kept of the religion of suicides. However, since different Indian communities use quite distinctive names it is possible in the majority of cases to determine their nominal religious community. Nevertheless, since some converts to Christianity retain Hindu names, the possibility of misclassification of such individuals cannot be dismissed.

Notes

1 The paper on which this chapter is based was co-authored with Dr S. Vaidyanathan. It was presented to the International Society for Suicide Prevention Conference, Chennai, India, 22–26 September, 2001. We are indebted to Mr S. Radjagopalane, Director, Maitreyi, Befrienders India Centre, Pondicherry for giving us permission to use the data which Maitreyi collected.
2 We have no convincing explanation for the discrepancy.
3 See Chapter 8 for a discussion of these patterns.
4 We have utilised cases from 1996 in constructing this figure.
5 The exceptionally high rates of suicide in Karaikal were first drawn to our attention by Sri Sharda Prasad, IPS, Director of the National Crime Records Bureau.
6 The 1994 volume of *Accidental Deaths and Suicides in India* lists such family quarrels as the circumstance of 44.1 per cent of suicides in Pondicherry, the highest proportion for this cause in India.
7 Lester (1996) has examined the question using ecological data.

16 Conclusion

Introduction

Compared to major killers such as diseases of the lung or heart and cancer, suicides are a relatively minor cause of death in India. About 3 per cent of rural Indian male deaths and a far smaller percentage of female deaths are attributable to suicide (Registrar General 2002, Statements 8–16). In Andhra in 1991, nearly 4 per cent of female deaths and slightly over 3 per cent of male deaths were self-inflicted (Institute of Health Systems).

Yet among young people in India, suicide is the leading cause of death (Registrar General 2002, Statement 7). Young women in rural India aged between 15 and 19 are almost twice as likely to take their own lives as die from tuberculosis, the next most prevalent cause of death (Ramanakumar 2004, Table 4). Suicide is also the most common cause of death of rural women aged between 15 and 44 (Registrar General 2002, Statement 24: 34). Despite the very high rates of youth suicides, popular perceptions in India, if we judge by media attention, are much more likely to identify farmers at high risk of suicide.

Summary of findings of social causes

Trends

Rates of recorded death by suicide in India have risen steadily not only in the years since 1967 when systematic national records were first published but from the very first accounts we have in the 1870s. If we can extrapolate from the experience of West Bengal, the national suicide rate may have nearly trebled in the first twenty years of independence, from an estimated rate of 2 per 100,000 in 1947 to 7.6 in 1967. It grew by 142 per cent between 1967 and 2007 when it reached 10.8 in 100,000. Only in the two large northern states of Uttar Pradesh and Bihar was there evidence of declining rates over the period. If the overall trend of the last two decades of the twentieth century persists, India's national suicide rate may reach 12.1 per 100,000 in 2020, which would probably change its global suicide ranking from near the middle to a spot in the top 15–20 per cent. That is a rate already exceeded at the present by five of the larger Indian states.

The apparently inexorable rise in the number of suicide deaths and of the rate at which they occur force us to consider both whether there are broader social changes that may explain the rising trend and what may be done to restrain it.

Let us begin by recapitulating some of the key findings that have emerged from our examination in depth in earlier chapters.

Age

Unlike developed countries, but consistent with what we know of developing ones, suicide rates in India do not increase steadily with age. Rather, as we saw in Chapter 8, they are concentrated in young and middle-aged adults. The rates for females are higher than those for males until age 29, after which the rate of male suicides is higher. Women aged between 15 and 29 are at greatest risk of suicide, while the period of greatest risk for men is in the age groups between 30 and 59. For women and men aged between 15 and 34, suicide is the leading cause of death (Registrar General 2002, Statement 7). After the period of peak risk, suicide rates in India tend to decline with age.

The concentration of risk of suicide in India in young adults is the basis for the argument advanced in Chapter 8 that India is in the midst of an unperceived youth and young adult suicide crisis. For young Indian women the rates are so high, when compared with the experience of other nations, that urgent remedial action must be taken. Young female suicide rates for Pondicherry, Karnataka, West Bengal, Sikkim, Maharashtra, Kerala, Tamil Nadu, Madhya Pradesh, Goa, Tirpura, Gujarat, Andhra Pradesh and Orissa are higher than those for young women in 32 nations for which the WHO provides data. Young adult male rates are also very high when compared internationally. States with very high young adult male rates are Pondicherry, Kerala, Karnataka, Assam, Tripura, Goa, West Bengal, Maharashtra, Haryana, Tamil Nadu and Madhya Pradesh.

Gender

India confounds the general pattern in other countries – China excepted – that suicide is predominantly a male phenomenon where there are typically three to five male suicides for every female suicide. The very high levels of female suicides in India, especially among young females, makes the male–female suicide ratio much more nearly equal at roughly 7 males: 5 females. We saw in Chapter 7 that despite increases in suicide rates, there has been little change in the rate of male to female suicide deaths in India over a 40-year period since 1967, a result which suggests that the factors leading to increases in the incidence of suicide are having an equal impact on males and females. Female literacy – which we expected to be a significant cause of increasing suicides – was found to have little impact once we took the impact of time into account.

Region

One of the most striking and enduring characteristics of suicide in India is the very great difference in rates between the Indian states. Suicide rates appear to increase as we move from the north of India to the south. Suicides are lowest (less than 5 per 100,000) in the Gangetic Plain. Rates are higher (5 to 15 per 100,000) in central India (broadly construed to include Haryana, Rajasthan and Gujarat as well as Maharashtra, Madhya Pradesh, Orissa and Andhra Pradesh). The highest levels (over 15 per 100,000) are found in south India. As we have noted at many points in earlier chapters the most extreme rates are in Kerala and Pondicherry.

The exceptions to this broad categorisation occur in eastern India. West Bengal has high suicide levels similar to those in south India. There is no overall pattern to the suicide rates observed in the small hill states of northeastern India. Rates are very high in Tripura, moderately high in Arunachal Pradesh and Assam, but very low in Nagaland, Meghalaya and Mizoram.

Marital status

Unlike the situation in industrialised economies, in India, marriage does not confer general protection from suicide. Married men, in particular, are more likely to take their own lives than are unmarried men. Married women, by contrast, do have lower rates of suicide than single women. For both men and women, divorce – still a relatively rare phenomenon in India – is associated with highly elevated risks of suicide. Widowers and widows are at strikingly different risks of suicide. Men whose wives have died are at increased risk of suicide. For women, loss of a partner leads to decreased risk of suicide, a surprising finding.

When we compared the relationship between the suicide rates of the unmarried to the married in the larger states we find an interesting pattern. While in general unmarried men are less likely than married to take their own lives, this is not the case in Bihar, Goa, Madhya Pradesh, Rajasthan and Uttar Pradesh. Unmarried women are, in general, at greater risk than married women of suicide, but the comparative risks are considerably greater in Bihar, Madhya Pradesh, Rajasthan and Uttar Pradesh.

Education

There is a clear, but at the same time complex, relationship between levels of education and rates of suicide. In states where literacy rates are low, so are suicide rates. As people acquire higher levels of education their risk of suicide also increases, except for university graduates. At each level of education, the suicide risk for women is higher than for men.

When we look at the patterns in individual states we find, on the whole, the same broad regional pattern (low in the north, high in the south) that is characteristic of suicides generally. At relatively higher levels of education, these generalisations no longer hold true. In states – principally in the north – where relatively small percentages of women attain matriculation, their suicide rates are very high. Yet another pattern, one that also defies ready encapsulation, applies to those who have been educated to higher secondary level. Women with technical degrees are at what can only be described as an extraordinary level of risk of suicide.

Occupation

Although the extensive media coverage of farmer suicides leads us to be acutely aware of the risks they face, there are other groups that receive relatively little attention which appear to be at very high suicide risk. The unemployed in India are one prominent group. Elevated suicide rates among the unemployed are perhaps especially noticeable in states like the Punjab in which suicides are otherwise relatively rare. By contrast, they are relatively lower in high unemployment/high suicide states such as Kerala. Other occupation groups at very elevated risk of suicide are civil servants and retired individuals. By contrast, the suicide rates for housewives, farmers and students, while significant, are relatively lower than groups such as civil servants.

Human development

We noted in Chapter 4 that there were two broad clusters of precipitating causes of suicide: those we termed 'crises of human development' and those we termed 'crises of personal relationships'. The former included factors such as the levels of unemployment and bankruptcy as well as levels of female literacy and levels of civic engagement – but also cases clustered under the label 'family problems'. As we will note shortly, unemployment and the relative failure of economic growth to generate jobs appears to be a significant contributing cause to suicide deaths in India.

A dark window on society: interpretation/synthesis

How should we understand the dense mass of facts that constitute the portrait of suicide in India? The reasons that lead an individual to take their life are often unknowable. The decision to end life itself comes at the end of a long and complex chain of antecedent causes. In this book we are concerned primarily with the social forces, broadly understood, that condition the world in which the suicidal individual lives – but those forces also form the world of the tens of thousands of their neighbours whose individual circumstances, psychological states and brain chemistry never take them down the shadowed corridor to the final interior decision to end life. Because the social forces that seem to lead to the broad differences in the rates of suicide between regions and over time affect most individuals in society, we must be cautious when we draw causal inferences. For example, as we have seen, education is associated with higher rates of suicide. It would be a mistake, however, to suggest that education – which from almost every point of view contributes to human development and wellbeing – is responsible for elevated rates of suicide. Rather, we must seek to understand why increased levels of education lead a relatively miniscule fraction of a population to be at elevated risk of suicide. We cannot conclude, as has sometimes been done, that a growing sense of individualism and awareness of other life possibilities arising from education are *ipso facto* harmful; it is more fruitful to attempt to understand why a very small number of individuals, in a society that as a whole enjoys higher levels of human development, are at increased risk. Suicide, from this perspective, informs us about the stresses emerging as society changes. Exceptional, individual choices to end unsupportable lives appear to open a dark window on society and to give us insight into the hairline social fractures that inevitably occur as ordinary lives are caught up in change.

Let us begin to draw together the disparate threads of the many social dimensions we have considered up to this point. We have seen that there are important differences in the risk of suicide between men and women, between the unmarried and the married and it is these primary differences that we will seek to explain.

We have seen that most female suicides cluster in the years of late adolescence and early adulthood. We speculated that issues arising around marriage in a society where arranged marriage is the rule and patriarchal domination is strong may explain why this is a period of acute stress for some young women especially those whose education and other experiences may lead them to aspire to greater individual autonomy. We can attempt to measure the strength of these competing social forces by looking, on the one hand, at the average size of family groups in the Indian states – a possible proxy for the strength of patriarchy and the traditional family – and, on the other, at the ability of females to gain access to the media, in particular to films, which in India are the most powerful sources of images of romantic love – a proxy for independence, both physical and psychic.[1]

When we examined the occupational dimensions of suicide we found that those who are unemployed are at elevated risk of suicide. We can examine two dimensions of employment: levels of reported unemployment in a state, and the overall dynamism of a state in terms of its capacity to generate employment, that is, its 'employment elasticity'.[2]

These four variables when incorporated in a multiple regression equation explain most of the variance ($R^2 = 0.70$) in state suicide rates in India. When we create a polynomial transformation of the variable which measures female access to the cinema to reflect the 'inverted U'-shaped nature of the relationship with suicide and incorporate it in a backwards step-wise multiple regression model, three factors (female access to films, percentage unemployed and the log of employment elasticity) explain virtually all the variance in the differences between state suicide rates ($R^2 = 0.98$), a remarkable result. A single variable — the polynomial transformation of female access to films – explains 74 per cent of the variance in state suicide rates.

When we examine the factors that appear to have the greatest impact on different categories of Indians a slightly more complex picture emerges. The variable that is most closely associated with the suicide rates of unmarried females is that which reports the percentage that see at least one or more films each month. When we examine a scattergram we find, as noted above, an unexpected result: the result is curvilinear. That is, in states where fewer than 5 per cent of women see at least one film once per month, such as the Punjab, Bihar, UP and Haryana, unmarried female suicide rates are low (Figure 16.1); the curve rises to a peak when about 30 per cent of women in a state see films regularly, then falls as the percentage of women with exposure to films approaches 50 per cent. A polynomial transformation of the variable explains 62 per cent of the variance in the unmarried female suicide rates between states.

The freedom women have to see films is also strongly correlated with the unmarried male suicide rate, explaining 69 per cent of the variance. Differences in the elasticity of employment explain a further 7 per cent of the variance, a suggestive result, but not a statistically significant one.

For married women, the freedom to see films explains a remarkable 81 per cent of the variance in suicide rates. The percentage of the population who are unemployed explains a further 4 per cent of the variance; this is significant at the 0.08 level.

Female film access explains 62 per cent of the married male suicide rate. The elasticity of employment explains a further 14 per cent of the variance in the suicide rates of married men, and this is significant at the 0.03 level.

The curved nature of the relationship suggests that once a significant percentage of women see films on a regular basis, the impact on suicide rates begins to diminish, that is, it appears that the impact of seeing films is to be understood as a consequence of changing ideas that occurs in a period of transition. There are suggestive parallels here with Stack's finding, which we noted in Chapter 9, of a curvilinear pattern in urban suicide rates, which tend to increase in the early stages of industrialisation and then fall as populations adjust to urban life (1982).

One line of interpretation of these findings about the relationship between viewing films and suicide is suggested by studies of the history of marriage and family relations in Europe between the sixteenth and twentieth centuries. Stone

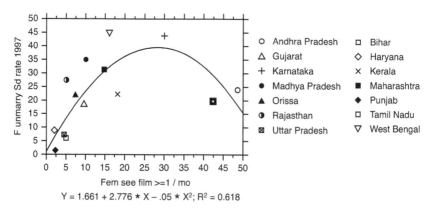

$$Y = 1.661 + 2.776 * X - .05 * X^2; R^2 = 0.618$$

Figure 16.1 Percentage of females who see at least one film per month vs female unmarried suicide rate.

and Shorter in influential studies suggested that over this period a major change in the nature of marriage occurred (Stone 1977; Shorter 1976). The traditional family, especially in sixteenth century France, says Shorter,

> ... was held firmly in the matrix of a larger social order. One set of ties bound it to the surrounding kin ... Another set fastened it to the wider community, and gaping holes in the shield of privacy permitted others to enter the household freely and, if necessary, preserve order. A final set of ties held this elementary family to generations past and future.
>
> (Shorter 1976: 3)

Traditional marital relations were relatively emotionless, says Shorter. A French farmer of the period would be more concerned at the sickness of his horse than his wife (Shorter 1976: 56):

> The surest evidence of emotionless courtship would be the arranged marriage. If the wishes of the young people were completely neglected and they were matched to whomever in the village best suited their parents' dynastic ambitions, affection and sentiment would by definition be absent.
>
> (Shorter 1976: 138)

Stone traces a slow process of transition from marital alliances based on parental concerns over property, status and power to ones increasingly reflecting a view that 'sentiment' should play a central role in the choice of marriage partner. He notes a rising trend of individualism and sentiment, which lasted from about 1670 up until the French revolution. This period was characterised by a tendency for the nuclear family to be the common form and for considerations of sentiment to enter into marital choices (Stone 1977: 666).

Stone offers a typology of mating arrangements that reflects a shift over time in the relations of power over marriage decisions between parents and children. In the first form, the decision over choice of marriage partner is made entirely by the parents 'without the advice or consent of the bride or groom' (Stone 1977: 270). In this form, concerns over property, social status and political power are the predominant concerns. In the second form, while parents select potential marriage partners, the children have an increasing right to veto an incompatible partner (Stone 1977: 270–71). In the third form, the children themselves make the choice, 'on the understanding that it will be made from a family of more or less equal financial and status positions, with the parents retaining the right of veto' (Stone 1977: 271). In the last form, the choice is made solely by the children themselves who 'merely inform their parents of what they have decided' (Stone 1977: 271).

One of the factors influencing the changing perceptions about the basis on which marriage should be founded was the rise of romantic ideas in literature. Stone traces the growth of romantic love as the 'principal theme of the novel' from the early eighteenth century (Stone 1977: 278). He argues that changing attitudes as well as changing economic structures appear to explain the shift in marriages alliances decided by parents to those increasingly influenced by 'sentiment'.

Watt, in his study of marriage in the French-speaking Neuchâtel region of Switzerland in the early modern period, notes a similar pattern of changes in marriage relations in the eighteenth century. In this period new courtship customs such as 'bundling' emerged; there were sharp increases in the number of prenuptial conceptions, and rapid increases in the number of divorces (Watt 1992: 174–193). He also found increasing evidence in the court records of a shift from marriages in which status and wealth were the primary concerns to ones in which affection between partners was evident (Watt 1992: 159–162, 210–218). Watt notes that besides philosophical writing, literature also promoted the idea of loving unions amongst equals. He quotes from Traer's *Marriage and the Family*:

> Increasingly during the [18th] century, imaginative literature proclaimed the importance of sentiment in human relationships. Dramatists and novelists portrayed happy marriages based on inclination or love and created by the free choice of the two spouses. They praised marriage as a source of emotional satisfaction and stressed the equality of the wife with her husband.
>
> (p. 78 in Traer quoted in Watt 1992: 270)

Like Stone, Watt identifies both changes in social ideas as well as the emergence of industrialisation as contributing to the increasing emphasis on affection in marriage.

> [T]he evidence from Neuchâtel suggests that the evolution of the *control* of marriage resulted primarily from ideological changes, as seen in the new decisions of judicial authorities. At the same time, transformations in the institution of marriage itself most likely were linked more to economic developments and most pronounced among members of the working classes. Far from being mutually exclusive, ideological and economic changes complemented and reinforced each other.
>
> (Watt 1992: 277–280)

In his subsequent study of suicide in Geneva, Watt discovered an interaction between changing forms of marriage and patterns of suicide. In the older form of arranged marriages, married individuals tended to have higher suicide rates relative to the unmarried. That changed significantly in the eighteenth century when the classical Western pattern of lower suicide rates among married people emerged.

> [W]hat was it about marriage [in the 18th century] that provided a degree of safety against suicide? The most plausible explanation is in the area of sentiment. The reason that the percentage of married people declined among suicides from the sixteenth and seventeenth centuries to the eighteenth was

because people were investing more of themselves emotionally in marriage and the nuclear family.

(Watt 2001: 222)

Watt also found that the emergence of ideas that marriages should be founded on affection increasingly led to conflicts between parents and children.

> Generational conflict . . . was more often a motive for suicide among Geneva's youth. . . . These suicides [arising from generational conflict] reflect a certain tension between the increasing independence that young people asserted, on the one hand, and the persistent efforts of parents to influence the major decisions in their children's lives, on the other. The growing importance of romantic love as a legitimate motive for marrying – at times conflicted with parents' interest in seeing their sons and daughters form advantageous matches. These suicides can also be explained in part by the growing importance of sentiment in the nuclear family. With the strengthening of the emotional bonds of the nuclear family, family dysfunction, like marital dysfunction, became less tolerable.

(Watt 2001: 236–237)

The relevance of the European experience in the seventeenth and eighteenth centuries to contemporary India is, we think, self-evident. India is undergoing profound social changes which exhibit some strong parallels with those which occurred in Europe: fewer children every year die before the age of five; increasing numbers of women are able to read and write, and at least in urban areas, increasing numbers of women make significant economic contributions to the welfare of their families (rural women have, of course, always played a significant economic role). And ideas about romantic love form a significant, perhaps the predominant theme, of popular culture as exemplified by India's enormous film industry.

We can see one aspect of the impact of these change with especial clarity in the reports of the experiences of suicidal adolescents in the Indian diaspora where expectations arising from Indian culture come into more direct clash with those current in the host country. Pillay and Wassenaar, for example, in their study of South African adolescents of Indian descent, found that 76 per cent of those who had attempted suicide had 'experienced conflict with their parents in the 12 hours preceding their self-destructive acts' (Pillay and Wassenaar 1997: 158).

> Conflicts with parents were found to revolve mainly around issues of individuation and developmental needs where adolescents reported that their parents opposed their requests to go on dates or have romantic or peer-group involvement.

(Pillay and Wassenaar 1997: 158)

Wassenaar and his colleagues note that for South African Indian women:

Socialized powerlessness, economic disadvantage, and increasing exposure to a 'Western' lifestyle perceived as more egalitarian and free contribute to 'acculturative stress' (Hovey and King, 1994: 35) and to the cycle of self-injury ... Where the patient is an adolescent ... the role conflict is heightened by the usual role conflicts of adolescence, which adds to the risk of suicidal expression.

(Wassenaar, van der Veen *et al.* 1998: 90)

As we saw in Chapter 14, similar factors have been identified in the Indian community in Fiji (Haynes 1984; Booth 1999a).

Bhugra *et al.*, in their study of suicidal behaviour in London, concluded:

[C]onflict with the family as a precipitant and life event in Asian females is a remarkable and important finding and deserves to studied further. These repetitions suggest that continuing conflict within the family needs to be understood and managed within the gender and cultural boundaries so that repetitions can be reduced.

(Bhugra, Baldwin *et al.* 1999)

Evidence for the emerging stresses in marriages emerges from anthropological studies of Indian society. Sylvia Vatuk, in a study of families in urban neighbourhoods in Meerut in the 1960s, found that arranged marriages were universal and that female subordination was greatest in larger families and where women were younger (Vatuk 1972: 66, Table XII). She noted the strong desire by young married women to escape from those positions of subordination and to create nuclear families in which the development of affectionate ties with their husbands might be enhanced:

Increasingly young people, particularly women, express a preference for living neologically, free to run a household as they see fit, without needing to defer to the older generation. Even urban parents of unmarried sons often speak of the time when their son's bride will leave them either before or soon after his marriage. 'The young people nowadays want to be free,' the old women lament; 'they don't know how to listen to their elders anymore.' They mourn the passing of the old-time daughter-in-law, replaced by the educated girl who dares to disagree with her mother-in-law and persuades her husband to separate from the parental household so she can socialize with neighbors, dress up in the latest styles, and go out to movies instead of staying home to do housework.

(Vatuk 1972: 69)

Vatuk also found evidence that as in Europe at an earlier time, very different ideas were emerging about what should be expected from a marriage partner:

Formal education is considered desirable in a bride, as long as it has not deflected her from the functions and duties of a woman. The demand for educated women as brides for white-collar young men is probably largely responsible for the high level of education reached by most girls in these mohallas, because few of them are seriously preparing for a career. Parents often say that educating one's daughter ensures her a 'good' match – and up to a point it does. The danger in education beyond the BA is that the range of acceptable men greatly narrows. Because her bridegroom must be equally well educated, parents often refuse to allow their daughter to pursue post-graduate studies. . . .

College-educated young men often explain their preference for educated wives in terms of social advantages. They speak of the greater sophistication of the educated girl, her awareness of things beyond the home and family, her knowledge of modern fashion and home decoration. More important, they praise her ability to entertain her husband's office colleagues in a refined manner, serving attractively prepared snacks or meals, perhaps even exchanging greetings and limited polite conversation. They admire the educated girl's ability to go out walking with her husband in public or to accompany him to the movies occasionally without feeling unduly embarrassed or shy. A gradual shift in the role of the wife – now seen as a companion in marriage – is clearly associated with the preference for educated brides.

Whatever reasons underlie the preference for educated girls, it is increasingly necessary, even in the lower middle class, for fathers to provide their daughters with at least a high school education, or even more, if they aspire to a son-in-law equal in status to themselves, or of higher status. If they want a man who can provide their daughter with the standard of living to which she is, or would like to become, accustomed, they have to encourage – or allow – her to continue studying, preferably to the BA level, before completing marriage arrangements.

(Vatuk 1972: 78–80)

Joanne Moller in her study of family relations in Kumaon in the early 1990s found similar tensions and tendencies emerging as different generational ideas about marriage come into conflict. As in Meerut in the 1960s, parents in Kumaon wanted to educate their daughters to ensure an advantageous match. For the groom's parents, the educated daughter is both desired – and feared.[3]

Extended schooling is . . . considered to have a detrimental impact on a female's disposition and conduct. Educated women are said to be obstinate, strong headed and outspoken (*tej*), and education is thought to develop a female's self-confidence and independence of spirit.

(Moller 2003: 110)

It is a well-known fact that in north India the in-marrying daughter-in-law is seen as a threat to the solidarity of the joint family and as a messenger of inauspiciousness and misfortune. . . . A main concern is that the new bride will win her husband's affection and convince him to set up an autonomous household unit, or, that after the birth of children, the tension and antagonism between sisters-in-law will intensify, resulting in premature and undignified partition.

(Moller 2003: 112)

[A]n educated daughter-in-law is deemed more likely to forge a strong alliance with her husband and persuade him to break off from his parents and set up a nuclear family on their own.

(Moller 2003: 115)

Fragments of evidence such as this appear to indicate that increasingly, while parentally arranged marriages remain the norm, the desire for 'companionate marriages' based on mutual affection and greater equality is clearly present.[4] It seems possible that, in a very small fraction of cases, the mismatch between arranged marriages in which the inclinations of the children play little part are coming into conflict with aspirations for relationships in marriage based on affection.

We have found a few fragments of evidence from urban India and from the Indian diaspora that indicate marriage arrangements have begun to pass to Stone's second stage in which children have some measure of veto over potential marriage partners, and have in some cases even passed to a stage which approaches his third form (for evidence from the diaspora, see Bellafante 2005; for a superficial summary of tends in India in the 1990s, see India Today 2000; for similar aspirations in Pakistan see Hasan 2004: 17–20).

We have inferred that where family size is largest the traditional family structure is strongest. One possible indicator that largely 'instrumental' views of marriage persist in these areas is to be found in the strong correlation between the average size of households and the reported rate of murders for dowry ($r = 0.68$, significant at 0.006). The converse holds for suicide rates, which are lowest for all gender and marital groups where households are largest. These are also the states where the smallest per cent of women see at least one film per month; the correlation between the two is strong and negative ($r = -0.76$; significant at 0.001). The relationship between family size and suicide rates in the Indian states is weakest for unmarried women ($r = -0.26$; not significant) and men ($r = -0.48$; not significant) but stronger for married men ($r = -0.58$, significant at 0.02) and strongest for married women ($r = -0.64$, significant at 0.01). This result suggests the hypothesis that it may be tensions arising within families that approach the nuclear family in size, arising perhaps from mismatches between the reality of marriages arranged without consideration of affection and the growing aspiration for companionate marriages, which lead in exceptional circumstances to suicide. Certainly this hypothesis is supported by the evidence presented in Chapters 4 and 16, which showed that conflict with kin is a major precipitating factor in suicides of both women and men.

The impact of the tensions arising from changed perceptions of the role of affection in marriage is, as we have already seen, a very profound one, if we may infer this from the relationship between exposure to films and suicide rates. It seems likely to us that the dreams of romantic love that are the staple of the Indian film industry play a very significant role changing attitudes towards relations with parents and spouses. Tensions within marriage arising from the misalignment between the way marriages are contracted and the changing aspirations of married couples may be one of the fracture lines in contemporary Indian society that we can perceive through the dark window of the incidence of suicide.

The lag between changes in systems of marriage arrangement and aspirations may also explain the finding which was presented in Chapter 9 that in states where suicide rates are generally low, urban rates are considerably higher than rural rates. It seems reasonable to hypothesize that the mismatch, which we believe is a significant causal factor, is lower in urban than rural areas in south India but is relatively higher in urban north India than in north Indian villages.

Attitudes toward marriage may also explain two other important findings reported in Chapter 12. The very low suicide rates we observed among widowed women may be the reverse side of elevated rates among the married. That is, if individuals obtain relatively little emotional support from marriage, then the death of a spouse may not lead to the emotional crisis found where companionate marriages are the prevalent form. Yip found a similar pattern in Hong Kong and concluded that women in particular may not have benefited as much from marriage as men (Yip 1998).

The other finding relates to the very high rates of suicide observed among those who are divorced. We observed in Chapter 12 that in states where divorce rates were low, the suicide rates of the divorced are higher than in states where divorce rates are relatively more common. Here again the result appears to show us the impact of social change. Divorce itself is an indicator of the disruption of traditional expectations that marriage is for life, which perhaps explains why suicide rates among the divorced are so high. Where divorce is less common – and presumably less socially acceptable – suicide rates are higher, and tend to be somewhat lower where divorce is more frequent.

Let us turn to another significant force that influences the incidence of suicide. Shorter, Stone and Watt all draw our attention to the mutual impact of both changes in social attitudes and in the structure of the economy on the changing nature of the family. In India, as we noted above, there is a strong relationship between unemployment, the elasticity of employment growth and the suicide rate. Where registered unemployment is highest and where economic growth produces only weak generation of employment, suicide rates are also highest. Aspects of employment show no significant correlation with unmarried female suicide rates in the Indian states. There is a moderately strong correlation between unmarried male suicide rates and unemployment ($r = 0.63$, significant at 0.01) and the natural log of the elasticity of employment ($r = -0.67$, significant at 0.007). The correlations are of almost equal strength for married women (unemployment: $r = 0.69$, significant at 0.005; ln elasticity of employment, $r = -0.67$, significant at 0.007). The strongest correlations are for married males (unemployment: $r = 0.75$, significant at 0.001; ln elasticity of employment: $r = -0.75$, significant at 0.001). This result appears to bear out at the all-India level Murphy Halliburton's suggestion that in Kerala the gap between the aspirations to employment, themselves the product of higher levels of education, and the realities of limited employment opportunities may be a significant cause of suicides. Our findings suggest that the relative failure of economic development to produce strong employment growth has consequences spread far wider than the more prominent examples of economic hardship in specific sectors such as weaving and farming. It is striking that in Kerala, where economic growth has the weakest impact on employment (employment elasticity = 0.013) and where unemployment in the 1990s was highest (21 per cent), suicide rates were also very high; at the other end of the distribution, in the Punjab, employment elasticity was high (0.43), and both unemployment rates (4 per cent) and suicide rates were low. We hypothesise that the relationship between unemployment and suicide may be the major explanation for the fact that male suicide rates tend to reach their peak between the ages of 30 and 40 when, for a small group of individuals, family responsibilities coupled with disappointment and failure in a highly competitive employment market may prove insurmountable. Unlike the situation common in the West, where the loss of identity following retirement is seen to be a contributor to elevated suicide rates among the over 60 age group, in India, the failure to establish what is perceived to be a suitable employment identity may explain the peak of male suicide rates in mid-adulthood. As we noted in Chapter 12, the comparatively carefree lives of young unmarried adult males may explain why their suicide rates are lower than those of married males.

Conclusion

India is being shaken by forces of social change. We have argued in this book that the fault-lines of those tectonic forces can in part be glimpsed through the lens of suicide statistics. India faces multiple suicide crises. We have seen that, while the media focuses, almost obsessively, on a few categories of suicide deaths such as those of farmers, there are profound issues of public health such as those involving young Indians, male and female, which must not continue to be ignored. There is urgent need in India for education programmes, counselling services and medical support. Such programmes have been effective in reducing needless suicide deaths in other countries. Dedicated NGOs in India in a few areas are showing what can be done. But concerted action by government is essential if the tragic toll of wasted lives is to be brought down.

Notes

1 Data on average household size come from the *Indian Human Development Report* (Shariff 1999: 70, Table 4.8). Data on women's access to the media come from (Kumar 1996). There is a moderately strong, statistically significant relationship between female literacy rates and the percentage of females who see one or more films per month ($r = 0.54$; $p = 0.04$). There are two notable clusters of outliers. Haryana and the Punjab have medium levels of female literacy but low levels of access to films. At the opposite pole are Karnataka and West Bengal in which high percentages of females view films regularly, but which have medium levels of female literacy.

2 Data on unemployment and employment elasticity come from *Economic and Political Weekly* 2005: 1299.
3 Steve Derne makes useful parallel observations on attitudes to joint families, pressures to separate, etc. (Derne 1994).
4 For discussion of the emergence of 'companionate marriages' in early modern Europe, see (Shorter 1976, especially Chapters 4 & 6; Stone 1977, Chapter 8; Watt 2001: 251).

Appendix 1   Suicide prevention

In a workshop focused on suicide prevention in 2001, Dr C. Hendricks Brown made three observations about the challenges involved in suicide prevention:

(1) Suicide is a low base-rate behavior, approximately 12 per 100,000 in the [U.S.] population at large. Therefore, changes in numbers of suicides must be studied appropriately to ensure that any change is due to the intervention, and not to other factors. (2) Risk factors for suicide are non-specific, since they associated with other undesirable outcomes. Therefore study of simple causal relationships for suicide is not possible. (3) Risk factors can change in individuals over short periods of time, and across developmental life-stages, further complicating assessment of suicide risk and prevention.

(Goldsmith 2001: 1–2)

Despite the difficulties in identifying the risk factors in any individual case, there are useful guidelines available which outline major risk factors and which give guidance to individuals who may be concerned about their own suicidal thoughts, and for parents and friends who may be concerned about the behaviour of a child or friend.

Risk factors

The first step in preventing suicide is to identify and understand the risk factors. A risk factor is anything that increases the likelihood that persons will harm themselves. However, risk factors are not necessarily causes. Research has identified the following risk factors for suicide (DHHS 1999):

- Previous suicide attempt(s)
- History of mental disorders, particularly depression
- History of alcohol and substance abuse
- Family history of suicide
- Family history of child maltreatment
- Feelings of hopelessness

- Impulsive or aggressive tendencies
- Barriers to accessing mental health treatment
- Loss (relational, social, work, or financial)
- Physical illness
- Easy access to lethal methods
- Unwillingness to seek help because of the stigma attached to mental health and substance abuse disorders or suicidal thoughts
- Cultural and religious beliefs – for instance, the belief that suicide is a noble resolution of a personal dilemma
- Local epidemics of suicide
- Isolation, a feeling of being cut off from other people

Source: http://www.cdc.gov/ncipc/factsheets/suifacts.htm
accessed 6 January 2006.

The path that leads from risk factors to action is different in every case. One conceptualisation of that path is presented in Figure A1.1

Important advice concerns the behaviours that are typical in individuals seriously contemplating suicide. In the majority of cases of youth suicide, the individual has made an attempt to communicate their thoughts and feelings to someone they know before attempting to take their own life.

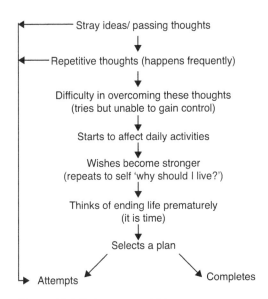

Figure A1.1 Pathways to suicide.

Source: Adapted from WHO Southeast Asia http://w3.whosea.org/en/Section1174/Section1199/
Section1567/Section1824_8080.htm, accessed 11 May 2002.

What are the warning signs of suicide risk?

Classroom behaviour

- Marked decline in school performance and levels achieved
- Skipping classes and opting out of school activities generally
- Poor concentration, sleepiness, inattentiveness
- Unusually disruptive or rebellious behaviour
- Death or suicide themes dominate written, artistic or creative work
- Loss of interest in previously pleasurable activities
- Inability to tolerate praise or rewards

Interpersonal behaviour

- Giving away prized possessions.
- Sudden changes in relationships, for example, exhibiting disruptive behaviour.
- Withdrawing from friends and social involvements
- Not wanting to be touched by others

Other behavioural signs

- Apathy about dress and appearance
- Sudden change in weight
- Running away from home
- Risk-taking and careless behaviour
- 'Accident proneness'
- Sudden and striking personality changes and changes in mood
- Overt signs of mental illness (for example, hallucinations)
- Loss of sense of humour or sudden compulsive joking
- Sleeping pattern changes
- Self-mutilation behaviours
- Noticeable increase in compulsive behaviour
- Development of extreme dependency
- Sudden happiness after a prolonged period of depression
- Impulsive tendencies
- Depressive tendencies
- Unrealistic expectations held of self

Verbal expression of suicidal intent or depression

- Direct statements, for example/'I wish I were dead', 'I'm going to end it all'
- Indirect statements, such as, 'No one cares if l live or die', 'Does it hurt to die?'

Episodic stressful precipitants (stressful episodes)

School and society

- In trouble with school authorities or police
- Loss or disappointment in school
- Change of school and/or address
- Strong demands from adults for show of strength, competence and effectiveness

Interpersonal and physical problems

- Loss of an important person through death or divorce
- Recent suicide of friend or relative
- Breaking up with boyfriend or girlfriend
- Exposure to violence, incest, rape
- Abusing drugs or alcohol
- Feared pregnancy
- Refusal by significant other to provide anticipated help, support or love
- Major disappointment or humiliation
- Major family dysfunction

Chronic stressful life situations

Home life

- Chronic depression or mental illness in parent(s)
- Incest or child abuse
- Severe parental conflict
- Family involvement with drug or alcohol abuse
- Poor communication with parents
- Pressures for high achievement to gain parental approval or acceptance
- Exposure to suicide, suicidal behaviour or violent death of relative or friend

Interpersonal relations

- Involvement in physical violence
- Inability to relate well to peers
- Sexual promiscuity
- Inability to enjoy or appreciate friendships or to express affection openly
- Mood swings and occasional outbursts
- Feelings of worthlessness, being a burden or having let parents or others down

• Feelings of guilt, failure. having no control over their lives

Source: http://www.infoxchange.net.au/dhs/youth/suicide/hs5.htm, accessed 6 January 2006.

Lastly, there is valuable advice about the most effective ways to respond to an individual who appears to entertain thoughts of suicide.

If someone is feeling depressed or suicidal, our first response is to try to help. We offer advice, share our own experiences, try to find solutions.

We'd do better to be quiet and listen. People who feel suicidal don't want answers or solutions. They want a safe place to express their fears and anxieties, to be themselves.

Listening – really listening – is not easy. We must control the urge to say something – to make a comment, add to a story or offer advice. We need to listen not just to the facts that the person is telling us, but to the feelings that lie behind them. We need to understand things from their perspective, not ours.

Here are some points to remember if you are helping a person who feels suicidal.

What do people who feel suicidal want?

• Someone to listen. Someone who will take time to really listen to them.
• Someone who won't judge, or give advice or opinions, but will give their undivided attention.
• Someone to trust. Someone who will respect them and won't try to take charge. Someone who will treat everything in complete confidence.
• Someone to care. Someone who will make themselves available, put the person at ease and speak calmly. Someone who will reassure, accept and believe. Someone who will say, 'I care.'

What do people who feel suicidal not want?

• To be alone. Rejection can make the problem seem ten times worse. Having someone to turn to makes all the difference. Just listen.
• To be advised. Lectures don't help. Nor does a suggestion to 'cheer up', or an easy assurance that 'everything will be okay.' Don't analyze, compare, categorize or criticize. Just listen.
• To be interrogated. Don't change the subject, don't pity or patronize.
• Talking about feelings is difficult. People who feel suicidal don't want to be rushed or put on the defensive. Just listen.

Source: http://www.befriendersindia.org/worryasf.htm.

Suicide prevention organisations in India

There are a number of voluntary organisations in India that offer counselling and help for individuals contemplating suicide. Most are located in major cities. Unfortunately, given the magnitude of the problem, there appears to be relatively little assistance available to those living in rural areas and those without access to telephones or the Internet.

Table A1.1 Suicide prevention organisations in India

NORTH	**Sumaitri**	Telephone, face to face and letter befriending
	Aradhana Hostel Complex No. 1, Bhagwan Das Lane Bhagwan Das Road Near National School of Drama New Delhi Phone: 011-23389090 Website: http://www.sumaitri.org *Monday to Friday 2pm to 10pm* *Saturday & Sunday 10am to 10pm*	
EAST	**Lifeline** Phone: 24637401/7432 Email: reach@lifelinekolkata.org Website: http://www.lifelinekolkata.org/home.html	Telephone befriending
WEST	**Samaritans (Bombay)**	Telephone, face to face and letter befriending
	C/o Naju K. Bhabha 49, Cuffe Parade, Colaba, Mumbai – 400005. Helpline – 022 32473267 Phone: +91 022 32410822 & +91 022 32410838 E-mail: smaritns@vsnl.com. Website: http://samaritansbombay.com/page1.htm *Monday to Friday 3pm to 9pm* *Saturday & Sunday 10am to 4pm*	
	Aasra	Telephone, face to face and letter befriending
	104, Sunrise Arcade, Plot No.100, Sector 16, Koparkhairane, Navi Mumbai Helpline : 27546669 (24 hrs) Phone: 27546667(3pm to 9pm) Dir: Johnson Thomas (9820466726) Email: aasrahelpline@yahoo.com Website: http://www.aasra.info/	

(*Continued Overleaf*)

Saath Suicide Prevention Rehabilitation Centre
B-12 Nilamber Complex
H.L. Commerce College Road
Navrangpura H.O.
Ahmedabad 380 009
Helpline 1: +91 79 2630 5544
Helpline 2: +91 79 2630 0222
Email: saakul@wilnetonline.net
Open daily 1pm to 7pm

Telephone, face to face and letter befriending

SOUTH   **Sneha**

11 Park View Road
(Near Chennai Kaliappa Hospital)
R.A. Puram 600 028 Chennai
Tamil Nadu
Website: www.snehaindia.org
Helpline 1: +91 (0) 44 2464 0050
Helpline 2: +91 (0) 44 2464 0060
Email Helpline: help@snehaindia.org
24 hour service

Telephone, face to face, letter and email befriending

Maitreyi

225, Thiagumudali Street,
Pondicherry 615 001.
Phone: 0413-2339999
Email: bimaitreyi@rediffmail.com
Website: www.maitreyi.org.in
Open daily 2pm to 8pm

Telephone, face to face and letter befriending

Maithri-Kochi

ICTA Shantigram,
Changampuzha Nagar (P.O.),
Kalamassery, Kochi – 682 033, Kerala
Phone: 91-0484-2540530
E-mails
maithrihelp@gmail.com
maithrikochi@gmail.com (only for
official correspondence)
Website: http://www.maithrikochi.org
Open daily 10am to 7pm

Telephone, face to face and letter befriending

Roshni

1-8-303/48/21
Kalavathy Nivas
Sindhi Colony
S.P. Road,
Secunderabad 500 003

Telephone, face to face and letter befriending

Helpline 1: 9166202000
Helpline 2: 9127848584
Email Helpline: help@roshnihyd.org
Monday to Saturday 11am to 9pm

Prateeksha	Telephone, face to face and letter befriending

Near Ambedkar Park
Peruvaram Road
North Paravur 683 513
Kerala
Phone: 0484 244 8830

Prathyasa	Telephone, face to face and letter befriending

Vidya Jothi
Cathedral Junction
IrinjalaKuda
Kerala 680 685
Telephone: 0480 282 0091

Thanal	Face to face, phone, letter

Iqra Hospital
Malamparamba
Calicut 673009 Kerala
Helpline 1: 0495 237 1100
Email: thanal.calicut@gmail.com
Open 10am to 6pm

Maiithri	Face to face, phone, letter

Kess Bhavan 1st Floor
Round West
Thrissur 680001 Kerala
Helpline 1: 0487 233 0300
Monday to Saturday: 1pm to 5pm
Sunday: 11am to 7pm

Sahai	Telephone, face to face

47 Pottery Road
Frazer Town
Bangalore 560005 Karnataka
Helpline 1: 2549 7777
Website: www.mpa.org.in
Monday to Saturday 10am to 6pm

ALL-INDIA	**Befrienders India** Website:http://www.befriendersindia.org/main.htm	Website of suicide prevention information and resources

Sources: http://www.snehaindia.org, http://www.maithrikochi.org, http://www.befrienders.org/helplines/helplines.asp?c2=India, http://maitreyi.org.in/documents/network.htm.

Appendix 2 Guidelines for the media

India's daily newspapers are principal source of information about suicide for many citizens. As we saw in the Introduction and other chapters, journalists tend to utilise a limited range of genres. In media coverage of farmer suicides, in particular, reporting of a shocking suicide has become an almost mandatory journalistic device, bordering on cliché, to frame a story about economic distress in the Indian countryside: no suicide, no story. Since the real focus of these articles is economic distress, or failure of government policy, or the harmful policies of international agencies, articles that report suicides almost never interview psychiatrists or others with expertise in suicide prevention. Only the most exceptional articles provide readers with the names and contact information of agencies working to prevent suicides. Similarly the warning signs of suicidal intention are almost never provided in the coverage of suicides in India's English-language press.

The British suicide-prevention society, The Samaritans, in their useful *Media Guidelines* argue that journalists must tread:

> . . . a fine line . . . between sensitive, intelligent reporting . . . and sensationalising the issue. The focus should be on educating and informing the public.
>
> Perhaps the most important guiding principle is to consider the reader, listener or viewer who might be in crisis when they read, hear or see the piece. Will this piece make it more likely that they will attempt suicide or more likely that they will seek help?
>
> (Samaritans, 2002: 9)

The Samaritans offer a number of recommendations that, with minor adjustments, are of general applicability.

Table A2.1 Recommendations on phraseology

Use phrases like:
- A suicide
- Die by suicide
- A suicide attempt
- A completed suicide
- Person at risk of suicide
- Help prevent suicide

Avoid phrases like:

- A successful suicide attempt
- An unsuccessful suicide attempt
- Commit suicide (since suicide was decriminalised in 1961, we prefer not to talk about 'committing suicide', but use 'take one's life', or 'die by suicide' instead)
- Suicide victim
- Just a cry for help
- Suicide-prone person
- Stop the spread/epidemic of suicide

Encourage public understanding of the complexity of suicide

People do not decide to take their own life in response to a single event, however painful that event may be. Nor can social conditions alone explain suicide. The causes of an individual suicide are manifold, and suicide should not be portrayed as the inevitable outcome of serious personal problems.

Seek expert advice
The Samaritans' Press Office can help put you in contact with acknowledged experts on suicide and offer advice about depiction based on an overview of previous cases.

Debunk the common myths about suicide

There is an opportunity to educate the public by challenging these.

Consider the timing
The coincidental deaths by suicide of two or more people makes the story more topical and newsworthy, but additional care is required in the reporting of 'another suicide, just days after . . .', which might imply a connection. There are 17 suicides every day, most of which go unreported.

Include details of further sources of information and advice
Listing appropriate sources of help or support at the end of an article or a programme shows the person who might be feeling suicidal that they are not alone and that they have the opportunity to make positive choices.

Remember the effect on survivors of suicide – either those who have attempted it or who have been bereaved
It might be helpful to be able to offer interviewees some form of support such as information about The Samaritans, or for those who are bereaved by suicide, information about The Compassionate Friends or Cruse.

Look after yourself
Reporting suicide can be very distressing in itself, even for the most hardened news reporter, especially if the subject touches something in your own experience. Talk it over with colleagues, friends, family or The Samaritans.

Encourage discussion by health experts on the possible contributory causes of suicide

(*Continued Overleaf*)

Encourage explanation of the risk factors of suicide

Avoid explicit or technical details of suicide in reports

Reporting that a person died from carbon monoxide poisoning is not in itself harmful, however providing details of the mechanism and procedure used to carry out the suicide may lead to the imitation of suicidal behaviour by other people at risk. Particular care should be taken in specifying the type and number of tablets used in an overdose.

Avoid simplistic explanations for suicide

Suicide is never the result of a single factor or event although a catalyst may seem obvious. Accounts that try to explain a suicide on the basis of dashed romantic feelings or a single dramatic incident should be challenged. News features could be used to provide more detailed analysis of the reasons behind the rise in suicides.

Don't romanticise or glorify suicide

Reporting that highlights community expressions of grief may suggest that the local community is honouring the suicidal behaviour of the deceased person, rather than mourning their death.

Avoid brushing over the realities of a suicide

Depiction may be damaging if it shows a character who has attempted suicide immediately recovered or if it glosses over the grim reality of slow liver failure following a paracetamol overdose.

Don't overemphasise the 'positive' results of a person's suicide

A dangerous message from the media is that suicide achieves results; it makes people sorry or it makes people eulogise you. For instance, a soap opera story line or newspaper coverage where a child's suicide or suicide attempt seems to result in separated parents reconciling or school bullies being publicly shamed may offer an appealing option to a despairing child in similar circumstances.

Source: Samaritans 2002: 10–11.

Bibliography

Abraham, J. (1995) 'Impact of prohibition on state excise: Study of four southern states', *Economic and Political Weekly*, 30 (48): 3051–3053.

Agarwal, A., Sharma, A. and Roychowdhury, A. (1996) *Slow Murder. The deadly story of vehicular pollution in India*, New Delhi: Centre for Science and Environment.

Agrawal, A. N. and Om Varma, H. (eds) (1997) *Indian Economy Statistical Yearbook 1997*, New Delhi: National Publishing House.

Ahmed, Z. (2010) Alarm at Mumbai's teen suicide trend. BBC News, at http://news.bbc.co.uk/2/hi/south_asia/8473515.stm (accessed 1 February 2010).

Aleem, S. (1994) *The Suicide: Problems & Remedies*, New Delhi: Ashish Publishing House.

Andriolo, K. R. (1993) 'Solemn departures and blundering escapes: Traditional attitudes toward suicide in India', *International Journal of Indian Studies* 3: 1–68.

Ashe, G. (1968) Gandhi: A Study in Revolution, London: Heinemann.

Assadi, M. (1998) 'Farmers' Suicides: signs of distress in rural economy', *Economic and Political Weekly* 33 (19): 1120–1140.

—— (2000) 'Karnataka: Seed Tribunal: interrogating farmer's suicides', *Economic and Political Weekly*, 28 October.

B.M.G. (2002) 'The martyr of Telugu statehood', *The Hindu*, 11 November. Available http://www.hinduonnet.com/thehinduthscrip/print.pl?file=20021111... (accessed 16 August 2005).

Baechler, J. (1975) *Suicides*, New York: Basic Books.

Bagadia, V. N., Pradhan, P. V. and Shah, L. P. (1974) 'Ecology and psychiatry in Bombay – India', *International Journal of Social Psychiatry* 20 (3–4): 302–310.

Banerjee, G., Nandi, D. N., Nandi, S., Sarkar, S., Boral, G. C. and Ghosh, A. (1990) 'The vulnerability of Indian women to suicide: a field study', *Indian Journal of Psychiatry* 32 (4): 305–308.

Bardhan, K. and Bardhan, P. (1973) 'The green revolution and socio-economic tensions: the case of India', *International Social Science Journal* 25 (3): 285–292.

Basham, A. L. (1954) *The Wonder That Was India*, London: Sidgwick and Jackson.

Baweja, H., Singh, N. K. and Sandhu, K. (1990) 'Mandal Commission Fall-Out: Pyres of Protest' *India Today*, 31 October:10–14.

Becker, C. B. (1990) 'Buddhist views of suicide and euthanasia', *Philosophy East and West* 40 (4): 543–556.

Bellafante, G. (2005) 'Courtship ideas of South Asians Get a U.S. touch'. *New York Times*, 23 August. Available http://www.nytimes.com/2005/08/23/national/23india.html (accessed 25 August 2005).

Bennett, R. and Daniel, M. (2002) 'Media reporting of Third World disasters: the journalist's perspective', *Disaster Prevention and Management* 11 (1): 33–42.

Beratis, S. (1986) 'Suicide in southwestern Greece 1979–1984', *Acta Psychiatrica Scandinavica* 74: 433–439.

Beskow, J. (1979) 'Suicide and mental disorder in Swedish men', *Acta Psychiatrica Scandinavica Supplementum* 277: 1–138.

Bhaktivedanta, A. C. (1969) *Sri Isopanisad*, Los Angeles: Iskon Books.

Bhalla, G. S., Sharma, S. L., Wig, N. N., Mehta, S. and Kumar, P. (1998) Suicides in Rural Punjab, Chandigarh: Institute for Development and Communication.

Bhatia, M. S. (2002) 'Stigma, suicide and religion', *British Journal of Psychiatry* 180: 188–189.

Bhatia, M. S., Aggarwal, N. K. and Aggarwal, B. B. L. (2000) 'Psychosocial profile of suicide ideators, attempters and completers in India', *International Journal of Social Psychiatry* 46: 155–163.

Bhugra, D. (1991) 'Politically motivated suicides', *British Journal of Psychiatry* 159 (4): 594–595.

Bhugra, D., Baldwin, D. S., Desai, M. and Jacob, K. S. (1999) 'Attempted suicide in West London, II: Inter-group comparisons', *Psychological Medicine* 29: 1131–1139.

Bhugra, D., Desai, M. and Baldwin, D. S. (1999) 'Attempted suicide in West London, I: rates across ethnic communities', *Psychological Medicine* 29 (5): 1125–1130.

Bilimoria, P. (1992) 'A report from India: the Jaina ethic of voluntary death', *Bioethics* 6 (4): 331–355.

—— (1995) 'Legal rulings on suicide in India and implications for the Right to Die', *Asian Philosophy* 5 (2): 159–180.

Boor, M. (1981) 'Methods of suicide and implications for suicide prevention', *Journal of Clinical Psychology* 37 (1): 70–75.

Booth, H. (1999a) 'Pacific Island suicide in comparative perspective', *Journal of Biosocial Science* 31 (4): 433–448.

—— (1999b) 'Patterns of suicide: factors affecting age–sex distributions of suicide in Western Samoa and Fiji Indians', Working papers in Demography, Australian National University, Research School of Social Sciences, Demography Program (77): 34 pp.

Booth, N. J. and Lloyd, K. (1999) 'Stress in farmers', *International Journal of Social Psychiatry* 46 (1): 67–73.

Bose, N. K. (1962) *Studies in Gandhism*. Third Edition (revised), Calcutta: Nirmal Kumar Bose.

Brass, P. R. (1994) *The Politics of India since Independence*, Cambridge: Cambridge University Press.

Breault, K. D. (1986) 'Suicide in America: A test of Durkheim's theory of religious and family integration, 1933–1980', *American Journal of Sociology* 92 (3): 628–56.

Brennan, L. (1998) 'Across the Kala Pani: An introduction', *South Asia XXI* (Special Issue): 1–18.

Brennan, L., McDonald, J. and Sholomowitz, R. (1998) 'The geographic and social origins of Indian indentured labourers in Mauritius, Natal, Fiji, Guyana and Jamaica', *South Asia XXI* (Special Issue): 39–71.

Brent, D. A. (1989) 'The psychological autopsy: methodological considerations for the study of adolescent suicide', *Suicide & Life-Threatening Behavior* 19 (1): 43–57.

Britton, A. and McPherson, K. (2001) 'Mortality in England and Wales attributable to current alcohol consumption', *Journal of Epidemiology and Community Health* 55 (6): 383–388.

Burrows, G. D. (1994) 'Editorial', *Mental Health in Australia* 6: 2–3.

Burvill, P. W. (1995) 'Suicide in the multiethnic elderly population of Australia, 1979–1990', *International Psychogeriatrics* 7 (2): 319–333.

Butler, D., Lahiri, A. and Roy, P. (1995) *India Decides: Elections 1952–1995*, New Delhi: Books & Things.

Caces, F. and Harford, T. (1998) 'Time series analysis of alcohol consumption and suicide mortality in the United States, 1934–1987', *Journal of Studies on Alcohol* 59 (4): 455–461.

Camus, A. (1955) *The Myth of Sisyphus and Other Essays*, Translated by J. O'Brien, New York: Vintage Books.

Capstick, A. (1960) 'Urban and rural suicide', *Journal of Mental Science* 60: 1327–1336.

Census of India Census of India 1991 Office of the Registrar General and Census Commissioner, India, New Delhi, 1991. Available http://www.bsos.umd.edu/socy/vanneman/districts/files/index.html (accessed 27 February 2008).

(2002) *Census of India 2001*. Office of the Registrar General and Census Commissioner, India, New Delhi. Available http://www.censusindia.net/ (accessed 10 October 2002).

—— (2007) *Census and You. Census of India*. Available http://censusindia.gov.in/Census_And_You/economic_activity.aspx (accessed 7 February 2010).

Centers for Disease Control (1990) 'Alcohol-related mortality and years of potential life lost: United States, 1987', *MMWR* 39 (11): 173–178.

Chakrabarti, P. (1979) 'Dharna: A dying ritual', *Journal of the Indian Anthropological Society* 14: 119–130.

Chandra, P. S., Ravi, V., Desai, A. and Subbakrishna, D. K. (1998) 'Anxiety and depression among HIV-infected heterosexuals: A report from India', *Journal of Pychosomatic Research* 45 (5): 401–409.

Charlton, J. (1995) 'Trends and patterns in suicide in England and Wales', *International Journal of Epidemiology* 24 (3 (Suppl. 1)): ss 45–52.

Chauhan, S. K. (1984) 'Suicide in India', *Social Change* 14 (3): 17–29.

Chen, M. and Drèze, J. (1995) 'Recent research on widows in India', *Economic and Political Weekly* 30 (39): 2435–2450.

Chen, M. A. (1997) 'Listening to widows in rural India', *Women: A Cultural Review* 8 (3): 311–318.

Cheng, A. T. A. and Lee, C.-S. (2000) 'Suicide in Asia and the Far East', in K. Hawton and K. van Heeringen, eds *The International Handbook of Suicide and Attempted Suicide*. Chichester: John Wiley & Sons, Ltd.

Chopra, R. N. and Chopra, I. C. (1965) *Drug Addiction with Special Reference to India*. New Delhi: Council of Scientific and Industrial Research.

Choudhary, S. (2009) *The Truth about Farmer Suicides in Chhattisgarh.* Infochange India. Available http://infochangeindia.org/200901057558/Agriculture/Features/The-truth-about-farmer-suicides-in-Chhattisgarh.html (accessed 7 February 2010).

Christian Aid (2005) *The Damage Done: Aid Death and Dogma*, London: Christian Aid. Available http://www.christian-aid.org.uk/indepth/505caweek/index.htm (accessed 18 May 2005).

Chynoweth, R., Tonge, J. I. and Armstrong, J. (1980) 'Suicide in Brisbane – A retrospective psychosocial study', *Australian and New Zealand Journal of Psychiatry* 14 (1): 37–45.

Clark, D. C. and Horton-Deustch, S. L. (1992) 'Assessment in absentia: The value of the psychological autopsy method for studying antecedents of suicide and predicting future suicides', in R. W. Maris, A. L. Berman, J. T. Maltsberger and R. I. Yufit, eds, *Assessment and Prediction of Suicide.* New York: Guildford Press.

Clarke, C., Peach, C. and Vertovec, S. (1990) 'Introduction: Themes in the study of the South Asian diaspora', in C. Clarke, C. Peach and S. Vertovec, eds *South Asians Overseas: Migration and Ethnicity.* Cambridge: Cambridge University Press.

Clinard, M. B. and Abbott, D. J. (1973) *Crime in Developing Countries: A Comparative Perspective. New York*: John Wiley & Sons.

Cohen, J. (1992) 'A power primer', Psychological Bulletin 112 (1): 155–159.

Connell, J., Dasgupta, B., Laishley, R. and Lipton, M. (1976) *Migration from Rural Areas. The Evidence from Village Studies.* Delhi: Oxford University Press.

Crombie, I. K. (1991) 'Suicide among men in the highlands of Scotland', *British Medical Journal* 302: 761–762.

Crooke, W. (1896) *The Popular Religion and Folk-Lore of Northern India.* Vol. I, Westminster: Archibald Constable & Co.

Dale, S. F. (1988) 'Anticolonial Terrorism in India, Indonesia, and the Philippines', *Journal of Conflict Resolution* 32: 37–59.

Dandekar, A., Narawade, S., Rathod, R., Ingle, R., Kulkarni, V. and Sateppa, Y. D. (2005) Causes of Farmer Suicides in Maharashtra: An Enquiry: Final Report Submitted to the Mumbai High Court, Tuljapur, Dist. Osmanabad: Tata Institute of Social Sciences.

Das, A. (2001) 'After farmers: Andhra students on suicide spree'. *Hindustan Times,* 12 February, Available http://www.hindustantimes.com/nonfram/120201/detNAT17.asp.

Datta, S. (2003) 'How many votes for a suicide?' *Indian Express*, 16 September, Available http://www.indianexpress.com/full_story.php?content_id=31565 (accessed 29 July 2004).

David, S. (1998) 'Karnataka: seeds of sorrow: a pest attack and unseasonal rains damage Tur Dal Crops in Bidar district forcing farmers to end their lives', *India Today* on the Net.

Day, T. P. (1982) *The Concept of Punishment in Early Indian Literature*, Waterloo, Ontario: Wilfrid Laurier University Press.

Dayashankar, K. M. (2001) 'Weavers – woes loom still: The suicides may have stopped for the moment but the plight of Andhra Pradesh's powerloom weavers has not improved'. *The Hindu.*

—— (2001) 'Weavers resort to Suicide in Sircilla'. *The Hindu,* 7 March.

de Bary, W. T., Hay, S. N., Weiler, R. and Yarrow, A. (1964) *Sources of Indian Tradition.* New York: Columbia University Press.

Deccan Herald (2002) 'B'lore model found dead in Mumbai'. *Deccan Herald,* 11 December, Available http://www.deccanherald.com/deccanherald/dec11/imodel.asp (accessed 29 January 2003).

Derne, S. (1994) 'Violating the Hindu norm of husband–wife avoidance', *Journal of Comparative Family Studies* 25 (2): 249–267.

Deshpande, V. (2003) 'When debts add up, death is still the only way out', *Indian Express*, 17 October, Available http://www.indianexpress.com/full_story.php?contentid+33587 (accessed 20 July 2004).

—— (2004) 'Pick-up delay triggers farmer suicide: death underlies cotton procurement turmoil after a dismal season in Vidarbha', *Indian Express*, 2 December, Available http://www.indianexpress.com/archive_full_story.php? (accessed 8 December 2004).

Desjarlais, R., Eisenberg, L., Good, B. and Kleinman, A. (1995) *World Mental Health: Problems and Priorities in Low-Income Countries.* New York: Oxford University Press.

Dhar, A. (2002) '"Auctioned" girl commits suicide', *The Hindu*, 20 August, Available http://www.thehindu.com/2002/08/20/stories/2002082004131100.htm (accessed 20 August 2002).

Diekstra, R. F. W. (1989) 'Suicide and the attempted suicide: An international perspective', *Acta Psychiatrica Scandinavica* 80 (Supp. 354): 1–24.

—— (1992) 'Suicide & attempted suicide: an international perspective', *Acta Psychiatrica Scandinavica* 354 (suppl.): 1–24.

Dikshitar, V. R. (1951) *Prehistoric South India*, Madras: N. S. Press.

Directorate of Economics and Statistics (2003) Statistical Abstract of Maharashtra State 1995–96 & 1996–97, Mumbai: Directorate of Economics and Statistics, Government of Maharashtra.

Douglas, J. D. (1967) *The Social Meanings of Suicide*, Princeton, New Jersey: Princeton University Press.

Drèze, J. and Sen, A. (1998) *India: Economic Development and Social Opportunity*, Delhi: Oxford University Press.

—— eds (1995), *India: Economic Development and Social Opportunity*. Delhi: Oxford University Press.

Dubois, J. A. (1906) *Hindu Manners, Customs and Ceremonies*. Third Edition, Delhi: Oxford University Press.

Durkheim, E. (1951) Suicide: *A Study in Sociology*, Translated by J. A. Spaulding and G. Simpson. Edited by G. Simpson, New York: Free Press.

—— (1964) The Division of Labor in Society, New York: Free Press.

Dyson, T. and Moore, M. (1983) 'On Kinship Structure, Female Autonomy, and Demographic Behavior in India', *Population and Development Review* 9 (1): 35–60.

Economic and Political Weekly (2005) 'Employment Trends in India', *Economic and Political Weekly* 1299.

Elwin, V. (1991 [1943]) *Maria Murder and Suicide*. Vanya Prakashan, 2nd impression, Bombay: Oxford University Press.

Escobedo, L. G. and Ortiz, M. (2002) 'The relationship between liquor outlet density and injury and violence in New Mexico', Accident Analysis and Prevention 34 (5): 689–695.

Farooq, O. 'Indian weavers driven to suicide'. BBC. Available http://news.bbc.co.uk/hi/english/world/south_asia/newsid_1281000/1281408.stm (accessed 22/8/2001).

Ferrada-Noli, M. (1997) 'Social psychological variables in populations contrasted by income and suicide rate: Durkheim revisited.' *Psychological Reports* 81 (1): 307–317.

Flisher, A. J. and Parry, C. D. H. (1994) 'Suicide in South Africa: An analysis of nationally registered mortality data for 1984–1986', *Acta Psychiatrica Scandinavica* 90: 348–353.

Freed, R. S. and Freed, S. A. (1989) 'Beliefs and practices resulting in female deaths and fewer females than males in India', *Population and Environment: A Journal of Interdisciplinary Studies* 10 (3): 144–161.

Gajalakshmi, V. and Peto, R. (2007) 'Suicide rates in rural Tamil Nadu, South India: Verbal autopsy of 39,000 deaths in 1997–98', *International Journal of Epidemiology* 36 (1): 203–7.

Ganapathi, M. N. and Venkoba Rao, A. (1966) 'A study on suicide in Madurai', *Journal of Indian Medical Association* 46: 18–23.

Gautami, S., Sudershan, R. V., Bhat, R. V., Suhasini, G., Bharati, M. and Gandhi, K. P. C. (2001) 'Chemical poisoning in three Telengana districts of Andhra Pradesh', *Forensic Science International* 122: 167–171.

Gehlot, P. S. and Nathawat, S. S. (1983) 'Suicide and family constellation in India', *American Journal of Psychotherapy* 37 (2): 273–278.

George, S. E. (2002) 'The last resort'. *The Hindu*, 12 May, Available http://www.hinduonnet. com/thehindu/mag/2002/05/12/stories/2002051200290500.htm (accessed 27 September 2002).

Gibbs, J. P. and Martin, W. T. (1964) *Status Integration and Suicide*, Eugene: University of Oregon Press.

Gillis, A. R. (1994) 'Literacy and the civilization of violence in 19th century France.' *Sociological Forum* 9 (3): 371–401.

Girard, C. (1993) 'Age, gender, and suicide: A cross-national analysis', *American Sociological Review* 58 (4): 553–574.

Goldney, R. D. and Schioldann, J. A. (2000) 'Pre-Durkheim Suicidology', *Crisis* 21 (4): 181–186.

Goldsmith, Sara K. (2001) 'Suicide Prevention and Intervention: Summary of a Workshop,' Committee on Pathophysiology and Prevention of Adolescent and Adult Suicide, Board on Neuroscience and Behavioral Health, Institute of Medicine. Washington, D.C.: National Academy Press.

Gruenewald, P. J., Ponicki, W. R. and Mitchell, P. R. (1995) 'Suicide rates and alcohol consumption in the United States, 1970–1989', *Addiction* 90 (8): 1063–1075.

Gruère, G., Mehta-Bhatt, P. and Sengupta, D. (2008) *Bt Cotton and Farmer Suicides In India: Reviewing the Evidence.* Washington, D.C.: International Food Policy Research Institute (IFPRI).

Gurr, T. R. (1980) 'Development and decay: their impact on public order in Western History', in J. A. Inchiardi and C. E. Faupel, eds *History and Crime: Implications for Criminal Justice Policy.* Beverly Hills: Sage Publications.

Gururaj, G. and Isaac, M. K. (2001) Epidemiology of Suicides in Bangalore, Bangalore: National Institute of Mental Health & Neuro Sciences.

Habil, M. H., Ganesvaran, T. and Agnes, L. S. (1992/1993) 'Attempted suicide in Kuala Lumpur', *Asia-Pacific Journal of Public Health* 6 (2): 5–7.

Hajicek-Dobberstein, S. (1995) 'Soma siddhas and alchemical enlightenment: Psychedelic mushrooms in Buddhist tradition.' *Journal of Ethnopharmacology* 48 (2): 99–110.

Halbwachs, M. (1978) *The Causes of Suicide*, translated by H. Goldblatt, London: Routledge & Kegan Paul.

Hallen, G. C. (1989) 'Studies in the sociology of suicides in India', *Indian Journal of Social Research* 30 (1): 37–68.

Halliburton, M. (1998) 'Suicide: A paradox of development in Kerala', *Economic and Political Weekly* 33 (36 & 37): 2341–2345.

Harlankar, S. (2003) 'Agriculture: harvest of death: Impoverished farmers switch to lucrative cash crops, little realising that it will trap them in a cycle of crop-failure and debt', *India Today* on the Net. Available http://www.indiatoday.com/itoday/ itoday/08061988/agri.html (accessed 31 January 2003).

Harrison, S. S. (1960) *India: The Most Dangerous Decades*, Princeton: Princeton University Press.

Hasan, A. (2004), 'The process of socio-economic change in Pakistan', 8 November, at Johns Hopkins University, School of Advanced International Studies (SAIS), Washington, D.C.

Hassan, R. (1983) *A Way of Dying: Suicide in Singapore*, Kuala Lumpur: Oxford University Press.

—— (1995) *Suicide Explained: The Australian Experience*, Melbourne: Melbourne University Press.

Hassan, R. and Tan, G. (1989) 'Suicide trends in Australia, 1901–1985: An analysis of sex differentials', *Suicide and Life-Threatening Behavior* 19 (4): 362–380.

Hawton, K., Appleby, L., Platt, S., Foster, T., Cooper, J., Malmberg, A. and Simkin, S. (1998) 'The psychological autopsy approach to studying suicide: a review of methodological issues', *Journal of Affective Disorders* 50 (2–3): 269–276.

Hawton, K., Fagg, J. and McKeown, S. (1989) 'Alcoholism, alcohol and attempted suicide', *Alcohol and Alcoholism* 24 (1): 3–9.

Hawton, K., Harriss, L., Hodder, K., Simkin, S. and Gunnell, D. (2001) 'The influence of the economic and social environment on deliberate self-harm and suicide: an ecological and person-based study', *Psychological Medicine* 31 (5): 827–836.

Haynes, R. H. (1984) 'Suicide in Fiji: a preliminary study', *British Journal of Psychiatry* 145: 433–438.

Heber, R. (1828) Narrative of a Journey through the Upper Provinces of India, from Calcutta to Bombay, 1824–1825, with *Notes upon Ceylon, an Account of a Journey to Madras and the Southern Provinces*, 1826, and *Letters Written in India*. 2 volumes, London: John Murray.

Hegde, R. S. (1980) 'Suicide in rural community', *Indian Journal of Psychiatry* 22 (4): 368–370.

Henry, A. F. and Short, J. F. (1954) *Suicide and Homicide*, Glencoe, IL: Free Press.

High Level Committee Report of the High Level Committee (2001) 'Non Resident Indians & Persons of Indian Origin Division', Ministry of External Affairs, Government of India. Available http://indiandiaspora.nic.in/part1-est.pdf (accessed 7 December 2005).

Hindu, The (1998) 'One more farmer commits suicide in Karnataka', *The Hindu*, 12 April. Available http://www.indiaserver.com/thehindu/1998/04/12/thb04.htm#Story2 (accessed 10 November 1999).

—— (2001a) '9 members of family commit suicide'. *The Hindu*, 25 February. Available http://www.hinduonnet.com/thehindu/2001/02/25/stories/0425210m.htm.

—— (2001b) 'India: "Family counselling centres must to check suicides". *The Hindu*, July 30.

—— (2001c) 'India: farmers' suicide: panel to study reasons'. *The Hindu*, Available LexisNexis (accessed 13 September 2001).

—— (2002a) 'Alleged suicide by three'. *The Hindu*, 9 April. Available http://www. hinduonnet.com/2002/04/09/stories/2002040902100300.htm (accessed 27 January 2004).

—— (2002b) 'Five of family commit suicide'. *The Hindu*, 17 September. Available http:// www.thehindu.com/2002/09/17/stories/2002091704310600.htm.

—— (2002c) 'Couple's bid to end life'. *The Hindu*, 27 September. Available http://www. thehindu.com/2002/09/27/stories/2002092709290300.htm (accessed 27 September 2002).

—— (2005) 'Fasting ascetic passes away'. *The Hindu*, 24 July. Available http://www. hindu.com/2005/07/24/stories/2005072413341000.htm (accessed 25 July 2005).

Hunter, W. W. (1872) 'Orissa under Indian rule', in N. K. Sahu, ed. *A History of Orissa.* Calcutta: Susil Gupta (India) Ltd.

India, T. o. (2003) 'TV Artist Revathisree commits suicide'. *Times of India*, 17 January, Available http://timesofindia.com/cms.dll/html/uncomp/articleshow?artid=34684447&s T. . . (accessed 29 January 2003).

India Today (2000) 'I, me, myself', *India Today* on the Net, 3 January. Available http:// www.indiatoday.com/itoday/20000103/cover3.html (accessed 31 January 2003).

Indian Express (1998) 'Failed girl says sorry, commits suicide'. *Indian Express*, 10 June. Available http://www.expressindia.com/ie/daily/19980610/16150624.htm (accessed 29 January 2003).

Institute of Health Systems, 'Cause of Death'. Available http://www.ihsnet.org.in/BurdenOfDisease/CauseofDeath.htm (accessed 18 August 2005).

Isometsä, E. T. (2001) 'Psychological autopsy studies – a review', *European Psychiatry* 16: 379–385.

Isometsä, E. T., Heikkinen, M., Henriksson, M., Marttunen, M., Aro, H. and Lonnqvist, J. (1997) 'Differences between urban and rural suicides', *Acta Psychiatrica Scandinavica* 95: 297–305.

Iyer, K. G. and Manick, M. S. (2000) *Indebtedness, Impoverishment and Suicides in Rural Punjab,* Delhi: Indian Publishers Distributors.

Iyer, L. (1998) 'Killing Men, Not Pests', *The Week*, 18 January. Available http://www.the-week.com/98jan18/events4.htm (Google cache accessed 22 August 2001).

Jagadeesan, N. (1983) 'Self-immolation vis-à-vis religion in the Tamil Society', in N. Subrahmanian, ed. *Self-Immolation in Tamil Society*. Madurai: International Institute of Tamil Historical Studies.

James, C. J. (1983) 'Self-immolation in Tamil Society', in N. Subrahmanian, ed. *Self-Immolation in Tamil Society*. Madurai: International Institute of Tamil Historical Studies.

Jarosz, M. (1985) 'Suicides in Poland as an indicator of social disintegration', *Social Indicators Research* 16: 449–464.

Jeffrey, P. (2003) 'A uniform customary code? Marital breakdown and women's economic entitlements in rural Bijnor', in R. Jeffrey and J. Lerche, eds *Social and Political Change in Uttar Pradesh: European Perspectives.* New Delhi: Manohar.

Jena, K. (1960) 'Modern impact of Urbanism on rural life', *Indian Journal of Social Work* 21 (2): 177–179.

Ji, J., Kleinman, A. and Becker, A. E. (2001) 'Suicide in Contemporary China: a review of China's distinctive suicide demographics in their sociocultural context', *Harvard Review of Psychiatry* 9: 1–12.

John, C. J. (1995) 'Psychiatric disorders and suicide', in G. Joseph and P. O. George, eds, *Suicide in Perspective: With Special Reference to Kerala. Rajagiri, Kerala & Secunderabad,* Andhra Pradesh: Centre for Health Care Research and Education (CHCRE) Health Accessories for All (HAFA).

Johnson, B. D. (1965) 'Durkheim's one cause of suicide', *American Sociological Review* 30: 875–886.

Kala, A. K. (2001), 'Law against attempted suicide: deterrent to prevention'. Paper read at International Association for Suicide Prevention, 22–26 September, at Chennai.

Kalidas, S. (1999) 'Death of a dancer' *India Today* on the Net, 15 November Available http://www.indiatoday.com/itoday/19991115/mfeature.html (accessed 31 January 2003).

Kant, A. (2000) 'Stress and suicide: identifying distress signals'. *Times of India*, Available http://www.healthlibrary.com/news/23-29jan/stress.htm (accessed 29 January 2003).

Karp, J. (1998) 'Deadly debts: As crops fail, farmers resort to suicide in India'. *Asian Wall Street Journal*, 19 February.

Katakam, A. (2005) 'The roots of a tragedy', *Frontline*, 2–15 July. Available http://www.frontlineonnet.com/fl2214/stories/20050715002104300.htm (accessed 15 August 2005).

Kaur, A. (1998) 'Tappers and weeders: South Indian plantation workers in peninsular Malaysia, 1880–1970', *South Asia* XXI (Special Issue): 73–102.

Keith, A. B. (1914) 'Suicide (Hindu)', in J. Hastings, ed. *Encyclopaedia of Religion and Ethics*. Edinburgh: T & T Clark.

Kishwar, M. and Vanita, R. (1984) *In Search of Answers: Indian Women's Voices from Manushi*, London: Zed Books Ltd.

Klerman, G. L. (1987) 'Clinical epidemiology of suicide', *Journal of Clinical Psychiatry* 48 (Suppl.): 33–38.

—— (1988) 'Depression and related disorders of mood', *New Harvard Guide to Psychiatry*. Cambridge, MA: Belknap Press.

Kowalski, G. S., Faupel, C. E. and Starr, P. D. (1987) 'Urbanism and suicide: A study of American counties', *Social Forces* 66 (1): 85–101.

Krishan, G. (1993) 'The slowing down of Indian urbanisation', *Geography* 78 (338): 80–84.

Krishnakumar, A. (2001a) 'The collapse of APCO', *Frontline*, 14–17 April Available http://www.hinduonnet.com/fline/fl1808/18080180.htm (accessed 9 August 2005).

—— (2001b) 'The crisis in Sircilla', *Frontline*, 14–17 April. Available http://www.hinduonnet.com/fline/fl1808/18080050.htm (accessed 9 August 2005).

—— (2001c) 'For the weavers', *Frontline*, 23 June–6 July. Available http://www.hinduonnet.com/fline/fl1813/18130800.htm (accessed 9 August 2005).

—— (2001d) 'Perilous policies', *Frontline*, 14–17 April. Available http://www.hinduonnet.com/fline/fl1808/18080170.htm (accessed 9 August 2005).

—— (2001e) 'Silence of the looms', *Frontline*, 14–17 April. Available http://www.hinduonnet.com/fline/fl1808/18080130.htm (accessed 9 August 2005).

—— (2001f) 'Warped policies', *Frontline*, 14–17 April. Available http://www.hinduonnet.com/fline/fl1808/18080090.htm (accessed 9 August 2005).

—— (2001g) 'Weavers in distress', *Frontline*, 14–17 April. Available http://www.hinduonnet.com/fline/fl1808/18080050.htm (accessed 9 August 2005).

Krishnan, K. G. (1983) 'On self-immolation from inscriptions', in N. Subrahmanian, ed. *Self-immolation in Tamil Society*. Madurai: International Institute of Tamil Historical Studies.

Krug, E. G., Dahlberg, L. L., Mercy, J. A., Zwi, A. B. and Lozano, R., eds (2002), *World Report on Violence and Health*. Geneva: World Health Organisation.

Krull, C., and Trovato, F. (1994) 'The quiet revolution and the sex differential in Quebec's suicide rates: 1931-1986', *Social Forces* 72 (4): 1121–1147.

Kua, E. H. and Ko, S. M. (1992) 'A cross-cultural study of suicide among the elderly in Singapore', *British Journal of Psychiatry* 160: 558–559.

Kua, E. H. and Tsoi, W. F. (1985) 'Suicide in the island of Singapore', *Acta Psychiatrica Scandinavica* 71: 227–229.

Kumar, K. A. (1995) 'Suicide in Kerala from a mental health perspective', in G. Joseph and P. O. George, eds Suicide in Perspective: With Special Reference to Kerala. Rajagiri, Kerala & Secunderabad, Andhra Pradesh: Centre for Health Care Research and Education (CHCRE) Health Accessories for All (HAFA).

Kumar, K. G. (1996) 'Media: female fancy', *Business India*, 33–34.

Kurosu, S. (1991) 'Suicide in rural areas: the case of Japan 1960–1980', *Rural Sociology* 56 (4): 603–618.

Kushner, H. I. (1984) 'Immigrant suicide in the United States: toward a psycho-social history', *Journal of Social History* 18 (1): 3–24.

—— (1985) 'Women and suicide in historical perspective', *Signs* 10: 537–552.

—— (1993) 'Suicide, gender, and the fear of modernity in nineteenth-century medical and social thought', *Journal of Social History* 26 (3): 461–476.

Labovitz, S. and Brinkerhoff, M. B. (1977) 'Structural changes and suicide in Canada', *International Journal of Comparative Sociology* 18 (3–4): 254–267.

Lal, B. V. (1983) 'Girmitiyas: The origins of Fiji Indians', Canberra: *Journal of Pacific History*.

—— (1998) 'Understanding the Indian indenture experience', *South Asia XXI* (Special Issue): 215–237.

Lal, V. (1990) 'The Fijian Indians: marooned at home', in C. Clarke, C. Peach and S. Vertovec, eds, *South Asians Overseas: Migration and Ethnicity*. Cambridge: Cambridge University Press.

Lane, R. (1980) 'Urban homicide in the nineteenth century: Some lessons for the twentieth', in J. A. Inciardi and C. E. Faupel, eds, *History and Crime: Implications for Criminal Justice Policy*. Beverly Hills: Sage Publications.

Lannoy, R. (1975) *The Speaking Tree*, London: Oxford University Press.

Latha, K. S., Bhat, S. M. and D'Souza, P. (1996) 'Suicide attempters in a general hospital unit in India: their socio-demographic and clinical profile – emphasis on cross-cultural aspects', *Acta Psychiatrica Scandinavica* 94 (1): 26–30.

Lester, D. (1982) 'The distribution of sex and age among completed suicides: A cross-national study', *International Journal of Social Psychiatry* 28: 256–260.

—— (1987) 'The stability of national suicide rates in Europe', *Sociological and Social Research* 71: 208.

—— (1989) *Suicide from a Sociological Perspective*, Springfield, Illinois: Charles C. Thomas Publisher.

—— (1992) *Why People Kill Themselves*, Springfield, IL: Charles Thomas.

—— (1995) 'The association between alcohol consumption and suicide and homicide rates: A study of 13 nations', *Alcohol & Alcoholism* 30 (4): 465–468.

—— (1996) *Patterns of Suicide and Homicide in the World*, Commack, NJ: Nova Science Publishers Inc.

—— (1996) 'Suicide in Indian states and religion', Psychological Reports 79 (1): 342.

—— (1997) 'Part III. International perspectives: Suicide in an international perspective', Suicide and Life Threatening Behavior 27 (1): 104–111.

—— (2000) 'Suicide in emigrants from the Indian subcontinent', Transcultural Psychiatry 37 (2): 243–254.

Lester, D., Agarwal, K. and Natarajan, M. (1999) 'Suicide in India', Archives of Suicide Research 5: 91–96.

Lester, D. and Natarajan, M. (1995) 'Predicting the time series suicide and murder rates in India', Perceptual and Motor Skills 80: 570.

Lubell, K. M., Swahn, M. H., Crosby, A. E. and Kegler, S. R. (2004) 'Methods of suicide among persons aged 10–19 years – United States 1992–2001', Morbidity and Mortality Weekly Report 53 (22): 471–474.

Mackinnon, I. (2000) 'Luck runs out for India's Hindu widows'. The Australian, 10 February.

Mahal, A. (2000) *What Works in Alcohol Policy? Evidence from Rural India,* New Delhi: National Council of Applied Economic Research.

Malmberg, A., Simpkin, S. and Hawton, K. (1999) 'Suicide in farmers', *British Journal of Psychiatry* 175: 103–105.

Maniam, T. (1988) 'Suicide and parasuicide in a hill resort in Malaysia', *British Journal of Psychiatry* 153: 222–225.

—— (1995) 'Suicide and undetermined violent deaths in Malaysia, 1966–1990: Evidence for the misclassification of suicide statistics', *Asia-Pacific Journal of Public Health* 8 (3): 181–185.

—— (2001), 'Why do Malaysian Indians have the highest suicide rate?' Paper read at XXII Congress of the International Association for Suicide Prevention, at Chennai, India.

Mayer, P. (2000) 'Development, gender equality and suicide rates', *Psychological Reports* 87: 367–372.

—— (2001) 'Human development and civic community in India', *Economic and Political Weekly* 36 (8): 684–692.

—— (2003) 'Female equality and suicide in the Indian States', *Psychological Reports* 92: 1022–1028.

Mayer, P. and Ziaian, T. (2002) 'Indian suicide and marriage: A research note', *Journal of Comparative Family Studies* 23 (2): 297–305.

Mayr, G. v. (1917) 'Selbstmordstatistik'Statistik und Gesellschaftslehre. Tübingen: Verlag von I. C. V. Mohr (Paul Siebeck).

McLeod, K. (1878) 'On the statistics and causes of suicide in India', in B. D. Gupta, ed. *Sociology in India: An Enquiry into Sociological Thinking & Empirical Social Research in the Nineteenth Century – with Special Reference to Bengal.* Calcutta: Centre for Sociological Research.

McMichael, A. J. (2000) 'The urban environment and health in a world of increasing globalization: issues for developing countries', *Bulletin of the World Health Organisation* 78 (9): 1117–1126.

Menon, L. (2002) 'Ending lives the easy way'. *The Hindu*, 10 June. Available http://www.hinduonnet.com/thehindu/mp/2002/06/10/stories/2002061000890200.htm (accessed 1 August 2002).

Menon, P. (2001a) 'A farm crisis and suicides', *Frontline*, 14–17 April. Available http://www.hinduonnet.com/fline/fl1808/18080210.htm (accessed 9 August 2005).

—— (2001b) 'Little evidence of relief', *Frontline*, 14–17 April. Available http://www.hinduonnet.com/fline/fl1808/18080240.htm (accessed 9 August 2005).

Micciolo, R., Willams, P., Zimmermann-Tansela, C. and Tansella, M. (1991) 'Geographical and urban–rural variation in the seasonality of suicide: some further evidence', *Journal of Affective Disorders* 21: 39–43.

Miner, J. R. (1922) 'Suicide and its relation to climatic and other factors', *American Journal of Hygiene (Monographic Series)* 2: 72–112.

Mishra, S. (2006a) 'Farmers' suicides in Maharashtra', *Economic and Political Weekly* 41 (16): 1538–1545.

—— (2006b) 'Suicide mortality rates across states of India, 1975–2001: A statistical note', *Economic and Political Weekly* 41 (16): 1566–1569.

—— (2006c) *Suicide of Farmers in Maharashtra.* Mumbai: Indira Gandhi Institute of Development Research.

—— (2008) 'Risks, farmers' suicides and agrarian crisis in India: Is there a way out?' *Indian Journal of Agricultural Economics* 63 (1): 38–54.

Mitra, A. (1952) Vital Statistics West Bengal 1941–5. Edited by A. Mitra, *Census of India*, 1951. Calcutta: Manager of Publications, Delhi.

Mitra, S. (1998) 'Unlovingly Yours', *India Today* on the Net. Available http://www.indiatoday.com/itoday/13071998/behave.html (accessed 31 January 2003).

Moller, J. (2003) 'Responses to modernity: female education, gender relations and regional identity in the hills of Uttar Pradesh', in R. Jeffrey and J. Lerche, eds, *Social and Political Change in Uttar Pradesh: European Perspectives.* New Delhi: Manohar.

Morris, P. and Maniam, T. (2001) 'Ethnicity and suicidal behaviour in Malaysia: a review of the literature', *Transcultural Psychiatry* 38 (1): 51–63.

Morselli, H. M. D. (1881) *Suicide*, London: C. Kegan Paul & Co.

Murugesan, G. and Yeoh, O. H. (1978) 'Demographic and psychiatric aspects of attempted suicide', *Medical Journal of Malaysia* 36: 39–46.

Mutatkar, R. K. (1995) 'Public health problems of urbanization', *Social Science and Medicine* 41 (7): 977–981.

Nagaraj, K. (2008) 'Farmers' Suicide in India: Magnitudes, Trends and Spatial Patterns'. Preliminary Report. Madras: Madras Institute of Development Studies. Available http://www.macroscan.com/anl/mar08/pdf/Farmers_Suicides.pdf (accessed 7 February 2010).

Nair, A. (2004) 'Suicide fury trashes Kerala & a few facts'. *Indian Express*, 29 July. Available http://www.indianexpress.com/full_story.php?content_id=51993 (accessed 29 July 2004).

National Crime Records Bureau (1995) *Accidental Deaths and Suicides in India 1994*, New Delhi: Ministry of Home Affairs Government of India.

—— (1997) *Accidental Deaths and Suicides in India 1995*, New Delhi: Ministry of Home Affairs Government of India.

National Crime Records Bureau (1999) *Accidental Deaths and Suicides in India 1997*, New Delhi: Ministry of Home Affairs Government of India.

—— (2001a) *Accidental Deaths and Suicides in India 1999*, New Delhi: Ministry of Home Affairs Government of India.

—— (2001b) *Crime in India 1999*, National Crime Records Bureau, Ministry of Home Affairs.

Nautiyal, S. (2002) 'Drought means death'. *Sunday Express*, 18 August.

Neeleman, J. and Wessely, S. (1999) 'Ethnic minority suicide: a small area geographical study in South London', *Psychological Medicine* 29 (2): 429–436.

Neeleman, J., Wilson-Jones, C. and Wessely, S. (2001) 'Ethnic density and deliberate self harm: a small area study in South East London', *Journal of Epidemiology and Community Health* 55 (2): 85–90.

Niven, C., Honan, M., Cannon, T., Mayhew, B., Collins, D., Plunkett, R. *et al.* (1999), India, Lonely Planet. Melbourne: Lonely Planet Publications.

Norström, T. (1988) 'Alcohol and suicide in Scandinavia', *British Journal of Addiction* 83: 553–559.

Our Principal Correspondent (1998) '110 AP Cotton farmers "commit suicide"', *Hindu Business Line* (Online Edition), 5 February, Available http://www.indiaserver.com/businessline/1998/02/05/stories/1405003u.htm (accessed 10 November 1999).

Our Staff Reporter (2001) 'Suicide by weavers continues'. *The Hindu*, 8 April. Available at Dow Jones Interactive accessed 7 February 2002.

—— (2002) 'Another college girl commits suicide'. *The Hindu*, 26 August. Available http://www.thehindu.com/2002/08/26/stories/2002082604980600.htm (accessed 27 July 2002).

—— (2002) 'Two of family commit suicide'. *The Hindu*, 27 September. Available http://www.thehindu.com/2002/09/27/stories/2002092709300300.htm (accessed 27 July 2002).

Pachauri, P., George, P., Ahmed, F. and Awasthi, D. (1990) 'Mandal commission: a tragic price', *India Today*, 15 October: 14–17.

Padma, T. V. (2002) *Debts and Poverty Drive Weavers to Suicide*, Dow Jones Interactive: Inter Press Service. Available at http://ptg.djnr.com/ccroot/asp/publib/story_clean_cpy.asp?articles=IPRS0120000002'INTE (accessed 7 February 2002).

Page, A., Morrell, S. and Taylor, R. (2002) 'Suicide and political regime in New South Wales and Australia during the 20th century', *Journal of Epidemiology and Community Health* 56 (10): 766–772.

Pampel, F. C. (1998) 'National context, social change, and sex differences in suicide rates', *American Sociological Review* 63: 744–758.

Pandey, R. (1985) 'The aetiology of suicide in India today', *Indian Journal of Social Work* 45 (4): 429–439.

Pandey, R. E. (1968) 'The suicide problem in India', *International Journal of Social Psychiatry* 14 (3): 193–200.

Pape, R. A. (2003) 'The strategic logic of suicide terrorism', *American Political Science Review* 97 (3): 343–361.

Parker, G. and Yap, H. L. (2001) 'Suicide in Singapore: A changing sex ratio over the last decade', *Singapore Medical Journal* 42 (1): 11–14.

Patton, W. M. (1914) 'Suicide (Muhammadan)', in J. Hastings, ed. *Encyclopaedia of Religion and Ethics.* Edinburgh: T & T Clark.

Pearson, B. (2003) 'Tamil coin crunch leads to suicide'. *Variety*, 19 May.

Peng, K. L. and Choo, A. S. (1990) 'Suicide and parasuicide in Singapore (1986)', *Medicine, Science and the Law* 30 (3): 225–233.

Pescosolido, B. A. and Mendelsohn (1986) 'Social causation or social construction of suicide? An investigation into the social organization of official rates', *American Sociological Review* 51: 80–100.

Phal, S. R. (1978) 'Suicide in Panaji (Goa)', *Indian Journal of Social Work* 39 (1): 41–26.

Phillips, D. P. and Ruth, T. E. (1993) 'Adequacy of official suicide statistics for scientific research and public policy', *Suicide and Life-Threatening Behavior* 23 (4): 307–319.

Phillips, M. R., Li, X. and Zhang, Y. (2002) 'Suicide rates in China, 1995–99', *Lancet* 359 (March 9): 835–840.

Phillips, M. R., Liu, H. and Zhang, Y. (1999) 'Suicide and social change in China', *Culture, Medicine and Psychiatry* 23: 25–50.

Pillay, A. L. and Wassenaar, D. R. (1997) 'Recent stressors and family satisfaction in suicidal adolescents in South Africa', *Journal of Adolescence* 20: 155–162.

Platt, S. (1984) 'Unemployment and suicidal behaviour: a review of the literature', *Social Science and Medicine* 19 (2): 93–115.

—— (1986) 'Parasuicide and unemployment', *British Journal of Psychiatry* 149: 401–405.

Ponnudurai, R. and Jeyakar, J. (1980) 'Suicide in Madras', *Indian Journal of Psychiatry* 22: 203–205.

Pope, W. (1976) *Durkheim's Suicide: A Classic Analyzed*, Chicago: University of Chicago Press.

Pope, W. and Danigelis, N. (1981) 'Sociology's "One Law"', *Social Forces* 60 (2): 495–516.

Pope, W., Danigelis, N. and Stack, S. (1983), 'The effect of modernization on suicide: A time series analysis, 1900–1974.' Paper read at American Sociological Association, at Detroit, MI, U.S.A.

Porter, A. E. (1933) Bengal & Sikkim. Edited by A. E. Porter. Vol. V, Part I – Report, *Census of India,* 1931, Calcutta: Government of India.

Pounder, D. J. (1993) 'Why are the British hanging themselves?' *American Journal of Forensic Medicine and Pathology* 14 (2): 135–140.

Pritchard, C. (1996) 'New patterns of suicide by age and gender in the United Kingdom and the western world 1974–1992: An indicator of social change?' *Social Psychiatry and Psychiatric Epidemiology* 31 (3–4): 227–234.

Prosser, D. (1996) 'Suicides by burning in England and Wales', *British Journal of Psychiatry* 168 (2): 175–182.

Radhakrishnan, S. (1953) *The Principal Upanisads*, New York: Harper & Brothers Publishers.

Raguram, R., Weiss, M. G., Channabasavanna, S. M. and Devins, G. M. (1996) 'Stigma, depression, and somatization in South India', *American Journal of Psychiatry* 15 (8): 1043–1049.

Rai, U. (1993) 'Escalating violence against adolescent girls in India', *The Urban Age*, 10.

Ramanakumar, A. V. (2004) 'Reviewing disease burden among rural Indian women', *Online Journal of Health and Allied Sciences* 2 (1).

Ramaswamy, S. (1997) *Passions of the Tongue: Language Devotion in Tamil India*, 1891–1970, Berkeley: University of California Press.

Ramesh, J. (1998) 'Killer cotton: reform cotton policy and rural credit – or face more farmer suicides'. *India Today* on the Net, 18 May. Available www.indiatoday.com/itoday/18051998/jairam.html (accessed 31 January 2003).

Ramstedt, M. (2001) 'Alcohol and suicide in 14 European countries', *Addiction* 96 (Supp. 1): S59–S75.

Rancans, E., Salander Renberg, E. and Jacobsson, L. (2001) 'Major demographic, social and economic factors associted to suicide rates in Latvia 1980–98', *Acta Psychiatrica Scandinavica* 103: 275–281.

Rao, R. (1998) 'Pesticide suicide: Radhakrishna Rao records an ironic end to a tragic episode in India', *New Internationalist* (302): 13.

Ratnayeke, L. (1998) 'Suicide in Sri Lanka', in R. J. Kosky, H. S. Eshkevari, R. D. Goldney and R. Hassan, eds, *Suicide Prevention: The Global Context*. New York: Plenum Press.

Reddy, C. P. (1998) 'Cotton farmers' suicide may be major poll issue'. *Business Line*, 18 January. Available http://www.indiaserver.com/businessline/1998/01/18/stories/14180229.htm (accessed 10 November 1999).

Reddy, S. G. (2002) 'AP Weavers' misery spins out of control'. *Indian Express*, 29 April. Available http://www.indianexpress.com/full_story.php?content_. . . (accessed 8 December 2004).

Registrar General (2002) *Survey of Causes of Death (Rural), 1998,* New Delhi: Office of the Registrar General, India, Vital Statistics Division.

Reporter, O. S. (2000) 'AIADMK volunteer immolates himself'. *The Hindu*, 4 February. Available http://www.hinduonnet.com/thehindu/2000/02/04/stories/04042239.htm (accessed 16 August 2005).

Rossow, I. (2000) 'Suicide, violence and child abuse: a review of the impact of alcohol consumption on social problems', *Contemporary Drug Problems* 27 (3): 397–433.

Rudolph, L. I. and Rudolph, S. H. (1987) *In Pursuit of Lakshmi: The Political Economy of the Indian State, Hyderabad*: Orient Longman Limited.

Russell, R. V. and Lal, H. (1916 [1969]) *The Tribes and Castes of the Central Provinces of India*. Reprinted as 4 vols. Vol. 2, Oosterhout: Anthropological Publications. Original edition, 1916.

Ruzicka, L. T. and Choi, C. Y. (1993) 'Suicide mortality in Australia, 1970–1991', *Journal of the Australian Population Association* 10 (2): 101–117.

Sainath, P. (1999) *Everybody Loves a Good Drought: Studies from India's Poorest Districts,* London: Review.

—— (2001a) 'Where stomach aches are terminal: I'. *The Hindu*, April 29, Available <LexisNexis> (accessed 12 September 2001).

—— (2001b) 'Where stomach aches are terminal: II'. *The Hindu*, May 6, Available <LexisNexis> (accessed 12 September 2001).

—— (2002) ' "Have tornado, will travel" '. *The Hindu*, 18 August 2002, Available http://www.hinduonnet.com/thehindu/thscrip/print.pl?file=20020818. . . (accessed 12 August 2005).

—— (2005a) 'As you sow, so shall you weep'. *The Hindu*, 30 June. Available http://www.hinduonnet.com/thehindu/thscrip/print.pl?file=20050630. . . (accessed 12 August 2005).

—— (2005b) 'Health as someone else's wealth'. *The Hindu*, 1 July, Available http://www.hinduonnet.com/thehindu/thscrip/print.pl?file=20050701. . . (accessed 12 August 2005).

—— (2005c) 'No free power link to farmers' suicides'. *The Hindu*, 28 June 2005, Available http://www.hinduonnet.com/thehindu/thscrip/print.pl.?file=2005062. . . (accessed 8 July 2005).

—— (2005d) 'Rural russian roulette in Vidharba'. *The Hindu*, 23 June 2005. Available http://www.hinduonnet.com/thehindu/thscrip/print.p.?file=20050623. . . (accessed 12 July 2005).

—— (2005e) 'Vidharba: Whose Suicide is it, Anyway?' *The Hindu*, 25 June. Available http://www.hinduonnet.com/thehindu/thscrip/print.pl?file=20050625. . . (accessed 12 July 2005).

—— (2007) 'Nearly 1.5 lakh farm suicides from 1997 to 2005'. *The Hindu*, 12 November. Available http://www.hindu.com/2007/11/12/stories/2007111257790100.htm (accessed 8 February 2010).

Sainsbury, P. and Barraclough, B. (1968) 'Differences between suicide rates', *Nature* 220: 1252.

Saldanha, I. M. (1995) 'On drinking and "drunkenness": History of liquor in colonial India', *Economic and Political Weekly* 30 (37): 2323–2331.

Samaritans, *The Media Guidelines: Portrayals of Suicide 2002*. Available http://www.samaritans.org/know/pdf/media.pdf (accessed 21 November 2005.

Saran, A. B. (1974) *Murder and Suicide among the Munda and the Oraon*, Delhi: National Pulishing House.

Sathyavathi, K. (1977) 'Suicide among unemployed persons in Bangalore', *Indian Journal of Social Work* 37 (4): 385–392.

Saucer, P. (1993) 'Education and suicide: the quality of life among modern Americans', *Psychological Reports* 73 (2): 637–638.

Saxena, S. (1999) 'Country profile on alcohol in India', in L. Riley and M. Marshall, eds *Alcohol and Public Health in 8 Developing Countries*. Geneva: Substance Abuse Department, Social Change and Mental Health, World Health Organization.

Schmidtke, A. (1997) 'Perspective: Suicide in Europe', *Suicide and Life-Threatening Behavior* 27 (1): 127–136.

Schroeder, W. W. and Beegle, J. A. (1953) 'Suicide: an instance of high rural rates', *Rural Sociology* 18: 45–52.

Selkin, J. (1994) 'Psychological autopsy: scientific psychohistory or clinical intuition?' *American Psychologist* 49 (1): 74–75.

Service, E. N. (2000) 'Anju Illyasi contemplated suicide in March 1999'. *Indian Express*, 21 January. Available http://www.indianexpress.com/ie/daily/20000121/ina21056.html (accessed 29 January 2003).

Sethi, H. (1991) 'Many unexplained issues: The anti-Mandal "suicides" spate', *Manushi* 63–64: 69–72.

Sethi, N. and Anand, K. (1988) 'A life of humiliation', *Manushi* 45: 19–20.

Shah, J. H. (1960) 'Causes and prevention of suicides', *Indian Journal of Social Work* 21 (2): 167–175.

Shamasastry, R. (1929) *Kautilya's Arthashastra*, Mysore: Wesleyan Mission Press.

Shariff, A. (1999) *India: Human Development Report – A Profile of Indian States in the 1990s*, New Delhi: Oxford University Press.

Sharma, A. (2002) 'Farmer commits suicide on Jogi turf'. *Indian Express*, 11 November. Available http://www.indianexpress.com/print.php?content+id=12845 (accessed 8 December 2004).

Sharma, D. (2005) 'Indian Farmer's Final Solution', zmag. Available http://www.countercurrents.org/gl-sharma290604.htm (accessed 26 May 2005).

Sharma, R. (1998) 'Farmers in distress' *Frontline* (online edition), 4–7 April.

Shaw, M., Dorling, D. and Davey Smith, G. (2002) 'Mortality and political climate: how suicide rates have risen during periods of Conservative government 1901–2000', *Journal of Epidemiology and Community Health* 56 (10): 723–725.

Shiang, J. E. (1998) 'Does culture make a difference? Racial/ethnic patterns of completed suicide in San Francisco, CA 1987–1996 and clinical applications', *Suicide and Life Threatening Behavior* 28 (4): 338–354.

Shiva Kumar, A. K. (1996) 'UNDP's Gender-Related Development Index: A computation for Indian states', Economic and Political Weekly 31 (14): 887–895.

Shiva, V. (2000) *Respect for the Earth*. BBC. Available http://news.bbc.co.uk/hi/english/static/events/reith_2000/lecture5.stm (accessed 17 July 2000).

—— (2004a) 'The Suicide Economy of Corporate Globalisation' zmag. Available http://www.zmag.org/sustainers/content/2004-02/19shiva.cfm (accessed 15 August 2005).

—— (2004b) To India's Finance Minister: An Open Letter Available http://www.countercurrents.org/eco-shiva010204.htm (accessed 15 August 2005).

Shiva, V., Jafri, A. H., Emani, A. and Pande, M. (2002) 'Seeds of Suicide: The Ecological and Human Costs of Globalisation of Agriculture', New Delhi: Research Foundation for Science, Technology and Ecology. Available http://citeseerx.ist.psu.edu/viewdoc/download;jsessionid. . .?doi=10.1.1.112.2992&rep1&type=pdf (accessed 17 February 2010).

Shorter, E. (1976) *The Making of the Modern Family*, London: Collins.

Shridharani, K. (1972) *War Without Violence: A Study of Gandhi's Method and its Accomplishments*, New York & London: Garland Publishing, Inc.

Shukla, S. (2003) *India Abroad: Diasporic Cultures of Postwar America and England*, Princeton: Princeton University Press.

Siddiq, M. (2000) 'Crop failures drive Andhra farmers to suicide again'. *India Abroad News Service*, October 4.

Siegel, J. (1998) 'Indian languages in Fiji: past, present and future', *South Asia XXI* (Special Issue): 181–214.

Simpson, M. E. and Conklin, G. H. (1989) 'Socioeconomic development, suicide and religion: a test of Durkheim's theory of religion and suicide', *Social Forces* 67 (4): 945–965.

Singh, D., Jit, I. and Tyagi, S. (1999) 'Changing trends in acute poisoning in Chandigarh zone', *American Journal of Forensic Medicine and Pathology* 20 (2): 203–210.

Singh, G. K. and Siahpush, M. (2002) 'Increasing rural–urban gradients in US suicide mortality, 1970–1997', *American Journal of Public Health* 92 (7): 1161–1167.

Singh, P. (2000) 'In-laws behind 80 percent of suicides'. *Indian Network News Digest*, August 9. Available http://www.indnet.org/demog/0039.html (accessed 29 January 2003).

Sinha-Kerkhoff, K. (2003) 'Practising Rakshabandhan: brothers in Ranchi, Jharkhand', *Indian Journal of Gender Studies* 10 (3): 431–455.

Skog, O.-J. (1991) 'Alcohol and suicide – Durkheim revisited', *Acta Sociologica* 34 (3): 193–207.

—— (1993) 'Alcohol and suicide in Denmark 1911–24 – experiences from a "natural experiment"', *Addiction* 88: 1189–1193.

Skog, O.-J. and Elekes, Z. (1993) 'Alcohol and the 1950–1990 Hungarian suicide trend – is there a causal connection?' *Acta Sociologica* 36: 33–46.

Skog, O.-J., Teixeira, Z. and Barrias, J. (1995) 'Alcohol and suicide – the Portuguese experience', *Addiction* 90 (8): 1053–1061.

Sleeman, W. H. (1844) *Rambles and Recollections of an Indian Official*. London: J. Hatchard and Son.

Soman, S. (2005) 'Work no worship for stressed out souls'. *The Hindu*, 13 December, Available http://www.hindu.com/2005/12/13/stories/2005121319240100.htm (accessed 14/12/2005).

Somasundaram, O. S., Babu, C. K. and Geelthayan, I. A. (1989) 'Suicide behaviour in ancient civilization with special reference to the families', *Indian Journal of Psychiatry* 31: 208–212.

Soni Raleigh, V. and Balarajan, R. (1992) 'Suicide and self-burning among Indians and West Indians in England and Wales', *British Journal of Psychiatry* 161: 365–368.

Soni Raleigh, V., Bulusu, L. and Balarajan, R. (1990) 'Suicides among immigrants from the Indian Subcontinent', *British Journal of Psychiatry* 156: 46–50.

Soni Raleigh, V. S. (1996) 'Suicide patterns and trends in people of Indian Subcontinent and Caribbean origin in England and Wales', *Ethnicity and Health* 1 (1): 55–63.

Spodek, H. (1970) 'On the origins of Gandhi's political methodology: the heritage of Kathiawad and Gujarat', *Journal of Asian Studies* 30 (2): 361–372.

Staal, F. (2001) 'How a psychoactive substance becomes a ritual: the case of Soma', *Social Research* 68 (3): 745–80.

Stack, S. (1978) 'Suicide: A comparative analysis', Social Forces 57 (2): 644–653.

—— (1982) 'Suicide: A decade review of the sociological literature', *Deviant Behavior* 4: 41–66.

—— (1987). The effect of female participation in the labor force on suicide: A time series analysis, 1948–1980. *Sociological Forum* 22: 257–277.

—— (1993) 'The effect of modernization on suicide in Finland: 1800–1984', *Sociological Perspectives* 36 (2): 137–148.

—— (2000) 'Suicide: A 15-year review of the sociological literature Part I: cultural and economic factors', *Suicide and Life-Threatening Behavior* 30 (2 Summer): 145–162.

—— (2000) 'Suicide: A 15-year review of the sociological literature Part II: Modernization and social integration perspectives.' *Suicide and Life-Threatening Behavior* 30 (2 Summer): 163–176.

—— (2001) 'Occupation and suicide', Social Science Quarterly 82 (2): 384–396.

Stack, S. and Danigelis, N. (1985) 'Modernization and the sex differential in suicide, 1919–1972', *Comparative Social Research* 8: 203–216.

Steen, D. M. and Mayer, P. (2003) 'Patterns of suicide by age and gender in the Indian states: A reflection of human development?' *Archives of Suicide Research* 7: 1–18.

—— (2004) 'Modernization and the male–female suicide ratio in India 1967–1997: divergence or convergence?' *Suicide and Life-Threatening Behavior* 34 (2): 147–159.

Steffensmeier, R. H. (1984) 'Suicide and the contemporary woman: Are male and female suicide rates converging?', *Sex Roles: A Journal of Research* 10: 613–631.

Stietencron, H. v. (1967) 'Suicide as a religious institution', *Bharatiya Vidya* XXVII: 7–24.

Stone, L. (1977) *The Family, Sex and Marriage in England 1500–1800*, London: Weidenfeld and Nicolson.

Subramanyam, C. (2004) 'Crime time host'. *Indian Express*, 16 May, Available http://www.indianexpress.com/full_story.php?content_id=46976 (accessed 20 July 2004).

Sundar, M. (1999) 'Suicide in farmers in India', *British Journal of Psychiatry* 175: 585–586.

Swami, P. (1998) 'Tales of life and death' *Frontline* (online edition), 21 November–4 December. Available http://www.indiaserver.com/frontline/1998/11/21/15240420.htm (accessed 8 April 2002).

Tata Services (1999) *Statistical Outline of India, 1999–2000*, Mumbai: Tata Services.

Thakkar, H. (2005) '644 Farmer Suicides in Maharashtra, says TISS Report'. Info Change India. Available http://www.infochangeindia.org/bookandreportsprint89.jsp (accessed 15 August 2005).

Thakur, U. (1963) *The History of Suicide in India: An Introduction*, Delhi: Munshi Ram Manohar Lal.

Thornton, M. (1991) *The Economics of Prohibition*, Salt Lake City: University of Utah Press.

Time International (1998) 'Death in the countryside: Poverty and poor harvests cause some Indian farmers to commit suicide', *Time International* 150 (43): 30.

Tinker, H. (1974) *A New System of Slavery: The Export of Indian Labour Overseas, 1830–1920*, London: Oxford University Press.

—— (1976) *Separate and Unequal: India and the Indians in the British Commonwealth, 1920–1950*, London: C. Hurst & Company.

Tod, J. (1829) *Annals and Antiquities of Rajast'han: or, the Central and Western Rajpoot States of India*. India (reproduction, 1972, no original publisher), London: Routledge & Kegan Paul.

Trovato, F. and Lalu, N. M. (2001) 'Narrowing sex differences in life expectancy: Regional variations, 1971–1991', *Canadian Studies in Population* 28 (1): 89–110.

Trovato, F. and Vos, R. (1992) 'Married female labor force participation and suicide in Canada', *Sociological Forum* 7 (4): 661–677.

Tsoi, W. F. (1974) 'Suicides and attempted suicides (with special reference to Singapore)', *Annals of the Academy of Medicine*, Singapore 3 (2): 125–30.

UNICEF (1996) *The Progress of Nations*, available at http://www.unicef.org/pon96/insuicid.htm.

upperstall.com M.G. Ramachandran. upperstall.com. Available http://www.upperstall.com/people/mgr.html (accessed 16 August 2005).

Vaidyanathan, A. (2006) 'Farmers' suicides and the agrarian crisis', *Economic and Political Weekly* 41 (38): 4009–4013.

Valmiki (1959) *The Ramayana of Valmiki*. Uttara Kanda, London: Shanti Sadan.

Varma, P. (1976) *Suicide in India and Abroad*. Agra: Sahitya Bhawan.

Varma, S. C. (1972) 'Some features of suicide in India', *Eastern Anthropologist* 25 (3): 227–234.

Vatuk, S. (1972) *Kinship and Urbanization: White Collar Migrants in North India*. Berkeley: University of California Press.

Venkatraman, R. (1983) 'Religious suicide in Tamil Society as revealed in sculpture', in N. Subrahmanian, ed. *Self-Immolation in Tamil Society*. Madurai: International Institute of Tamil Historical Studies.

Venkoba Rao, A. (1975) 'Suicide in India', in N. L. Farberow, ed. *Suicide in Different Cultures*. Baltimore: University Park Press.

—— (1991) 'Suicide in the elderly: A report from India', Crisis 12 (2): 33–39.

Venkoba Rao, A. and Chinnian, R. (1972) 'Attempted suicide and suicide in "students" in Madurai', *Indian Journal of Psychiatry* 14: 389–394.

Venkoba Rao, A., Mahendran, N., Gopalakrishnan, C., Kota Reddy, T., Prabhakar, E. R., Swaminathnan, R., Belinda, C., Andal, G., Baskaran, S., Rashme, P., Kumar, N., Luthra, U. K., Aynkaran, J. R. and Catherine, I. (1989) 'One hundred female burns cases: a study in suicidology', *Indian Journal of Psychiatry* 31 (1): 43–50.

Venugopal, D. and Jagadisha (2000) 'An Indian perspective of farmer stress – a priority area for future research', *International Journal of Social Psychiatry* 46 (3): 231–235.

Vidyasagar, R. M. and Suman Chandra, K. (2003) 'Debt trap or suicide trap? [Excerpts from Chapter IV "Summary, Conclusions and Suggestions for Future Interventions"]', *Farmers' Suicides in Andhra Pradesh and Karnataka*. Hyderabad: National Institute of Rural Development.

—— (2003) *Farmers' Suicides in Andhra Pradesh and Karnataka*, Hyderabad: National Institute of Rural Development.

Vijayakumar, L. and Rajkumar, S. (1999) 'Are risk factors for suicide universal? A case-control study in India', *Acta Psychiatrica Scandinavica* 99: 407–411.

Visaria, P. (1997) 'Urbanization in India: An overview', in G. W. Jones and P. Visaria, eds *Urbanization in Large Developing Countries*. China, Indonesia, Brazil and India. Oxford: Clarendon Press.

Wagle, S. A., Wagle, A. C. and Apte, J. S. (1999) 'Patients with suicidal burns and accidental burns: a comparative study of socio-demographic profile in India', *Burns* 25: 158–161.

Wai, B. H. K., Hong, C. and Heok, K. E. (1999) 'Suicidal behavior among young people in Singapore', *General Hospital Psychiatry* 21: 128–133.

Wai, B. H. K. and Kua, E. H. (1998) 'Parasuicide: A Singapore perspective', *Ethnicity and Health* 3 (4): 255–264.

Waldman, A. (2004) 'Heavy debt and drought drive India's farmers to desperation'. *New York Times*, 6 June, Available http://www.nytimes.com/2004/06/06/international/asia/... (accessed 7 June 2004).

Walker, B. (1983) *Hindu World: An Encyclopedic Survey of Hinduism*. Two volumes, volume II M–Z, New Delhi: Manshiram Manoharal Publishers.

Washington Report on Middle East Affairs (2002) 'Academic pressure leads Indian students to suicide', *Washington Report on Middle East Affairs* 21 (7): 41.

Wassenaar, D. R., van der Veen, M. B. W. and Pillay, A. L. (1998) 'Women in cultural transition: Suicidal behavior in South African Indian women', *Suicide and Life Threatening Behavior* 28 (1): 82–93.

Wasserman, D. and Värnik, A. (1998) 'Reliability of statistics on violent death and suicide in the former USSR, 1970–1990', *Acta Psychiatrica Scandinavica* 98 (Suppl. 394): 34–41.

Wasserman, I. M. (1989) 'The effects of war and alcohol consumption patterns on suicide: United States, 1910–1933', *Social Forces* 68: 513–30.

Watanabe, N., Hasegawa, K. and Yoshinaga, Y. (1995) 'Suicide in later life in Japan: urban and rural differences', *International Psychogeriatrics* 7 (2): 253–261.

Waters, A. B. (1999) 'Domestic dangers: approaches to women's suicide in contemporary Maharashtra, India', *Violence Against Women* 5 (5): 525–547.

Watt, J. R. (1992) *The Making of Modern Marriage: Matrimonial Control and The Rise of Sentiment in Neuchatel, 1550–1800*. Ithaca: Cornell University Press.

—— (2001) *Choosing Death: Suicide and Calvinism in Early Modern Geneva*, Kirksville, MO: Truman State University Press.

WHO Southeast Asia http://w3.whosea.org/en/Section1174/Section1199/Section1567/Section1824_8080.htm, accessed 11 May 2002.

WHO, 'Suicide rates and absolute numbers of suicide by country'. Available http://www.who.int/mental_health/prevention/suicide/suicideprevent/en/.

Wilhelmsen, L., Elmfeldt, D. and Wedel, H. (1983) 'Causes of death in relation to social and alcohol problems among Swedish men aged 35–44 years', Acta Medica Scandinavica 213: 263–268.

Wilkinson, K. P. (1984) 'Rurality and patterns of social disruption', *Rural Sociology* 49 (1): 23–36.

Wilkinson, K. P. and Israel, G. D. (1984) 'Suicide and rurality in urban society', *Suicide and Life-Threatening Behavior* 14 (3): 187–200.

World Health Organisation (1998) *World Health Statistics Annual, 1996, Volume 1,* Geneva, Switzerland: World Health Organization.

—— (1999) 'Figures and Facts about Suicide', Geneva: Department of Mental Health, Social Change and Mental Health, World Health Organisation.

—— (2001) 'Burden of Mental and Behavioural Disorders', Chapter 2 in *World Health Report 2001 – Mental Health: New Understanding, New Hope.* Available at http://www.who.int/whr/2001/en/whr01_ch2_en.pdf.

—— (2003) World Health Report, Geneva. Available http://www.who.int/whr/2003/chapter1/en/index3.html.

—— (2004) 'Suicide rates and absolute numbers of suicide by country'. Available http://www.who.int/mental_health/prevention/suicide/suicideprevent/en/.

—— (2005) Suicide Prevention. Available http://www.who.int/mental_health/prevention/suicide/suicideprevent/en/ (accessed 5 August 2005).

Yeoh, O. H. (1981) 'Attempted suicide in Penang – preliminary observations', *Medical Journal of Malaysia* 36 (1): 39–46.

Yip, P. S. F. (1996) 'Suicide in Hong Kong, Taiwan and Beijing', *Journal of Psychiatry* 169: 495–500.

—— (1998) 'Age, sex, marital status and suicide – an empirical study of East and West', *Psychological Reports* (1): 311–322.

Yip, P. S. F., Callanan, C. and Yuen, H. K. (2000) 'Urban/rural and gender differentials in suicide rates: East and West', *Journal of Affective Distress* 57: 99–106.

Yule, H. and Burnell, A. C. (1886) Hobson–Jobson: *A Glossary of Colloquial Anglo-Indian Words and Phrases.* New edition ed. William Crooke, London: Routledge & Kegan Paul. Original edition, 1886.

Zacharakis, C. A., Madianos, M. G., Papadimitiou, G. N. and Stefanis, C. N. (1998) 'Suicide in Greece 1980–1995: patterns and social factors', *Social Psychiatry and Psychiatric Epidemiology* 33: 471–476.

Zehr, H. (1976) *Crime and the Development of Modern Society: Patterns of Criminality in Nineteenth Century Germany and France,* London: Croom Helm, Rowman and Littlefield.

Ziaian, T. and Mayer, P. (2002) 'Gender, marital status and suicide in India', *Journal of Comparative Family Studies* 33: 297–305.

Index

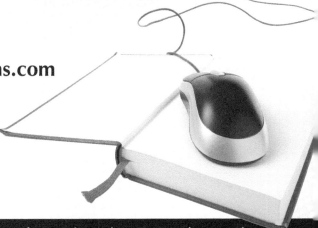

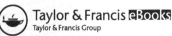

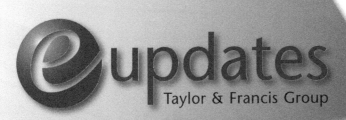
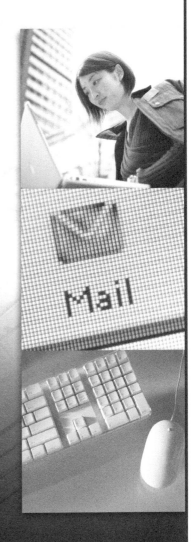

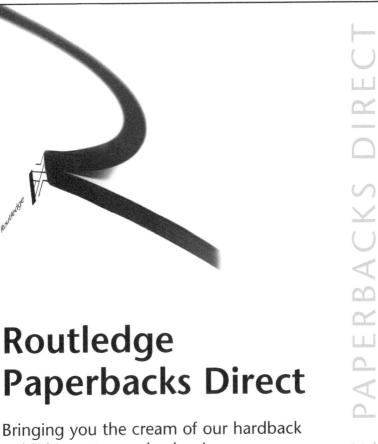
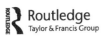